Communications
in Computer and Information Science 1710

More information about this series at https://link.springer.com/bookseries/7899

Claudine Gehin · Bruno Wacogne ·
Alexandre Douplik · Ronny Lorenz ·
Bethany Bracken · Cátia Pesquita · Ana Fred ·
Hugo Gamboa (Eds.)

Biomedical Engineering Systems and Technologies

14th International Joint Conference, BIOSTEC 2021
Virtual Event, February 11–13, 2021
Revised Selected Papers

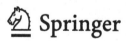 Springer

Editors
Claudine Gehin
INSA-Lyon
Villeurbanne, France

Alexandre Douplik
Toronto Metropolitan University
Toronto, ON, Canada

Bethany Bracken
Charles River Analytics, Inc.
Cambridge, MA, USA

Ana Fred
Instituto de Telecomunicações
Aveiro, Portugal

University of Lisbon
Lisbon, Portugal

Bruno Wacogne
FEMTO-ST
Besancon, France

Ronny Lorenz
University of Vienna
Vienna, Austria

Cátia Pesquita 🅘
University of Lisbon
Lisbon, Portugal

Hugo Gamboa
Universidade Nova de Lisboa
Caparica, Portugal

ISSN 1865-0929   ISSN 1865-0937 (electronic)
Communications in Computer and Information Science
ISBN 978-3-031-20663-4   ISBN 978-3-031-20664-1 (eBook)
https://doi.org/10.1007/978-3-031-20664-1

This Springer imprint is published by the registered company Springer Nature Switzerland AG
The registered company address is: Gewerbestrasse 11, 6330 Cham, Switzerland

Preface

The present book includes extended and revised versions of a set of selected papers from the 14th International Joint Conference on Biomedical Engineering Systems and Technologies (BIOSTEC 2021), exceptionally held as an online event, due to COVID-19, during February 11–13, 2021.

BIOSTEC is composed of co-located conferences, each specialized in a different knowledge area, namely BIODEVICES, BIOIMAGING, BIOINFORMATICS, BIOSIGNALS and HEALTHINF.

BIOSTEC 2021 received 265 paper submissions from authors in 52 countries, of which 4.9% were included in this book.

The papers were selected by the event chairs and their selection is based on a number of criteria that include the classifications and comments provided by the Program Committee members, the session chairs' assessment and also the program chairs' global view of all papers included in the technical program. The authors of selected papers were then invited to submit revised and extended version of their papers having at least 30% innovative material.

The purpose of BIOSTEC is to bring together researchers and practitioners, including engineers, biologists, health professionals and informatics/computer scientists, interested in both theoretical advances and applications of information systems, artificial intelligence, signal processing, electronics and other engineering tools in knowledge areas related to biology and medicine.

The papers selected to be included in this book contribute to the understanding of relevant trends of current research on biomedical engineering systems and technologies, including pattern recognition and machine learning, application of health informatics in clinical cases, evaluation and use of healthcare IT, medical signal acquisition, analysis and processing, data mining and data analysis, decision support systems, e-health, e-health applications, mobile technologies for healthcare applications and medical devices design.

We would like to thank all the authors for their contributions and also the reviewers who helped ensure the quality of this publication.

February 2021

Claudine Gehin
Bruno Wacogne
Alexandre Douplik
Ronny Lorenz
Bethany Bracken
Cátia Pesquita
Ana Fred
Hugo Gamboa

Organization

Conference Co-chairs

Ana Fred	Instituto de Telecomunicações and University of Lisbon, Portugal
Hugo Gamboa	Nova University of Lisbon, Portugal

Program Co-chairs

BIODEVICES

Claudine Gehin	INSA-Lyon, France
Bruno Wacogne	FEMTO-ST, CNRS, France

BIOIMAGING

Alexandre Douplik	Ryerson University, Canada

BIOINFORMATICS

Ronny Lorenz	University of Vienna, Austria

BIOSIGNALS

Bethany Bracken	Charles River Analytics Inc., USA

HEALTHINF

Cátia Pesquita	Universidade de Lisboa, Portugal

BIODEVICES Program Committee

Carlos Abreu	Instituto Politécnico de Viana do Castelo, Portugal
Andreas Bahr	University of Kiel, Germany
Steve Beeby	University of Southampton, UK
Wenxi Chen	University of Aizu, Japan
JungHun Choi	Georgia Southern University, USA
Seokheun Sean Choi	State University of New York, Binghamton, USA
Youngjae Chun	University of Pittsburgh, USA

Alberto Cliquet Jr.	University of São Paulo and University of Campinas, Brazil
Pedro Estrela	University of Bath, UK
Maria Evelina Fantacci	University of Pisa and INFN, Italy
Mireya Fernández Chimeno	Universitat Politècnica de Catalunya, Spain
Juan Carlos Garcia	University of Alcala, Spain
Miguel García Gonzalez	Universitat Politècnica de Catalunya, Spain
Javier Garcia-Casado	Universitat Politècnica de València, Spain
Leonid Hrebien	Drexel University, USA
Bozena Kaminska	Simon Fraser University, Canada
Ondrej Krejcar	University of Hradec Kralove, Czech Republic
Dean Krusienski	Virginia Commonwealth University, USA
Vladimir Kublanov	Ural Federal University, Russia
Hiroshi Kumagai	Kitasato University, Japan
Anita Lloyd Spetz	Linköpings Universitet, Sweden
Carlos Maciel	University of São Paulo, Brazil
Jarmo Malinen	Aalto University, Finland
Dan Mandru	Technical University of Cluj Napoca, Romania
Ana MoitaIN+	Instituto Superior Tecnico and Academia Militar, Portugal
Raimes Moraes	Universidade Federal de Santa Catarina, Brazil
Robert Newcomb	University of Maryland, USA
Abraham Otero	Universidad San Pablo, Spain
Lionel Pazart	CHU Besançon, France
Wim Rutten	University of Twente, Netherlands
Seonghan Ryu	Hannam University, South Korea
Michael Schöning	FH Aachen, Germany
Mauro Serpelloni	University of Brescia, Italy
Dong Ik Shin	Asan Medical Center, South Korea
Filomena Soares	University of Minho, Portugal
Marco Tatullo	University of Bari, Italy
John Tudor	University of Southampton, UK
Duarte Valério	Universidade de Lisboa, Portugal
Renato Varoto	University of Campinas, Brazil
Richard Willson	University of Houston, USA
Hakan Yavuz	Çukurova Üniversity, Turkey
Alberto Yufera	Universidad de Sevilla, Spain

BIOIMAGING Program Committee

Ahmet Ademoglu	Bogazici University, Turkey
Peter Balazs	University of Szeged, Hungary
Virginia Ballarín	Universidad Nacional de Mar del Plata, Argentina

Richard Bayford	Middlesex University, UK
Alpan Bek	Middle East Technical University, Turkey
Obara Boguslaw	University of Durham, UK
Alberto Bravin	Università degli Studi di Milano-Bicocca, Italy
Heang-Ping Chan	University of Michigan, USA
Mostafa Charmi	University of Zanjan, Iran
Chung-Ming Chen	National Taiwan University, Taiwan
Jyh-Cheng Chen	National Yang-Ming University, Taiwan
Miguel Coimbra	University of Porto, Portugal
Christos Constantinou	Stanford University, USA
Carlos Geraldes	Universidade de Coimbra, Portugal
Tzung-Pei Hong	National University of Kaohsiung, Taiwan
Jae Youn Hwang	DGIST, South Korea
Xiaoyi Jiang	University of Münster, Germany
Jin Kang	Johns Hopkins University, USA
Algimantas Krisciukaitis	Lithuanian University of Health Sciences, Lithuania
Roger Lecomte	Université de Sherbrooke, Canada
Hongen Liao	Tsinghua University, China
Ivan Lima Jr.	North Dakota State University, USA
Hua Lin	Shanghai Institute of Optics and Fine Mechanics, Chinese Academy of Sciences, China
Siyu Ma	Massachusetts General Hospital, USA
Lucia Maddalena	ICAR, National Research Council (CNR), Italy
Jan Mares	University of Chemistry and Technology, Czech Republic
Vaidotas Marozas	Kaunas University of Technology, Lithuania
Konstantinos Moutzouris	University of West Attica, Greece
Subhash Narayanan	Sascan Meditech Pvt. Ltd., India
Joanna Isabelle Olszewska	University of West Scotland, UK
Kalman Palagyi	University of Szeged, Hungary
Tae Jung Park	Chung-Ang University, South Korea
Gennaro Percannella	University of Salerno, Italy
Vadim PerezInstituto	Mexicano del Seguro Social, Mexico
Wan Qin	University of Washington, USA
Olivier Salvado	CSIRO, Australia
Gregory Sharp	Massachusetts General Hospital, USA
Leonid Shvartsman	Hebrew University, Israel
Magdalena Stoeva	Medical University of Plovdiv, Bulgaria
Piotr Szczepaniak	Lodz University of Technology, Poland
Arkadiusz Tomczyk	Lodz University of Technology, Poland

Carlos Travieso-González	Universidad de Las Palmas de Gran Canaria, Spain
Benjamin Tsui	Johns Hopkins University, USA
Vladimír Ulman	Masaryk University, Czech Republic
Sandra Ventura	Politécnico do Porto, Portugal
Yuanyuan Wang	Fudan University, China

BIOINFORMATICS Program Committee

Mohamed Abouelhoda	Nile University, Egypt
Carlos Abreu	Instituto Politécnico de Viana do Castelo, Portugal
Tatsuya Akutsu	Kyoto University, Japan
Payam Behzadi	Shahr-e-Qods Branch, Islamic Azad University, Iran
Shifra Ben-Dor	Weizmann Institute of Science, Israel
Gilles Bernot	Université Côte d'Azur, France
Pawel Blazej	Wroclaw University, Poland
Rita Casadio	University of Bologna, Italy
Matthias Chung	Virginia Tech, USA
Jean-Paul Comet	Univesité Côte d'Azur, France
Keith Crandall	George Washington University, USA
Thomas Dandekar	University of Würzburg, Germany
Maria Evelina Fantacci	University of Pisa and INFN, Italy
Alexandru Floares	SAIA, Romania
Liliana Florea	Johns Hopkins University, USA
Dmitrij Frishman	Technical University of Munich, Germany
Ronaldo Hashimoto	University of São Paulo, Brazil
Volkhard Helms	Universität des Saarlandes, Germany
Asier Ibeas	Universitat Autònoma de Barcelona, Spain
Giuseppe Jurman	Fondazione Bruno Kessler, Italy
Jirí Kléma	Czech Technical University in Prague, Czech Republic
Ivan Kulakovskiy	IPR RAS, Russia
Yinglei Lai	George Washington University, USA
Man-Kee Lam	Universiti Teknologi PETRONAS, Malaysia
Antonio LaTorre	Universidad Politécnica de Madrid, Spain
Carlile Lavor	University of Campinas, Brazil
Pawel Mackiewicz	Wroclaw University, Poland
Elena Marchiori	Radboud University, Netherlands
Johnny Marques	Instituto Tecnológico de Aeronáutica, Brazil
Giancarlo Mauri	Università degli Studi di Milano-Bicocca, Italy
Paolo Milazzo	Università di Pisa, Italy
Jason Miller	Shepherd University, USA

Chilukuri Mohan	Syracuse University, USA
José Molina	Universidad Carlos III de Madrid, Spain
Jean-Christophe Nebel	Kingston University, UK
Hakan Orer	Koc University School of Medicine, Turkey
Oscar Pastor	Universidad Politécnica de Valencia, Spain
Matteo Pellegrini	University of California, Los Angeles, USA
Gianfranco Politano	Politecnico di Torino, Italy
Javier Reina-Tosina	University of Seville, Spain
Laura Roa	University of Seville, Spain
Vincent Rodin	UBO, LabSTICC/CNRS, France
Ulrich Rückert	Bielefeld University, Germany
J. Cristian Salgado	University of Chile, Chile
Alessandro Savino	Politecnico di Torino, Italy
Andrew Schumann	University of Information Technology and Management in Rzeszow, Poland
Noor Akhmad Setiawan	Universitas Gadjah Mada, Indonesia
João Setubal	Universidade de São Paulo, Brazil
Anne Siegel	CNRS, France
Christine Sinoquet	University of Nantes, France
Sylvain Soliman	Inria Saclay, France
Peter F. Stadler	University of Leipzig, Germany
Peter Sykacek	University of Natural Resources and Life Sciences, Vienna, Austria
Piotr Szczepaniak	Lodz University of Technology, Poland
Y-h. Taguchi	Chuo University, Japan
Arkadiusz Tomczyk	Lodz University of Technology, Poland

BIOINFORMATICS Additional Reviewers

| Eugene Baulin | Institute of Mathematical Problems of Biology, Russia |
| Dmitry Penzar | Russia |

BIOSIGNALS Program Committee

Eda Akman Aydin	Gazi University, Turkey
Raul Alcaraz	University of Castilla-La Mancha, Spain
Robert Allen	University of Southampton, UK
Jesús B. Alonso	Universidad de Las Palmas de Gran Canaria, Spain
Eberhard Beck	Brandenburg University of Applied Sciences, Germany
Philipp Beckerle	TU Darmstadt, Germany

Pedro Rodrigues	Universidade Católica Portuguesa, Portugal
Heather Ruskin	Dublin City University, Ireland
Giovanni Saggio	Tor Vergata University of Rome, Italy
Andrews Samraj	Mahendra Engineering College, India
Gerald Schaefer	Loughborough University, UK
Reinhard Schneider	Fachhochschule Vorarlberg, Austria
Lotfi Senhadji	University of Rennes 1, France
Zdenek Smekal	Brno University of Technology, Czech Republic
Jana Šnupárková	University of Chemistry and Technology, Czech Republic
H. So	City University of Hong Kong, China
Jordi Solé-Casals	University of Vic - Central University of Catalonia, Spain
Asser Tantawi	IBM, USA
Wallapak Tavanapong	Iowa State University, USA
António Teixeira	University of Aveiro, Portugal
Carlos Thomaz	Centro Universitário FEI, Brazil
Hua-Nong Ting	University of Malaya, Malaysia
Carlos Travieso-González	Universidad de Las Palmas de Gran Canaria, Spain
Athanasios Tsanas	University of Edinburgh, UK
Egon L. van den Broek	Utrecht University, Netherlands
Pedro Vaz	University of Coimbra, Portugal
Yuanyuan Wang	Fudan University, China
Rafal Zdunek	Politechnika Wroclawska, Poland

BIOSIGNALS Additional Reviewer

Lukas P. A. Arts	Utrecht University, The Netherlands

HEALTHINF Program Committee

Carlos Abreu	Instituto Politécnico de Viana do Castelo, Portugal
Luca Anselma	Università degli Studi di Torino, Italy
Payam Behzadi	Shahr-e-Qods Branch, Islamic Azad University, Iran
José Alberto Benítez-Andrades	Universidad de León, Spain
Jon Bird	University of Bristol, UK
Sorana Bolboaca	Iuliu Hatieganu University of Medicine and Pharmacy, Romania
Alessio Bottrighi	Università del Piemonte Orientale, Italy
Andrew Boyd	University of Illinois at Chicago, USA
Klaus Brinker	Hamm-Lippstadt University of Applied Sciences, Germany

Federico Cabitza	Università degli Studi di Milano-Bicocca, Italy
Andrea Campagner	University of Milano-Bicocca, Italy
Manuel Campos-Martinez	University of Murcia, Spain
Davide Ciucci	Università degli Studi di Milano Bicocca, Italy
Malcolm Clarke	Ondokuz Mayis University, UK
Miguel Coimbra	University of Porto, Portugal
Emmanuel Conchon	XLIM, France
Carlos Costa	Universidade de Aveiro, Portugal
Liliana Dobrica	University Politehnica of Bucharest, Romania
Ivan Donadello	Fondazione Bruno Kessler, Italy
George Drosatos	Athena Research Center, Greece
Farshideh Einsele	Berne University of Applied Sciences, Switzerland
Christo El Morr	York University, Canada
Gunnar Ellingsen	UIT - The Artic University of Norway, Norway
Daniela Fogli	Università degli Studi di Brescia, Italy
José Fonseca	UNINOVA, Portugal
Christoph Friedrich	University of Applied Sciences and Arts Dortmund, Germany
Sebastian Fudickar	University of Luebeck, Germany
Henry Gabb	Intel Corporation, USA
Luigi Gallo	National Research Council of Italy, Italy
Angelo Gargantini	University of Bergamo, Italy
Yves Gourinat	ISAE-SUPAERO, France
Alexandra Grancharova	University of Chemical Technology and Metallurgy, Bulgaria
David Greenhalgh	University of Strathclyde, UK
Tahir Hameed	Merrimack College, USA
Cristina Jácome	Centro de Investigação em Tecnologias e Serviços de Saúde, Portugal
Dragan Jankovic	University of Nis, Serbia
Bridget Kane	Karlstad University, Sweden
Spyros Kitsiou	University of Illinois at Chicago, USA
Josef Kohout	University of West Bohemia, Czech Republic
Haridimos Kondylakis	Foundation for Research and Technology - Hellas, Greece
Tomohiro Kuroda	Kyoto University Hospital, Japan
Elyes Lamine	University of Toulouse, IMT Mines Albi, CGI, France
Erwin Lemche	King's College London, UK
Lenka Lhotska	Czech Technical University in Prague, Czech Republic
Guillaume Lopez	Aoyama Gakuin University, Japan

Martin Lopez-Nores	University of Vigo, Spain
Chi-Jie Lu	Fu Jen Catholic University, Taiwan
Gang Luo	University of Washington, USA
Alessandra Macedo	University of São Paulo, Brazil
Alda Marques	University of Aveiro, Portugal
Juan Martinez-Romo	National University Distance Education, Spain
Ken Masters	Sultan Qaboos University, Oman
Stefania Montani	Piemonte Orientale University, Italy
Roman Moucek	University of West Bohemia, Czech Republic
Hammadi Nait-Charif	Bournemouth University, UK
Michelle Norris	Lero and University of Limerick, Ireland
Thomas Ostermann	Witten/Herdecke University, Germany
Nelson Pacheco da Rocha	University of Aveiro, Portugal
Rui Pedro Paiva	University of Coimbra, Portugal
Antonio Piccinno	University of Bari, Italy
Enrico Piras	Fondazione Bruno Kessler, Italy
Arkalgud Ramaprasad	Ramaiah Public Policy Center, India
Grzegorz Redlarski	Gdansk University of Technology, Poland
David Riaño	Universitat Rovira i Virgili, Italy
Alejandro Rodríguez González	Centro de Tecnología Biomédica, Spain
Valter Roesler	Federal University of Rio Grande do Sul, Brazil
George Sakellaropoulos	University of Patras, Greece
Ovidio Salvetti	National Research Council of Italy (CNR), Italy
Akio Sashima	AIST, Japan
Bettina Schnor	Potsdam University, Germany
Andrea Seveso	University of Milano-Bicocca, Italy
Carla Simone	University of Milano-Bicocca, Italy
Jan Sliwa	Bern University of Applied Sciences, Switzerland
Åsa Smedberg	Stockholm University, Sweden
Jiangwen Sun	Old Dominion University, USA
Chia-Chi Teng	Brigham Young University, USA
Francesco Tiezzi	University of Camerino, Italy
Marie Travers	University of Limerick, Ireland
Yi-Ju Tseng	National Yang Ming Chiao Tung University, Taiwan
Lauri Tuovinen	University of Oulu, Finland
Mohy Uddin	King Abdullah International Medical Research Center (KAIMRC), Saudi Arabia
Gary Ushaw	Newcastle University, UK
Bert-Jan van Beijnum	University of Twente, Netherlands
Egon L. van den Broek	Utrecht University, Netherlands
Sitalakshmi Venkatraman	Melbourne Polytechnic, Australia

Francisco Veredas   Universidad de Málaga, Spain
Chien-Chih Wang   Ming Chi University of Technology, Taiwan
Hsin-Hung Wu   National Changhua University of Education,
                                   Taiwan
Dimitrios Zarakovitis   University of Peloponnese, Greece

HEALTHINF Additional Reviewers

Vita Santa Barletta   University of Bari, Italy
Silvia Bonfanti   University of Bergamo, Italy
Kristina Sahlmann   University of Potsdam, Germany
Rafika Thabet   INPG, France

Invited Speakers

Athanasios Tsanas   University of Edinburgh, UK
Thomas Ostermann   Universität Witten/Herdecke, Germany
Mireya Fernández Chimeno   Universidade de Lisboa, Portugal

Contents

Systematic Design Procedure of CMOS Microelectrode-Arrays Based
on Analog Signal Processing Noise Figure 1
Marcello De Matteis, Andrea Baschirotto, Lorenzo Stevenazzi,
and Elia Vallicelli

LigityScore: A CNN-Based Method for Binding Affinity Predictions 18
Joseph Azzopardi and Jean Paul Ebejer

Chaotic Changes in Fingertip Pulse Waves and Psychological Effects
of Reminiscence Therapy Intervention 45
Eri Shibayama and Taira Suzuki

Determination of Charge Transfer Resistance from Randles Circuit
Spectra Using Elliptical Fitting 61
Norman Pfeiffer, Toni Wachter, Jürgen Frickel, Hamdi Ben Halima,
Christian Hofmann, Abdelhamid Errachid, and Albert Heuberger

Towards Segmentation and Labelling of Motion Data in Manufacturing
Scenarios 80
António Santos, João Rodrigues, Duarte Folgado, Sara Santos,
Carlos Fujão, and Hugo Gamboa

Evaluating the Performance of Diadochokinetic Tests in Characterizing
Parkinson's Disease Hypokinetic Dysarthria 102
Pedro Gómez-Vilda, Andrés Gómez-Rodellar, Daniel Palacios-Alonso,
and Athanasios Tsanas

Technology-Based Education and Training System for Nursing
Professionals 120
Conrad Fifelski-von Böhlen, Anna Brinkmann, Sebastian Fudickar,
Sandra Hellmers, and Andreas Hein

Evaluation of Algorithms to Measure a Psychophysical Threshold Using
Digital Applications 139
Silvia Bonfanti and Angelo Gargantini

Improving Teledermatology Referral with Edge-AI: Mobile App to Foster
Skin Lesion Imaging Standardization 158
Maria João M. Vasconcelos, Dinis Moreira, Pedro Alves,
Ricardo Graça, Rafael Franco, and Luís Rosado

Towards Interpretable Machine Learning Models to Aid
the Academic Performance of Children and Adolescents
with Attention-Deficit/Hyperactivity Disorder 180
    *Caroline Jandre, Marcelo Balbino, Débora de Miranda, Luis Zárate,
    and Cristiane Nobre*

Requirements for Implementing Digital Health Terminology Standards
in Uganda's Electronic Medical Records-Based Health Information
Systems 202
    Achilles Kiwanuka and Josephine Nabukenya

Multi-class Detection of Arrhythmia Conditions Through the Combination
of Compressed Sensing and Machine Learning 213
    *Giovanni Rosa, Marco Russodivito, Gennaro Laudato,
    Angela Rita Colavita, Luca De Vito, Francesco Picariello,
    Simone Scalabrino, Ioan Tudosa, and Rocco Oliveto*

DL-Assisted ROP Screening Technique 236
    *Vijay Kumar, Het Patel, Shorya Azad, Kolin Paul, Abhidnya Surve,
    and Rohan Chawla*

Author Index 259

Systematic Design Procedure of CMOS Microelectrode-Arrays Based on Analog Signal Processing Noise Figure

Marcello De Matteis$^{(\boxtimes)}$ ⓘ, Andrea Baschirotto ⓘ, Lorenzo Stevenazzi, and Elia Vallicelli ⓘ

Department of Physics, University of Milano Bicocca, Piazza Della Scienza 3, 20126 Milan, Italy
marcello.dematteis@unimib.it

Abstract. Microelectrode-Arrays (MEAs) allow neural recording of thousands of neurons/mm^2 by sensing: Extracellular Action Potentials (EAP) and Local Field Potentials (LFP). MEAs arrange several recording sites (or pixels) in a spatial grid/matrix, planarly and capacitively coupled with in-vitro cell cultures (growth above the chip surface) and/or integrated in electrocorticography grids. This paper focuses on Electrolyte-Oxide (C)MOS Field-Effect-Transistors MEAs for cell-level recording. In this type of biosensors, each single row of the matrix is composed of N planar metal electrodes and is scanned synchronously and regularly for N clock cycles, adopting Time-Division-Multiplexing (TDM) schemes. TDM approach generates an analogue output signal for each biosensor row, which includes in a single time track the information acquired by the N electrodes of the matrix.

It is therefore of fundamental importance to estimate the noise power of the output signal of the single row because this power defines the minimum detectable threshold of the neuro-potential signal power.

Noise in planar MEA is determined by the classical contributions of electronic noise (thermal and flicker, coming from both biological environment and semiconductor devices) and from the spurious corrupting signal due to multiplexing action (which behaves to all effects as a statistical noise signal following a Gaussian probability distribution).

This paper presents the complete procedure for designing an (active) biosensor matrix/array (embedding the analog signal processing channels) as a function of a specific Noise Figure requirement (that measures the Signal-to-Noise-Ratio (SNR) degradation and thus is defined as the ratio between the biosensor array input SNR and the output SNR of the analog acquisition channel).

This procedure is applied to a single row of the biosensor matrix, can be easily extended to 2D array, and allows to define all the design parameters (including electrode area, gain, bandwidth and noise power of the analog stages building the array) to obtain the specific Noise Figure.

Keywords: Biological neural networks · BiosEnsors · Neural engineering · Analog integrated circuits · Low-noise amplifier

© The Author(s), under exclusive license to Springer Nature Switzerland AG 2022
C. Gehin et al. (Eds.): BIOSTEC 2021, CCIS 1710, pp. 1–17, 2022.
https://doi.org/10.1007/978-3-031-20664-1_1

1 Introduction

There is a rather large lack of information between neuron membrane electrical activity of single neurons, and physiological or whole brain behavioral events. To fill this gap, we need to understand the activity of individual neurons and how it contributes to neural circuits functioning. Such ambitious perspective cannot be achieved by macroscale neural recording techniques (electroencephalogram, magnetic resonance, etc.), nor by patch clamps (monitoring single cell unit). One of the best options is to adopt Microelectrode-Arrays (MEAs, [1–3]) that allow monitoring thousands of neurons/mm^2 by sensing: extracellular Action Potential (EAP in 300 Hz–5 kHz bandwidth) and (in-vivo) Local Field Potential (LFP up to 300 Hz bandwidth). They are used as planar probes where the cell population is growth above, forming a cell-electrode capacitive coupling. Implanted MEAs are typically needle-shaped probes that deeply penetrate the cortex for tissues recording/stimulating and for increasing proximity and signals detection rate.

Both in-culture and implantable MEAs can be integrated in commercial CMOS silicon substrates with an additional post-processing step consisting of covering CMOS metal aluminum electrodes by noble metal films (Pt/Au [4]) or dedicated oxide layers (TiO2 [5]). Active MEAs embed both analog signal processing channels (by neural amplifier, low-pass filter for antialiasing and A-to-D conversion) and digital circuits synthesizing advanced Digital Spikes Detection ([6, 7], DSD) algorithms.

DSDs exploit the large array spatial resolution for separating relevant extracellular events from background noise by spatial correlation post-processing algorithms. They perform complex digital algorithms that require a certain computing power leading to a non-negligible dynamic power consumption and preventing integration in the same MEA silicon area.

Despite outstanding advancements in neural probes development, there are still many phenomena (as ultra-weak neuro-potentials) that state-of-the-art MEA technology cannot observe at high spatial resolution:

- at membrane level, subthreshold events, such as synaptic potentials can influence cell rest status without producing an action potential;
- propagation of the action potentials (AP) in axons, the backpropagation of AP in the dendrites and the generation of dendritic spikes, and weak extracellular synaptic field potential;
- traces of membrane oscillations in the extracellular space, never observed by planar probes since they require single-cell patch recording techniques.

Simply speaking, these events and phenomena cannot be observed because noise power floor in cell-electrolyte-electrode-electronics junctions, is to date higher than the signal power of those extracellular neuro-potentials carrying information coming from subthreshold or ultra-weak events.

In this context, to detect ultra-weak neuro-potential signals, it is essential to avoid significant degradation of the SNR at the electrolyte-electrode interface first and then at the electrode-electronics interface.

Given the physical and geometrical dimensions of the extracellular biological environment (cell-electrode adhesion or proximity, electrode area and coating material), the noise power at the interface is fully defined by the electrolyte resistance thermal noise power and coating material flicker noise power [3].

Hence, the goal of the analog signal processing channel driven by the electrode is to minimize the degradation of such biosensor input SNR, or in other words to minimize the Noise Figure. This is possible only using a systematic design approach that allows to clearly define all the parameters that contribute to the output SNR (electronic (thermal and flicker) noise, amplification stages gain and bandwidth, spurious disturbing signal power introduced by the operation of the TDM scheme).

This paper addresses these problems and proposes a model based on simple and efficient design equations that allow to set all the parameters of the biosensor analog signal processing stages starting from a minimum set of input specifications and, more importantly, satisfying the specific requirement of Noise Figure.

Section 2 presents both topology and architecture of a CMOS MEA and the general principles of operation. Section 3 introduces the equations that regulate the analog signal processing Noise Figure, including the electrolyte-electrode junction model and the effects of signal corruption due to TDM operation. Section 4 reports the noise Power Spectral Density (PSD) simulation results as a function of a given Noise Figure and the final design parameters to meet such Noise Figure. At the end of the paper conclusions will be drawn.

2 CMOS MEAs

Figure 1 shows the block scheme of a classical CMOS MEA chip implementation. The system is composed by two main sections: the Biological Sensitive Area and the Analog Signal Processing chains (one chain per row).

In state-of-the-art neural recording setups [8–16], the cells culture is typically placed above the biological sensitive area. $N_E x N_{CH}$ is the matrix resolution, i.e. the total electrodes count. More in detail, N_E is the row electrode count and N_{CH} is the column (or analog signal processing channels) count.

The electrodes are capacitively coupled by a biocompatible coating layer (TiO2 in this specific case of study) with the extracellular electrolyte bath (as illustrated in Fig. 2 for the case of a single electrode). The signals coming from the N_E electrodes that form a row of the matrix, converge in an Analog Bus that serves N_E Low Noise Amplifiers (LNA1 in Fig. 1). Such LNA1 stages drive the Analog Multiplexer (MUX) that implements the TDM scheme providing the single-line input signal for the second amplifier (LNA2). The LNA2 output voltage is then digitalized by the A-to-D converter (ADC).

The single electrode receives a signal coming from the extracellular environment which is composed of two main terms:

- extracellular/biological neuro-potentials ($v_{np,b}$, including EAP and LFP);
- noise signal introduced at two different levels at the electrolyte-electrode interface level;

Afterwards, the Analog Signal Processing chain (LNA1, TDM and LNA2) introduces additional noise contributions.

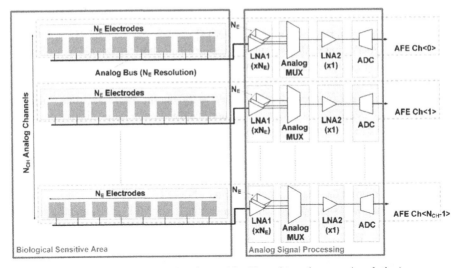

Fig. 1. CMOS MEA block scheme (N_ExN_{CH} electrodes count/resolution).

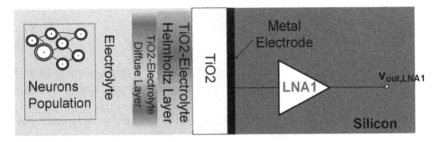

Fig. 2. Cells-electrolyte-electrode interface [16].

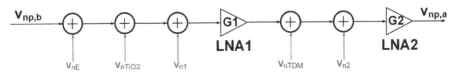

Fig. 3. CMOS MEA block scheme (N_ExN_{CH} electrodes count/resolution).

Obviously, the main aim of MEA neural recording operations is to maximize the acquisition SNR to provide accurate spatio-temporal imaging of the on-going neural electrical activity.

The neuro-potential electrical power at the electrolyte-electrode interface depends on specific factors which are not always under control of MEA designers, as cell-silicon adhesion, cell-electrode proximity, electrolyte bulk conductivity, etc. [18]. For instance, neural recording experiments reports 70 μV_{RMS} signal power in typical scenario of moderate proximity and/or adhesion between cell and electrodes [19]. Higher signal power can be observable if compatible with the output Dynamic Range of the Analog

Signal Processing stages (i.e. LNA2 output voltage is lower than supply voltage, avoiding output swing saturation/drop). Lower signal power can be critically corrupted by the interface noise power. On the other hand, noise power is, to all effects, a parameter that can be under certain conditions optimized, enhancing in this way the final output SNR. Figure 3 shows the signal flow block scheme in terms of both neuro-potentials and noise signal tracks. This scheme is referred to a single biosensor row and to the specific case of:

- TiO2 coating the MEA electrode (or chip surface);
- a single electrode in the row detecting a specific neuro-potential signal ($v_{np,b}$);
- all the remaining electrodes in the row detecting only noise, without any relevant neural activity above.

With reference to Fig. 3 scheme, $v_{np,b}$ and $v_{np,a}$ are neuro-potential signals coming from the biological environment (EAP and LFP) and at the LNA2 output, respectively. LNA1 and LNA2 have G1 and G2 passband amplification factors. Different noise contributions appear on different points of the signal flow block scheme, adding to the neuro-potential signal and influencing the final output SNR. More specifically:

- v_{nE} is the noise signal track coming from electrolyte resistance (R_E);
- v_{nTiO2} is the flicker noise signal track due to oxide layer coating the planar surface of the metal electrodes;
- v_{n1} and v_{n2} ar the equivalent input referred noise signal tracks of LNA1 and LNA2 stages, respectively;
- v_{nTDM} is the modulated noise signal track introduced by the TDM scheme.

3 Noise Figure and Noise Contributions in CMOS MEAs

The Noise Figure of an analog acquisition channel is typically defined as the ratio between the input SNR and the output SNR [20]. It is a fundamental parameter to measure not only noise power contributions to the final SNR, but also the effective degradation of the signal quality or SNR. The Noise Figure (NF) of the electrode/electronics interface with reference to the single biosensor row is:

$$NF = \frac{SNR_{IN}}{SNR_{OUT}} = \left(\frac{1}{G_1 \cdot G_2} \cdot \frac{v_{nout,RMS}}{v_{nin,RMS}} \right)^2 \tag{1}$$

where SNR_{IN} (SNR_{OUT}) is the input (output) SNR of the electrolyte/electrode (electrode/electronics) interface. SNR_{IN} noise power denominator ($v^2_{nin,RMS}$) is given by two main noise contributions: R_E thermal noise and TiO2 flicker noise power ($v^2_{nE,RMS}$ and $v^2_{nTiO2,RMS}$, respectively):

$$v^2_{nin,RMS} = v^2_{nE,RMS} + v^2_{nTiO2,RMS} \tag{2}$$

The total output noise power ($v^2_{nout,RMS}$) depends on how the individual noise power contributions propagate along the equivalent network in the Fig. 3, as follows:

$$v_{nout,RMS}^2 = \left(v^2_{nin,RMS} + v^2_{n1,RMS} \right) \cdot (G_1 \cdot G_2)^2 + \left(v^2_{nTMD,RMS} + v^2_{n2,RMS} \right) \cdot (G_2)^2 \tag{3}$$

Table 1. Neuron-silicon electrical model parameters [16].

Parameter	Explanation	Value
A_{ELE}	Metal electrode area	$100\ \mu m^2$
R_E	Electrolyte bulk resistance	$125\ k\Omega$
C_D	Stern capacitance	$35.9\ pF$
C_H	Helmotz capacitance	$17.3\ pF$
C_T	TiO2 capacitance	$3.3\ pF$
C_{HDT}	Total electrolyte-electrode capacitance	$2.58\ pF$

Thus, the final NF is:

$$NF = 1 + \frac{v_{n1,RMS}^2}{v_{nin,RMS}^2} + \frac{v_{nTMD,RMS}^2 + v_{n2,RMS}^2}{(G_1)^2} \cong 1 + \frac{v_{n1,RMS}^2}{v_{nin,RMS}^2} + \frac{v_{nTMD,RMS}^2}{(G_1)^2} \quad (4)$$

To minimize the NF (and/or to minimize the noise power at the output of the analog channel (LNA2)), the methodology presented in this paper is based on two fundamental pillars:

- to define the noise power due to the extracellular biological environment ($v^2_{nin,RMS}$) which cannot be eliminated because precisely due to the environment in which the neuro-potential signals are generated (electrolyte bath and electrode area);
- to define the target Noise Figure, or, in other words, the minimum acceptable amount (in dB) of degradation of the SNR.

Moreover, the noise power due to the LNA2, intervening after the first amplification (G_1 from LNA1) is in first approximation negligible (as expressed in Eq. 4). Hence the NF is purely function of $v^2_{n1,RMS}$ (input referred noise power of LNA1), G_1 (LNA1 passband gain) and the noise induced by the TDM operation (v^2_{nTMD}).

Following, Sects. 3.1 and 3.2 analytically define the noise PSD expressions of the electrolyte/electrode interface ($v_{nin,RMS}$ as a function of v_{nE} and v_{nTiO2}) and the the TDM operation (v_{nTDM}), respectively.

3.1 Noise Power at the Electrolyte-Electrode Interface

To fully understand and model the noise mechanisms at electrolyte-electrode interface level, it is worth to consider the simple case of a MEA single electrode feeding a voltage amplifier (LNA1) as illustrated in the physical cross-section view of Fig. 2.

The proposed model scheme (both physical and electrical views) is shown in Fig. 4. Table 1 resumes the main physical and electrical parameters of the neuron-electronics junction.

The neuron population and the silicon die are separated by an electrolyte bath (NaCL at 0.1 mol concentration). The TiO_2 post-processing layer [5] isolates the silicon circuits from the biological environment.

The extracellular ionic currents flow by the electrolyte equivalent resistance (R_E) inducing a small voltage variation. Thus, the voltage across R_E is coupled with the TiO_2 capacitance (C_{TiO2}) by the C_D-C_H series, where C_D and C_H are the double-layer region capacitances (Diffuse and Helmotz layers capacitances, respectively [18]). Just beneath the TiO_2 there is an on-chip Metal Electrode, whose area (A_{ELE}) is in this case 100 μm^2.

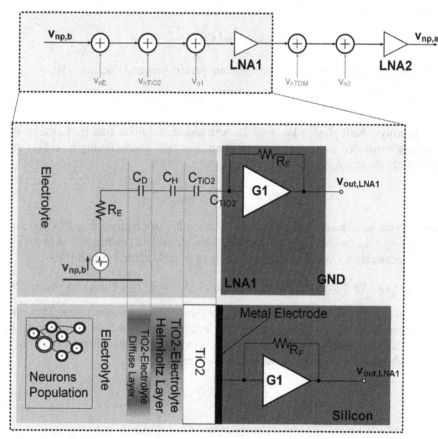

Fig. 4. Single electrode cross-section and equivalent electrical scheme [16].

This oxide layer has approximately 6 nm thickness and builds a specific series capacitance (C_{TiO2}). Notice that this scheme is referred to the worst-case scenario of scarce neuron-chip adhesion [18], where neuro-potentials signals are very weak and are spread across the electrolyte bath. Thus, the voltage source ($v_{np,b}$) models both EAP and LFP signals. The equivalent capacitance (C_{DHT}) between the cells and the input node of the LNA1 stage is:

$$C_{HDT} = \frac{1}{1/C_D + 1/C_H + 1/C_T} \tag{5}$$

C_D and C_H capacitances depend on the charge concentration at the electrolyte-oxide interface.

More specifically such Helmoltz and Diffuse Layers capacitances can be calculated using the metal electrode area (A_{ELE}), the water permittivity ($\varepsilon_w = 78.4 \cdot \varepsilon_0$ where ε_0 is the vacuum permittivity equal to 8.85 pF/m) and two physical lengths L_D (Deybe length, equal to 1 nm) and x_2 (Stern length, equal to 2 nm) depending on the electrolyte-oxide interface [21, 22].

$$C_D = \frac{\varepsilon_w}{L_D} \cdot A_{ELE} \text{ and } C_H = \frac{\varepsilon_w}{x_2} \cdot A_{ELE} \tag{6}$$

The TiO$_2$ layer capacitance has $45 \cdot \varepsilon_0$ and 6 nm permittivity and thickness [5]:

$$C_T = \frac{\varepsilon_{TiO2}}{x_{TiO2}} \cdot A_{ELE} \tag{7}$$

The electrolyte bulk plays a key role for both signal and noise transfer function. Its equivalent resistance R_E depends on the electrolyte bulk conductibility k' and on the metal electrode area A_{ELE} [22] as follows:

$$R_E = \frac{1}{k'} \cdot \sqrt{\pi / A_{ELE}} \tag{8}$$

Assuming the same number of carriers ($N_C = N_P = N_N$) for both positive (N_P, cations) and negative (N_N, anions) charges, then the bulk electrolyte conductivity depends on moles concentration (N_{MOL}) and water density ($\rho = 1000$ kg/m^3) as in Eq. 9:

$$k' = q \cdot (\mu_P \cdot N_P + \mu_N \cdot N_N) = q \cdot (\mu_P + \mu_N) \cdot N_C = q \cdot (\mu_P + \mu_N) \cdot \rho \cdot N_{MOL} \tag{9}$$

where μ_P-μ_N are the mobility coefficients for cations-anions, respectively. Thus, the bulk electrolyte conductivity is equal to 12.6 mA/(V·m) and the bulk resistance R_E is then 125 kΩ at 100 mM. The electrolyte resistance (R_E) generates a thermal noise (v_{nE}) whose in-band noise power spectral density is given by Eq. 10:

$$\frac{\langle v_{nE}^2 \rangle}{\Delta f} = 4 \cdot k \cdot T \cdot R_E \tag{10}$$

k ($= 13.8e{-}24$ J·K^{-1}) and T ($= 300$ K) are Boltzman constant and temperature, and R_E is 125 kΩ (Table 1). The $v_{out,LNA1}/v_{nE}$ transfer function (in Laplace domain) defines the transfer of the noise signal to the output as a function of C_{HDT} capacitance (C_H, C_D, and C_{TiO2} serie), the feedback pseudo-resistor (R_F) and the LNA1 passband gain ($G1$):

$$\frac{v_{out,LNA1}}{v_{nE}}(s) = \frac{s \cdot C_{HDT} \cdot R_F}{1 + s \cdot \frac{C_{HDT} \cdot R_F}{G_1}} \cdot \frac{1}{1 + s \cdot \tau_{LP}} = \frac{s \cdot \tau_{HP}}{1 + s \cdot \frac{\tau_{HP}}{G_1}} \cdot \frac{1}{1 + s \cdot \tau_{LP}} \tag{11}$$

The resulting transfer function has a passband corresponding frequency response limited by two frequency corners, f_{HP} ($=1/(2 \cdot \pi \cdot \tau_{HP})$) and f_{LP} ($=1/(2 \cdot \pi \cdot \tau_{HP})$). Electrolyte resistance noise PSD at the output of the LNA1 is thus given by:

$$v_{nE,OUTPSD}^2(f) = 4 \cdot k \cdot T \cdot R_E \cdot \left(\frac{\left(\frac{f}{f_{HP}}\right)^2}{1 + \left(\frac{1}{G_1} \cdot \frac{f}{f_{HP}}\right)^2} \cdot \frac{1}{1 + \left(\frac{f}{f_{LP}}\right)^2} \right) \tag{12}$$

TiO$_2$ film (to separate the biological environment from silicon chip) mainly generates flicker noise. Its noise PSD is inversely proportional to the frequency (f), as follows:

$$\frac{\langle v^2_{n,TiO2} \rangle}{\Delta f} = \frac{k_{pf,TiO2}}{C_{TiO2}} \cdot \frac{1}{f} \tag{13}$$

where $k_{pf,TiO2}$ is the specific flicker constant and C_{TiO2} is the equivalent TiO$_2$ capacitance. $v_{n,TiO2}$ signal has the same transfer function to the output as v_{nE} (Eq. 11). TiO2 Noise PSD at the output of the LNA1 stage is thus given by Eq. 14:

$$v^2_{nE,OUTPSD}(f) = \frac{k_{pf,TiO2}}{C_{TiO2}} \cdot \frac{1}{f} \cdot \left(\frac{\left(\frac{f}{f_{HP}}\right)^2}{1 + \left(\frac{1}{G_1} \cdot \frac{f}{f_{HP}}\right)^2} \cdot \frac{1}{1 + \left(\frac{f}{f_{LP}}\right)^2} \right) \tag{14}$$

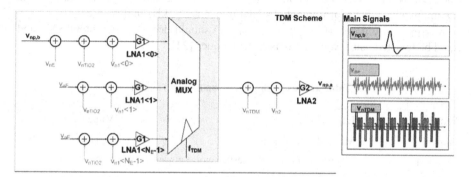

Fig. 5. TDM scheme Signal and Noise.

3.2 TDM Noise

Considering Fig. 3 signal flow scheme, the LNA2 features two relevant input referred noise contributions: the classical electronic noise coming from the input stage of the amplifier (v_{n2}, whose noise power has been hereby assumed in the same order of magnitude of LNA1 noise power and thus negligible for the purposes of Noise Figure calculation and modeling as in Eq. 4) and the noise induced by the TDM operation. This noise generates from statistical (static) offset voltage variation at the output of the N_E LNA1 that is converted into a statistical (dynamic) noise (v_{nTDM}) affecting final NF (and SNR$_{OUT}$) by the TDM sampling action (at f_{TDM} interrogation frequency).

To better explain this phenomenon of noise associated with TDM operation, consider the diagram in Fig. 5. The case in question assumes that there is a neuro-potential signal at the input of the first electrode of the biosensor (LNA1 <0>) and that all the other electrodes of the row have the input node connected to ground through the electrolyte resistance (R_E). In this specific case, the output static/dc voltage of each of the N_E LNAs that make up the row will vary by a certain amount which depends on the voltage offset statistic of the LNA1 stage. The output offset of a voltage amplifier has a standard deviation ($\sigma_{LNA1,OFFSET}$) in first approximation given by:

$$\sigma_{LNA1,OFFSET} = \frac{A_{VTH}}{\sqrt{W_1 \cdot L_1}} \tag{15}$$

where A_{VTH} is a CMOS process-dependent value (2 mV·μm [23]) and $W_1 \cdot L_1$ is the area of the MOST used for the input stage of the LNA1.

The sampling operation/interrogation frequency (f_{TDM}) of the TDM procedure converts such (static) voltage offset into a dynamic (time variant and frequency dependent) noise phenomenon, whose noise PSD spreads over the $f_{TDM}/2$ bandwidth as follows:

$$\frac{\langle v_{nTDM}^2 \rangle}{\Delta f} = 2 \cdot \frac{\left(\sigma_{LNA1,OFFSET}\right)^2}{f_{TDM}} = \frac{\left(\sigma_{LNA1,OFFSET}\right)^2}{N_E \cdot OVR \cdot f_0} \tag{16}$$

where N_E is the LNA1 row count, OVR is the ADC oversampling ratio and f_0 is the maximum detectable neuro-potential signal frequency (1 kHz in this case).

v_{nTDM}^2 noise power (i.e. $= \sigma_{LNA1,OFFSET}^2$) should decrease the output SNR and could be rejected using digitally assisted techniques [24].

Table 2. Design procedure input specifications.

Parameter	Explanation	Value
A_{ELE}	Metal electrode area	100 μm^2
$v_{nin,RMS}^2$	Electrolyte-electrode interface noise power	5.95 μV$_{RMS}$
$v_{nE,RMS}^2$	Electrolyte (R_E) noise power	3.4 μV$_{RMS}$
$v_{nTiO2,RMS}^2$	Electrolyte-electrode interface noise power	4.89 μV$_{RMS}$
$v_{nTDM,RMS}^2$	TDM noise power	200 μV$_{RMS}$
$v_{n2,RMS}^2$	LNA2 input referred noise power	10 μV$_{RMS}$
NF$_{[dB]}$	Target noise figure	1–6 dB

This approach requires an extra power budget to be allocated to the digital signal processing (DSP) stages driven from the ADC.

The alternative methodology adopted in this paper is to fix a certain LNA1 offset voltage ($\sigma_{LNA1,OFFSET}$) of 0.2 mV. This corresponding to 100 μm^2 MOST area, equal to the electrode area and thus satisfying the hypothesis to place the LNA1 input MOST just beneath the metal electrode, for improving electrode-LNA1 coupling.

Afterwards, the resulting v_{nTDM}^2 noise power is included in Eq. 4 Noise Figure.

Hence, the final $v_{n1,RMS}^2$-G_1 pair will satisfy the Noise Figure requirements even in presence of v_{nTDM} corrupting action, and, more importantly, without any necessity of embedding digitally assisted techniques compensating TDM noise and increasing computational power.

4 Noise Figure Based Design Procedure of CMOS MEAs

The Analog Signal Processing chain (single row in Fig. 1) and the Biological Sensitive Area are fully defined in terms of Noise Figure (Eq. 4) and in terms of equivalent electrical network (Fig. 4 and Table 1).

The starting point of the hereby proposed design procedure as a function of the required Noise Figure is to define a specific set of input parameters/specifications and to find the specific LNA1 parameters meeting the required Noise Figure.

The input specifications are: electrode area (A_{ELE}), electrolyte-electrode interface input noise power ($v^2_{nin,RMS}$, due to R_E thermal noise and TiO2 flicker noise power) and TDM induced noise power (at 200 μV LNA1 voltage offset ($v^2_{nin,RMS}$)).

The output results are: gain (G1), bandwidth (BW1) and input referred noise power ($v^2_{n1,RMS}$) of the first amplification stage (LNA1).

LNA2 gain will be then automatically set considering the total chain gain (G1·G2).

Such input specifications are listed in Table 2.

More specifically, $v^2_{nin,RMS}$ has been obtained by integrating the noise PSD functions in Eq. 13 and Eq. 15 into the specific neuro-potential signal bandwidth (1 Hz–5 kHz [18, 19]) and then quadratically summing the respective results. These operations gives 5.95 μV_{RMS} total input noise power for the electrolyte-electrode interface (with 3.4 μV_{RMS} and 4.89 μV_{RMS} for R_E and TiO2 noise contributions, respectively).

In this situation the Noise Figure in Eq. 4 is purely function of the noise power induced by the input stage of the LNA1 amplifier ($v^2_{n1,RMS}$) and of the amount of passband gain allocated to the first amplifier (G1).

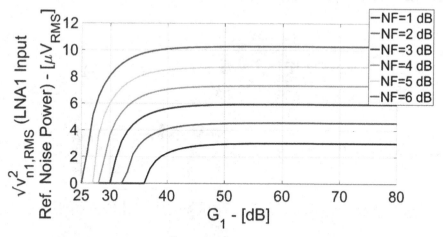

Fig. 6. $\sqrt{v^2_{n1,RMS}}$ vs. G1 at NF = 1–6 dB.

Figure 6 shows a group of curves where the LNA1 input referred noise power ($\sqrt{v^2_{n1,RMS}}$, in μV_{RMS}) is plotted vs. G1 gain (in dB) using a specific Noise Figure vinculum and for different possible Noise Figure values (in dB).

For each NF curve, there is lower region of G1 gain (from 0 to 25 dB at NF = 6 dB and from 0 to 36 dB at NF = 1 dB) in which the relation binding Noise Figure to LNA1 input noise power and G1 cannot be satisfied, because the noise power of the TDM alone saturates the Noise Figure.

For a given Noise Figure curve, when G1 increases then the maximum allowable noise power budget for LNA1 increases, because TDM noise power is more attenuated by the same G1 gain.

On the other hand, increasing Noise Figure for a given gain (G1) results in higher LNA1 input referred noise power because the level of the SNR degradation increases.

Considering the more aggressive Noise Figure of 1 dB curve, Fig. 6 finally aims to set a specific LNA1 gain-noise (G1-$\sqrt{v^2_{n1,RMS}}$) pair that allows to satisfy the specific required Noise Figure. The problem now arises of choosing a specific pair of G1-$\sqrt{v^2_{n1,RMS}}$ values. This choice is made according to the requirement of LNA1 static current consumption as follows.

The single row Analog Signal Processing in Fig. 7 has been modelled adopting a single MOST LNA1 stage. In this case the LNA1 input referred noise power is dominated by thermal and flicker noise contributions of M1 ($\gamma = 0.5$ is the MOST thermal noise coefficient, $k_{nf} = 25e-24$ V$^2\cdot$F/Hz is the flicker noise constant and C'$_{OX} = 19$ fF/μm^2 is the MOST gate oxide capacitance per unit area [25]):

$$\frac{\langle v^2_{n1,RMS}\rangle}{\Delta f} = 4 \cdot \gamma \cdot k \cdot T \cdot \frac{1}{g_{m1}} + \frac{k_{nf}}{C'_{OX}} \cdot \frac{1}{f} \qquad (17)$$

State-of-the-art CMOS MEAs [7-16] typically adopts few μA current consumption for LNA1 stages, in order to minimize the total grid power consumption. For this reason this case of study adopts 2 μA I1 dc current for LNA1 M1 MOST.

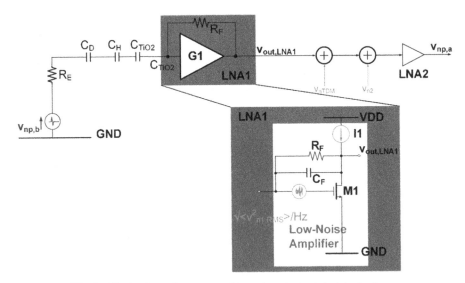

Fig. 7. Single electrode cross-section and equivalent electrical scheme.

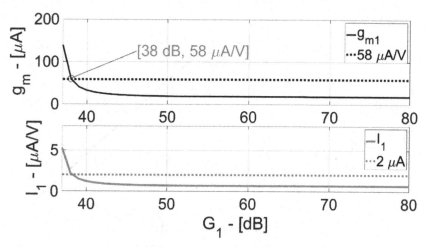

Fig. 8. M1 MOST dc Current (I1) and Transconductance (g_{m1}) vs. G1 at NF = 1 dB.

In these conditions of basing current, M1 MOST operates in subthreshold region with its proper transconductance (g_{m1}) approximately equal to $I1/(n \cdot k \cdot T/q)$, where I1 is the M12 dc current and n is the subthreshold slope factor [23].

Figure 8 shows the estimated M1 transconductance (g_{m1}) and current (I1) starting from $\sqrt{v^2_{n1,RMS}}$ vs. G1 curve at NF = 1 dB (Fig. 6) and assuming the same noise power for thermal and flicker contributions in Eq. 16.

$\sqrt{v^2_{n1,RMS}}$ at NF = 1 dB curve in Fig. 6 increases with G1, resulting in higher allowable noise. Thus, M1 transconductance and dc current must decrease for increasing G1 (as illustrated in Fig. 8).

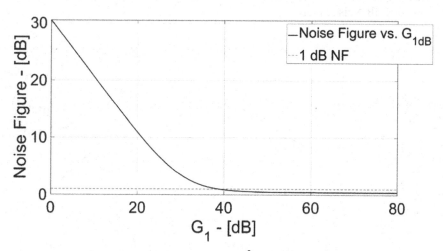

Fig. 9. Noise Figure vs. G1 at $\sqrt{v^2_{n1,RMS}} = 1.8\ \mu V_{RMS}$.

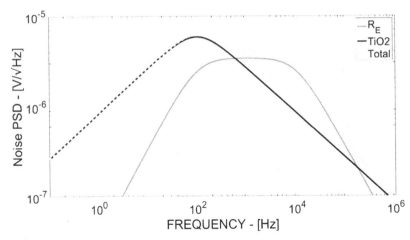

Fig. 10. V_{nin} Noise PSD (R_E and TiO2 Noise).

$I1 = 2$ μA M1 dc current results in 58 μA/V transconductance and 1.8 μV$_{RMS}$ LNA1 input referred noise power ($\sqrt{v^2}_{n1,RMS}$).

Figure 9 shows that it is possible to further improve the NF (at the same $\sqrt{v^2}_{n1,RMS} = $ 1.8 μV$_{RMS}$) by increasing the LNA1 passband gain, or in other words further attenuating the TDM noise power.

As a conclusion, the proposed model equations, simply based on Noise Figure expression (Eq. 4) and electrolyte-electrode electrical model (Fig. 4), allows to clearly set the most relevant design parameters meeting the required Noise Figure [6].

The output design parameters of the proposed model are listed in Table 2 and resumes the most important values to be used in LNA1, TDM and LNA2 implementation as a function of 1 dB Noise Figure.

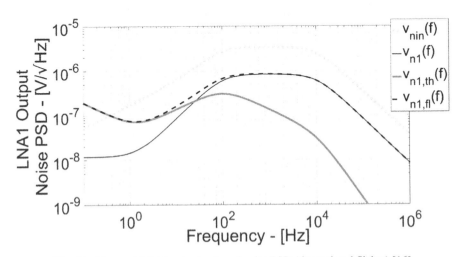

Fig. 11. V_{nin} and LNA1 output referred noise PSD (thermal and flicker) [16].

Table 3. Design procedure output results.

Parameter	Explanation	Value
G1	LNA1 passband gain	38 dB
$v^2_{n1,RMS}$	LNA1 input referred noise power	1.8 μV_{RMS}
BW1	LNA1 bandwidth	<10 kHz
RF	LNA1 feedback resistance	21 GΩ
I1	M1 MOST dc current	2 μA
g_{m1}	M1 MOST transconductance	58 μA/V
G2	LNA2 passband gain	22 dB

For sake of completeness, the model allows also to define the frequency behavior of the noise power (the noise PSD) for all relevant noise contributions in the single row MEA Analog Signal Processing channel. Figure 10 shows the noise PSD simulation results for what concerns the electrolyte-electrode interface noise. These PSD curves are plotted starting from Eq. 12 and Eq. 14, respectively, and are referred to the LNA1 output node at 37 dB G1 gain. TiO2 noise PSD (from flicker contribution) dominates at low frequency while R_E thermal noise PSD becomes more important from approximately 500 Hz intersecting frequency.

Figure 11 illustrates the noise PSD behavior of electrolyte-electrode interface (v_{nin}) and LNA1 (v_{n1}), respectively (again referred to LNA1 output node).

5 Conclusions

This paper has presented a complete design procedure for CMOS Microelectrode Arrays in neural recording experiments. The proposed procedure is based on two successive steps: the complete modelling of the electrical network composing the neural interface (starting from the biological electrolyte bath up to Analog Signal Processing stages) and an easy-to-use design equation that correlate the required Noise Figure with the first amplifier gain and noise and with the noise induced by the TDM operation. This approach produces accurate design parameters meeting the starting Noise Figure while including TDM noise/artifacts effects and then in principle enabling the use of MEAs with the target Noise Figure without adding specific calibration stages for TDM noise rejection.

Extensive simulation results at whole system level (noise and Noise figure vs. LNA1 gain) and at frequency domain level (noise PSD at the output of the LNA1 stage) have been proposed to validate the design methodology.

Starting from few numerical input specifications (Table 1), the proposed design procedure provides specific results to be used as design parameters, as listed in Table 3.

Acknowledgments. This work has been partially supported by the Brain28 PRIN Project.

References

1. Obien, M.E.J., et al.: Revealing neuronal function through microelectrode array recordings. Front. Neurosci. **8**, 423 (2015)
2. Thomas Jr., C.A., et al.: A miniature microelectrode array to monitor the bioelectric activity of cultured cells. Exp. Cell Res. **74**(1), 61–66 (1972)
3. Pine, J.: Recording action potentials from cultured neurons with extracellular microcircuit electrodes. J. Neurosci. Methods **2**(1), 19–31 (1980)
4. Gross, G.W., Williams, A.N., Lucas, J.H.: Recording of spontaneous activity with photoetched microelectrode surfaces from mouse spinal neurons in culture. J. Neurosci. Methods **5**(1–2), 13–22 (1982)
5. Cianci, E., et al.: Atomic layer deposited TiO2 for implantable brain-chip interfacing devices. Thin Solid Films **520**(14), 4745–4748 (2012)
6. Vallicelli, E.A., et al.: Neural spike digital detector on FPGA. Electronics **7**(12), 392 (2018)
7. Shahid, S., Walker, J., Smith, L.S.: A new spike detection algorithm for extracellular neural recordings. IEEE Trans. Biomed. Eng. **57**(4), 853–866 (2009)
8. DeBusschere, B.D., Kovacs, G.T.A.: Portable cell-based biosensor system using integrated CMOS cell-cartridges. Biosens. Bioelectron. **16**(7–8), 543–556 (2001)
9. Huys, R., et al.: Single-cell recording and stimulation with a 16k micro-nail electrode array integrated on a 0.18 μm CMOS chip. Lab Chip **12**(7), 1274–1280 (2012)
10. Frey, U., et al.: Switch-matrix-based high-density microelectrode array in CMOS technology. IEEE J. Solid-State Circ. **45**(2), 467–482 (2010)
11. Maccione, A., et al.: Sensing and actuating electrophysiological activity on brain tissue and neuronal cultures with a high-density CMOS-MEA. In: 2013 Transducers & Eurosensors XXVII: The 17th International Conference on Solid-State Sensors, Actuators and Microsystems (TRANSDUCERS & EUROSENSORS XXVII). IEEE (2013)
12. Eversmann, B., et al.: A 128/spl times/128 CMOS biosensor array for extracellular recording of neural activity. IEEE J. Solid-State Circ. **38**(12), 2306–2317 (2003)
13. Wang, S., et al.: A compact quad-shank CMOS neural probe with 5,120 addressable recording sites and 384 fully differential parallel channels. IEEE Trans. Biomed. Circ. Syst. **13**, 1625–1634 (2019)
14. Lopez, C.M., et al.: A multimodal CMOS MEA for high-throughput intracellular action potential measurements and impedance spectroscopy in drug-screening applications. IEEE J. Solid-State Circ. **53**(11), 3076–3086 (2018)
15. Dragas, J., et al.: In vitromulti-functional microelectrode array featuring 59 760 electrodes, 2048 electrophysiology channels, stimulation, impedance measurement, and neurotransmitter detection channels. IEEE J. Solid-State Circ. **52**(6), 1576–1590 (2017)
16. Tomasella, D., Vallicelli, E.A., Baschirotto, A., De Matteis, M.: Detection of <12 μVRMS extracellular action potential and local field potential by optimum design of a single pixel electrolyte-oxide-MOSFET interface in CMOS 28 nm. In: BIODEVICES, pp. 66–76 (2021)
17. Harrison, R.R., Charles, C.: A low-power low-noise CMOS amplifier for neural recording applications. IEEE J. Solid-State Circ. **38**(6), 958–965 (2003)
18. Massobrio, P., Massobrio, G., Martinoia, S.: Interfacing cultured neurons to microtransducers arrays: a review of the neuro-electronic junction models. Front. Neurosci. **10**, 282 (2016)
19. Vassanelli, S., Mahmud, M., Girardi, S., Maschietto, M.: On the way to large-scale and high-resolution brain-chip interfacing. Cogn. Comput. **4**(1), 71–81 (2012)
20. Razavi, B., Behzad, R.: RF Microelectronics, vol. 2, p. 39. Prentice Hall, New York (2012)
21. Hassibi, A., Navid, R., Dutton, R.W., Lee, T.H.: Comprehensive study of noise processes in electrode electrolyte interfaces. J. Appl. Phys. **96**(2), 1074–1082 (2004)

22. Deen, M.J., Shinwari, M.W., Ranuárez, J.C., Landheer, D.: Noise considerations in field-effect biosensors. J. Appl. Phys. **100**(7), 074703 (2006)
23. Sansen, W.M.: Analog Design Essentials, vol. 859. Springer, Heidelberg (2007). https://doi.org/10.1007/b135984
24. Uehlin, J.P., et al.: A single-chip bidirectional neural interface with high-voltage stimulation and adaptive artifact cancellation in standard CMOS. IEEE J. Solid-State Circ. **55**, 1749–1761 (2020). https://doi.org/10.1109/jssc.2020.2991524
25. Baschirotto, A., Delizia, P., D'Amico, S., Chironi, V., Cocciolo, G., De Matteis, M.: Low power analog design in scaled technologies. In: Proceedings of the Topical Workshop on Electronics for Particle Physics, TWEPP 2009, Paris, France, 21 September 2009, pp. 103–109 (2009)

LigityScore: A CNN-Based Method for Binding Affinity Predictions

Joseph Azzopardi[1]([⊠])🆔 and Jean Paul Ebejer[2]🆔

[1] Department of Artificial Intelligence, University of Malta, Msida MSD 2080, Malta
{joseph.azzopardi.06,jean.p.ebejer}@um.edu.mt
[2] Centre for Molecular Medicine and Biobanking, University of Malta, Msida MSD 2080, Malta

Abstract. Scoring functions are the heart of structure based drug design, where they are used to estimate how strongly the docked pose of a ligand binds to the target. Seeking a scoring function that can accurately predict the binding affinity is key for successful virtual screening methods. Deep learning approaches have recently seen a rise in popularity as a means to improve the scoring function having the key advantage to automatically extract features and create a complex representation of the data without feature engineering and expert knowledge.

In this study we present the LigityScore scoring functions – LigityScore1D and LigityScore3D. The LigityScore models are rotationally invariant scoring functions based on convolutional neural networks (CNN). LigityScore descriptors are extracted directly from the structural and interacting properties of the protein-ligand complex which are input to a CNN for automatic feature extraction and binding affinity prediction. This representation uses the spatial distribution of Pharmacophoric Interaction Points (PIPs), derived from interaction features from the protein-ligand complex based on pharmacophoric features conformant to specific family types (Hydrogen Bond Acceptor (HBA), Hydrogen Bond Donor (HBD), etc.) and distance thresholds. The data representation component and the CNN architecture together, constitute the LigityScore scoring function.

LigityScore1D considers a single distance from each combination of two PIPs from the extracted ligand and protein PIP pools, and generates a feature vector for each pharmacophoric family pair (example HBA-HBD) based on the distribution of the PIP pair distances in discretised space. The different pharmacophoric family pair combinations are grouped to construct a matrix representation of the complex. Similarly, LigityScore3D considers 3-PIP combinations to create a triangular structure with three distances between the PIPs. These are discretised to represent binning coordinates for a 3D feature cube for each pharmacophoric family set (example HBA-HBD-HBD) that describe the distribution of distances in 3D space. The cube from each pharmacophoric family set are grouped together to from a feature cube collection.

The main contribution for this study is to present a novel rotationally invariant protein-ligand representation for use as a CNN based scoring function for binding affinity prediction. The CNN model is used for automatic feature extraction from the LigityScore representations. LigityScore models are evaluated for scoring power on the latest two CASF benchmarks. The Pearson correlation coefficient, and the standard deviation in linear regression were used to compare LigityScore with the benchmark model, and also other models in literature published in recent years. LigityScore3D has achieved better results than LigityScore1D and showed

ⓒ The Author(s), under exclusive license to Springer Nature Switzerland AG 2022
C. Gehin et al. (Eds.): BIOSTEC 2021, CCIS 1710, pp. 18–44, 2022.
https://doi.org/10.1007/978-3-031-20664-1_2

similar performance in both CASF benchmarks. LigityScore3D ranked 5th place in the CASF-2013 benchmark, and 8th in CASF-2016, with an average Pearson correlation coefficient (R) performance of 0.713 and 0.725 respectively. LigityScore1D obtained best results when trained using the PBDbind v2018 dataset, and ranked 8th place in the CASF-2013 and 7th place in CASF-2016 with an R performance of 0.635 and 0.741 respectively. Our methods show relatively good performance that exceed the Pafnucy performance, as one of the best performing CNN based scoring function, on the CASF-2013 benchmark, using a less computationally complex model that can be trained 16 times faster.

Keywords: Virtual screening · Structure-based virtual screening · Scoring function · Pharmacophoric interaction point · Machine learning · Deep-learning · Convolutional neural networks · LigityScore

1   Introduction

Drug discovery is a process used to identify small molecules which elicit the desired biological response when they bind to target proteins. This bioactivity either activates or inhibits a biological function thus acting as a drug to the body. In recent years, Computer-Aided Drug Design (CADD) methods have seen a rise in popularity for drug discovery processes due to the unprecedented amount of data available together with the advent of powerful computational tools available such as cloud computing platforms [33].

Structure-based drug design is a virtual screening (VS) technique that employs computational methods on known 3D protein structures to measure the ability of a small molecule to bind to the target protein structure. A docking program is normally an integral part of structure based virtual screening (SBVS) which measures the ability of the small molecule to bind to the target structure in a typical *'lock and key'* fashion [6]. The docking process iteratively tests a huge number of ligand conformers, or docking poses to potentially find the ligand pose that yields the best binding affinity. The scoring function is considered the heart of the docking program as it estimates the binding affintity and the complementarity of a particular pose. The scoring function can be defined as "estimating how strongly the docked pose of a ligand binds to the target" [1] and it is therefore crucial for the success of docking programs in SBVS. Scoring functions are typically used for fast evaluation of protein-ligand interactions, so optimising the performance and the ability of the scoring function to assess the binding capability between a protein and a ligand, helps improve the performance of docking programs, which in turn improves the effectiveness of drug discovery in SBVS methods. The scoring function is considered the foundation in SBVS and used in the following areas for hit discovery and optimization [32]:

1. **Pose Prediction:** Predict the shape of the ligand which gives the best binding affinity.
2. **Ranking:** Ranking of molecules with known binding pose in order of the binding affinity for a given protein target.

3. **Classification:** Given the binding-pose, classify whether a small molecule is active or inactive for a given 3D structure of a target protein.

Intense research has been carried out over the years on scoring functions, however improving the accuracy for binding affinity prediction has proven to be a non-trivial task [1]. Despite several advances in binding affinity prediction, the current binding affinity estimates are still not accurate enough leading to high false positive rates [42]. The work presented in this paper describes in detail the LigityScore methods introduced in Azzopardi and Ebejer (2021) [2] highlighting the differences in the feature representation, CNN architecture and the results obtained.

The LigityScore methods focus directly on the scoring function layer of SBVS and tackle this problem by finding an alternative data representation of the protein-ligand complex and then apply a Convolutional Neural Network (CNN) regression model to implement the scoring function. The prediction of binding affinity is a regression problem where the model learns the salient information of the input features to output a value of binding affinity. The binding affinity prediction model can then be used in SBVS for classification of the small molecule as inactive or active. Although computational methods have been used in drug design for over three decades, accurate prediction of binding affinity still remains an open problem in computational chemistry [6].

Deep Learning (DL) has been recently applied for drug discovery, where multiple hidden layers are used to build a deep neural network (DNN). The key advantage of DNN is the ability to automatically extract features and create a complex representation of the data through the hidden layers without the need of applying feature engineering [31]. Feature extractions thus occur as a natural byproduct of fitting the input to the model's parameters. Deep learning models allow for further reduction in feature engineering and reliance on expert knowledge. On the other hand, conventional ML techniques such as Random Forests and Support Vector Machines, are limited to process raw data, require careful feature engineering and expert domain knowledge [19]. The first deep neural network used for VS was introduced by the winning team of the 2012 Kaggle Merck Molecular activity challenge [15], motivated by the remarkable success in various other areas such as computer vision [38] and natural language processing [9]. The team applied a multi-task deep feed-forward network for quantitative structure-activity (QSAR) LBVS. This work was later published by Ma *et al.* (2015) [26] which generated a lot of interest and excitement for the use of DL in this field.

The Convolutional Neural Network (CNN) is one of the most common DL architectures used for scoring functions [14,24,32,36,42]. The CNN uses a number of sequential layers of convolutions and pooling modules to encode the hidden features of the data, and then use a fully connected feedforward NN layers for classification or regression. Since protein-ligand complexes are 3D structures, their representation can include multi-dimensional tensors. CNNs are known to process multi-dimensional inputs, such as colour images, successfully to extract the relevant features and achieve remarkable accuracy [38]. Similarly, CNNs can be used to extract features for protein-ligand complexes that are represented by multi-dimensional tensors. CNNs are also able to capture the spatial placement of features as described by Goodfellow *et al.* (2016) [10], which can be an important factor to extract interactions features from 3D structures such as the protein-ligand complexes. For these reasons, and the success achieved with CNNs in the works of Jiménez *et al.* (2018) [14] and Stepniewska-Dziubinska *et al.* (2017) [36] we have chosen the CNN as the DL model to use for automatic features extraction from our multi-dimensional representation of the protein-ligand complexes. Due to the its natural feature extraction ability, the CNN applied in the SBVS domains, shift the importance from feature engineering to representation engineering. Therefore, our strategy is to allow deep learning models to *learn* the underlying molecular interactions from the LigityScore representation, so that this learned information can be reapplied to other protein targets for exploration of novel ligands, without the need to incorporate expert chemical knowledge. Our work is evaluated using the CASF-2013 [20] and CASF-2016 [37] benchmarks and is also compared to other recently-published scoring function methods that use the same benchmarks.

Ragoza *et al.* (2017) were the first to use CNNs to implement a DL scoring function for SBVS and pose prediction. Ragoza *et al.* (2017) [32] claim that their CNN scoring function outperforms Autodock Vina on the DUD-E [27] and CSAR [7] datasets for both screening and pose prediction tasks respectively. For the input of the CNN, Ragoza *et al.* (2017) have discretized the protein-ligand structure into a 3D grid of 24 Å for each side, centered at the binding site. The 3D grid is composed of multiple 2D grids— one for each heavy atom of the protein-ligand complex analogous to RGB channels in images. Each element in the grid at 0.5 Å resolution stores atom information using a density distribution function $A(d, r)$, dependent on the distance d from atom centre, and the van der Waals radius, r. However, Sieg *et al.* (2019) [34] later showed that their model was effected by non-causal bias. Sieg *et al.* (2019) reproduced the model and concluded that the CNN was not learning from the features of the protein-ligand but was instead just learning from the bias found in the small molecule features introduced while generating the DUD-E decoys.

Pafnucy proposed by Stepniewska-Dziubinska *et al.* (2017) is one of the most promising DL scoring function models where the authors achieved a Pearson Coefficient, R, for the predicted versus experimental binding affinity of 0.70 and 0.78 for the CASF-2013 and CASF-2016 benchmarks respectively. Pafnucy uses a 3D CNN model with a 4D tensor to represent 19 protein-ligand features in 3D space. The 4D tensor includes discretised atom locations in the first three dimensions, whilst the 19 features for the particular atom such as atom type, charge, and SMARTS are encoded in the fourth dimension. Jiménez *et al.* (2018) also utilise a 3D CNN model termed K_{deep} and achieved state of the art results on the CASF-2016 test with an R value of 0.82. Their input features use a 3D voxel representation with eight channels. Each channel, representing a different pharmacophoric feature of the protein-ligand structure, are stacked together to create a 4D input tensor. The pharmacophoric features used include hydrophobic, aromatic, hydrogen bond acceptor (HBA), hydrogen bond donor (HBD), cation, anion, metallic, and excluded volume.

A recent study proposed by Zheng *et al.* (2019) compares their model, OnionNet, to Stepniewska-Dziubinska *et al.* (2017) and criticize the Pafnucy model, and claim that the protein-ligand interactions in a 3D grid box of 20 Å are not sufficient to capture all the protein-ligand interactions, and suggest that other long-range interactions outside the 20 Å, termed *non-local* electrostatic interactions are also important. To capture all the interactions between protein-ligand complexes, Zheng *et al.* (2019) divide all the 3D space of the binding site into a number of shells or zones and count the number of different element-to-element interactions within each shell. [42] conducted tests that excluded one shell at a time during training to uncover which shells were contributing more to the Pearson Coefficient. The loss with the removed shell was compared with the loss of the best performing model. The larger the change in loss noticed, the more important is the feature. Their experiments show that the shells closer to the ligand are more important, as was intuitively expected, however they also show that non-local interactions have significant importance. This method is rotationally invariant since their representation is composed of element to element counts which do not change with the orientation of the complex. This simple element to element interaction count feature was inspired by the RF-score model [3].

Zheng *et al.* (2019) compare OnionNet to another recent model, AGL-Score by Nguyen and Wei (2019a), and comment that their algebraic sub-graphs coupled with a gradient boosting trees ML model implementation provides a more *complete* representation of the protein-ligand complex and manages to improve the R Pearson's correlation coefficient to 0.833. To date this represents the best performing ML scoring function.

A major challenge faced by Jiménez *et al.* (2018) [14] and Stepniewska-Dziubinska *et al.* (2017) [36] was the requirement of training a CNN model that can handle different views or snapshots of the same representation. If the orientation from where the snapshot is taken is changed, a different representation of the *same* structure is obtained, since the protein-ligand complex is a 3D structure. The authors have worked around this limitation by introducing different systematic rotations of the protein-ligand complex during training. However, rotations increase the data input and are therefore slower to train. These might also present additional challenges when testing novel complexes that can take different orientations. This limitation has led us to explore methods that are inherently rotationally invariant. One such method is Ligity [8], which is based on the spatial distance distribution between different set of pharmacophoric interactions points. Since these distances remain the same irrespective of the orientation of the structure, the Ligity method is inherently rotationally invariant. Ligity is a hybrid VS technique that collects key interaction features within the protein-ligand complexes, and was shown to be successful for a virtual screening exercises using similarity measures. These key interaction points, known as *hot-spots*, are defined by considering specific pharmacophoric features that lie within a predetermined distance threshold between the protein and ligand feature pairs. Each of these pharmacophoric features that *interact* together are termed *Pharmacophoric Interaction Points* or PIPs. Once these pairs are extracted, the Ligity descriptor for the ligand is created by considering only the PIPs from the ligand space. Three or four PIP combinations are considered in the original Ligity method. The Ligity descriptor is built using the spatial distribution of PIPs (*i.e.* the distance between PIPs), and is, therefore, rotationally invariant.

Ligity was used as the basis of our study and has inspired us to build a feature representation using *both* the protein and ligand PIPs, as opposed to Ligity that uses only ligand PIPs. In this study we present *LigityScore* – a novel rotationally invariant CNN based scoring function that utilises the interaction of pharmacophoric features of the protein and ligand for its data representation. In our approach we have therefore hypothesised that pharmacophoric interactions across different feature types contain key information to suitably represent the protein ligand structure and their binding properties. We have further hypothesised that this representation would be suitable to train a CNN model as a scoring function for binding affinity prediction. Our approach introduces two techniques, LigityScore1D and LigityScore3D, that make use of important structural features of both the protein and ligand to create a suitable data representation of the protein-ligand complex.

The novel protein-ligand representations employed by LigityScore1D and LigityScore3D for use in a CNN based scoring function for binding affinity prediction is our major contribution in the SBVS domain. The source code for LigityScore is available at https://gitlab.com/josephazzopardi/ligityscore.

2 LigityScore Overview

LigityScore is a CNN based scoring function that utilises a rotationally invariant data representation extracted from interacting pharmacophoric features in protein-ligand complexes. An overview of LigityScore is illustrated in Fig. 1, highlighting the parameters that can be changed for each module. The major functional parts for LigityScore (LigityScore1D and LigityScore3D) are detailed below:

1. **Pre-Processing.** A pre-processing module is used to process, extract and clean the required information from the PDBbind [23] protein-ligand complexes and build our PDBbind dataset that includes the binding affinity information. This module also validates that the required molecular files are available, and fixes molecular files that cannot be loaded by the RDKit cheminformatics software [17].
2. **PIP (Hot-spots) Generation.** The pharmacophoric features of the protein-ligand complex are extracted using the RDKit *BuildFeatureFactory* class (see Fig. 3). A cartesian product across all possible protein and ligand pharmacophoric feature pairs is constructed, and then filtering using a number of constraints (see Table 1). The filtered protein-ligand pharmacophoric feature represent the PIPs for the particular complex.
3. **Generation of LigityScore Descriptors.** The filtered pharmacophoric features (PIPs) are grouped into ligand and protein PIP pools for each complex. These PIP *pools* are used to extract all possible combination of PIPs and generate a feature descriptor for each complex. The name of our models is derived from the dimensionality of the spatial information used to generate the features. LigityScore1D considers combination of two PIPs at a time that correspond to one inter-PIP distance. For each pharmacophoric feature famility, these distances are encoded in a feature vector hence the name LigityScore1D. On the other hand, LigityScore3D uses combination of three PIPs at a time, that correspond to 3 inter-PIP distances. These distances are encoded in a features cube for each PIP family set example Acceptor-Acceptor-Acceptor). For each complex a feature matrix is generated for LigityScore1D, whilst a feature cube collection, grouped feature cubes for each PIP family set combination, is generated for LigityScore3D (see Figs. 5 and 6).

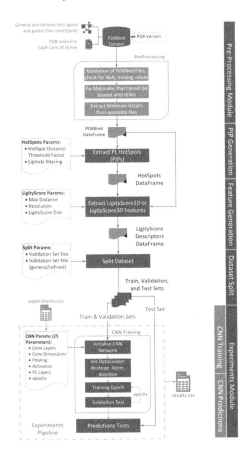

Fig. 1. LigityScore schematic representation of the major functional components used in our app-roach to develop a CNN based scoring function for virtual screening. The parameters used in each functional block are included as reference. For example PIP Hot-spots extraction can take two parameters – Lipinski filtering, and the hot-spots distance threshold factor. Reproduced from Azzopardi and Ebejer (2021) [2].

4. **CNN Training.** This module is built using the Pytorch library [30] and includes a dynamic model to construct a CNN in order to facilitate the testing and evaluation of different CNN architectures. The CNN module is used to train the network as a scoring function using the LigityScore descriptors. The CNN has one regression output neuron to predict the binding affinity of the complex. The convolution layers provide automatic feature extraction whilst the feed-forward layers are used to pre-dict he binding affinity. Each epoch is validated against the validation set, composed of 1,000 randomly sampled complexes from the PDBbind Refined set and the model with the lowest root means squared error (RMSE) is stored to disk.

5. **CNN Predictions.** The Predictions module loads the best performing CNN model and provides RMSE, MAE (Mean Absolute Error), SD (Standard Deviation in Regression), and R (Pearson Correlation Coefficient) values for the test sets to assess the performance of the model.

6. **Experiments Pipeline.** This module is used to automate the workflows for training, validation and testing. Experiments are defined as a csv file and are loaded in the pipeline to execute the experiments in sequence. The CSV file includes parameters such as number of convolution layers, layer filter dimensions, kernel size, training epochs, number of fully connected (FC) layers, and size of each FC layer. A total of 39 parameters are required to initialise one experiment. For each experiment the best epoch is chosen based on the lowest RMSE for the validation set.

3   Dataset

The PDBbind dataset [23] is regarded as a golden dataset for the development of scoring functions [23], and was therefore used for training and testing of LigityScore. The PDBbind v2016 dataset is primarily used as a means to evaluate our models with other models. The PDBbind v2018, which contains around 2,700 additional protein-ligand complexes, was also used as an additional experiment and to facilitate comparison with other models.

The PDBbind dataset [23] includes manually curated records of experimentally measured binding affinity data for biomolecular complexes taken from the Protein Data Bank (PDB) [4] using only direct original references [23]. The PDBbind dataset expresses binding affinity values in terms of dissociation (K_d), inhibition (K_i) or half-concentration (IC_{50}) constants. No distinction is made between these constants and they were converted into a negative log; $pK_a = -log_{10}K_x$, where K_x can be K_i, K_d or IC_{50}, and pK_a is the binding affinity [36,42]. The protein-ligand complexes defint in PDBbind (v2016 and v2018) are grouped into different sets which include:

1. **The General Set.** The general set is composed of 13,308 (v2016) protein-ligand complexes, and represents all the available protein-ligand complexes available in the dataset.
2. **The Refined Set.** The refined set is a subset of the general set and is composed of 3,689 protein-ligand complexes (v2016). It was constructed after quality controls on structural resolution and experimental precision of the binding data measurement.
3. **The Core Set.** The core sets are not defined in the grouping of the PDBbind dataset, but were established as part of the Comparative Assessment of Scoring Functions (CASF) benchmark. This CASF v2013 was defined by Li *et al.* (2016) [21], whilst CASF v2016 was defined in Su *et al.* (2018) [37]. The Comparative Assessment of Scoring Functions (CASF) benchmarks aim to provide an objective platform to assess scoring functions strengths and weaknesses using high-quality protein ligand complexes from the refined set, following a systematic, non-rendundant sampling procedure.

The CASF benchmarks were used to assess the *Scoring Power* of LigityScore1D and LigityScore3D. The scoring power is quantitatively measured for evaluation using the Pearson's correlation coefficient, R, and the standard deviation in linear regression (SD). The Scoring Power measures the ability of the model to map a linear correlation of the predicted and known experimental affinity values. This study is focused to predict the binding affinity and the scoring power CASF benchmarks will be used for objective assessment and evaluation of the proposed scoring function.

The relation between the PDBbind sets, core sets, and the training, validation, and test sets is summarised in Fig. 2. The core sets (2013 and 2016) were used entirely as the two test sets to simulate new and unseen protein-ligand complexes during the prediction stage. The complexes defined in the core sets were not used during training and validation. The validation is made up of 1,000 randomly sampled complexes from the refined set as it provides higher quality protein-ligand complexes that are more reliable for the development of scoring functions [23]. The remainder of the protein-ligand complexes were used as the training set.

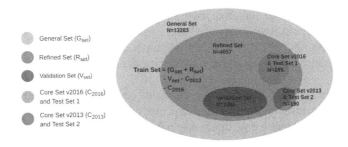

Fig. 2. PDBbind Venn-diagram showing the general, refined and cores sets, together with how these were split up for training, validation and testing. The core sets are reserved as test sets. The validation set is made up of 1,000 protein-ligand complexes from the refined set, whilst the remaining complexes are used for training. N represents the count of protein-ligand complexes in each set.

Dataset Preparation. A pre-processing module was used to process, extract and clean the required protein-ligand information from the PDBbind dataset. This module was used to create our molecular dataset, validate that the required molecular files are available, and fix molecular files that cannot be loaded using RDKit [17]. Preprocessing of the molecular files such as removal of water molecule, addition of hydrogens, and computation of partial charges, is not required for the LigityScore methods.

Some of the molecular files in the dataset have an incorrect mapping of atomic bonds and consequently fail to load with RDKit and therefore would be excluded from training. The ligand files generate most of the errors with 1,603 invalid ligand molecules for the PDBbind v2016, and 1,839 for the PDBbind v2018. To fix the ligand molecular files, the molecules were evaluated using different formats (.mol2 or .sdf) and then fetched directly using PyMol. This process minimised the discarded molecules to 172 and 207 for PDBbind v2016 and PDBbind v2018 respectively.

4   LigityScore Implementation

The LigityScore scoring function consists of the following two components:

1. Feature generation process to extract a representation of the protein ligand complex in LigityScore space

2. The CNN model for automatic feature extraction and representation for binding affinity predictions.

The LigityScore method considers six pharmacophore features: hydrophobic, hydrogen bond acceptor, hydrogen bond donor, aromatic, cation, and anion. Gund (1977) [11] describes a *pharmacophore* as "*a set of structural features in a molecule that are recognised at the binding site and is responsible for that molecule's biological activity*". Therefore a pharmacophore model represents a number of structural features such as aromatic or hydrophobic regions within the molecule, which are used to find strong molecular binding interactions or *hot-spots* in the protein-ligand complex. These features at the binding site are used to extract descriptors that represent the protein-ligand interaction attributes [18]. An example of pharmacophoric features are illustrated in Fig. 3 for the Acetylglutamate Kinase (3ZZF) protein, and *NLG* ligand. Each coloured mesh surrounding different groups of atoms represent a different pharmacophoric feature; for example the red atom mesh represent *Acceptors*, blue atom represent *Donor* atoms, whilst green atom mesh represent a *Lumped Hydrophobe*. This combination of fingerprints of both ligand and proteins was used as the basis of the feature representation of the LigityScore methods.

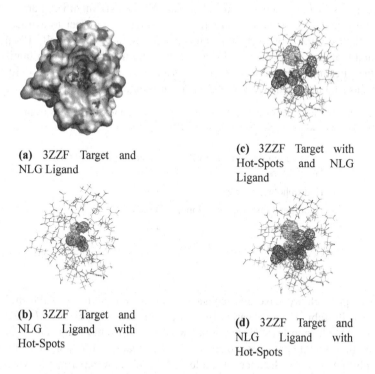

(a) 3ZZF Target and NLG Ligand

(c) 3ZZF Target with Hot-Spots and NLG Ligand

(b) 3ZZF Target and NLG Ligand with Hot-Spots

(d) 3ZZF Target and NLG Ligand with Hot-Spots

Fig. 3. Protein and Ligand Pharmacophore features used in LigityScore. Figure (b) ligand only, Figure (c) protein only. Their combination, as shown in Figure (d) will be used to extract unique combinations of Pharmacophoric Interaction Points (PIPs). Each coloured mesh represents a different pharmacophore family type. For example the blue mesh represents *Donor* atoms. (Color figure online)

4.1 Feature Generation

Once the pharmacophoric features are identified, the PIPs (or hotspots) of each individual protein-ligand complex need to be extracted to create the *PIP dataset* using all the PDBbind complexes. The algorithm used for PIP generation is based on the Ligity methodology described in Ebejer *et al.* (2019). The PIPs are extracted from the query protein-ligand complex using the open-source cheminformatics package *RDKit BuildFeatureFactory* class [17]. The BuildFeatureFactory uses SMARTS patterns to identify these pharmacophoric features within the molecule as shown in Fig. 3. Each BuildFeatureFactory stores a number of properties of the feature including its family, atom details, and coordinates. These pharmacophoric features from both the protein and the ligand, are then filtered by a set of rules constraining feature family-pairs at a specific distance threshold so as to capture only the stronger interactions. These filtered pharmacophoric features represent the PIPs or hotspots. For a hydrogen bond acceptor-donor PIP pair to be included in the PIP dataset, the hydrogen bond acceptor feature in the ligand requires a corresponding hydrogen bond donor at the protein side, or vice-versa, that has a distance which is less than 4.5 Å. The allowed feature family pairs and their corresponding distance thresholds are listed in Table 1 (taken from Ebejer *et al.* (2019)). The euclidean distances between the features are calculated using the centre of the atoms making up the feature. For example in a six-membered aromatic ring PIP, only the centre of the atomic structure is considered. In order to extract all conformant PIPs from the protein-ligand complex a cartesian product of all PIPs from the protein and ligand is performed, followed by the filtering of the allowed family pairs, and further filtering by the maximum distances allowed. PIP interactions are illustrated in Fig. 4 showing the calculated distances between centres of PIPs.

Table 1. Pharmacophoric features and distance thresholds used to extract PIPs from the protein-ligand complex, reproduced from Ebejer *et al.* (2019).

Interacting protein-ligand PIP family pairs	Distance threshold (Å)
Hydrophobic, hydrophobic	4.5
Hydrogen bond acceptor, donor	3.9
Cation, anion	4.0
Aromatic, aromatic	4.5
Cation, aromatic	4.0

In our approach we have also considered using longer distance thresholds than those stated in Table 1 which varies from the approach of Ebejer *et al.* (2019), and was inspired by the non-local electrostatic interactions used in Zheng *et al.* (2019). The PIP generation module provides a distance *threshold-factor* argument that can be used to multiply the baseline distance of Table 1. A number of experiments were carried out using a varying distance threshold-factor between 1.0 and 1.6 in order to capture additional PIP interactions in our feature representation. This additional information includes also other weaker interactions, since the protein and ligand features are further apart, which can lead to a more information-rich representation of the protein-ligand

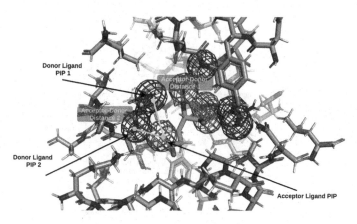

Fig. 4. PIP pair interaction between two hydrogen bond donor protein PIPs (blue mesh), and a hydrogen bond acceptor ligand PIP (red mesh). Other PIPs not shown for clarity. For each PIP interaction the distance between the geometric centres of the PIPs is calculated. (Color figure online)

complex. Considering a larger distance threshold factor implies that more PIPs are selected which in turn leads to a larger number of combinations that would be considered during the feature generation process. Our CNN model is then able to select the important interactions.

As a optional step the molecules can be filtered against the Lipinski Rule of Five [22]. These rules define an approach that suggests whether or not the molecule is likely to be poorly absorbed. When the molecular properties exceed the Lipinski thresholds, the molecule is regarded as non drug-like as it can lead to poor absorption in the body. The filtering of the dataset based on Lipinski rules is an optional paramater for the PIP generation script, and is used to determine if the "drug-likeness" property of molecules affects the scoring function prediction ability.

4.2 Feature Representation of Molecular Complex

The second phase of the protein-ligand complex representation uses the *PIP dataset* described in the previous section to create a feature matrix, or a *feature cube collection* for every complex for LigityScore1D or LigityScore3D respectively.

LigityScore1D. Each feature matrix is calculated using the PIPs from the *PIP-dataset* related to the particular protein-ligand complex. The PIPs for the ligand side and those of the protein side are extracted to obtain two separate sets—the ligand PIP set, and the protein PIP set.

The feature matrix is constructed by considering all the possible combinations when choosing one PIP from the ligand-PIP set, and one PIP from the protein-PIP set. LigityScore1D considers a combinations of 2-PIPs at a time, and hence one inter-PIP distance (1D). This contrasts with the approach used in Ebejer *et al.* (2019) where only the ligand PIP pool was considered to take 3-PIP and 4-PIP combinations. Our hypothesis

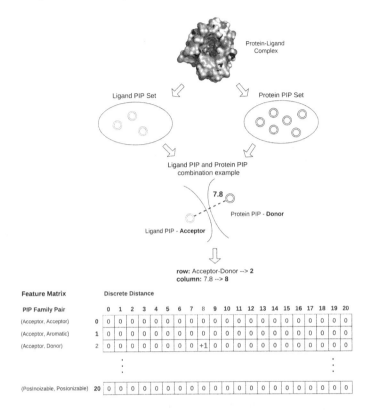

Feature Matrix	Discrete Distance																				
PIP Family Pair	0	1	2	3	4	5	6	7	8	9	10	11	12	13	14	15	16	17	18	19	20
(Acceptor, Acceptor) 0	0	0	0	0	0	0	0	0	0	0	0	0	0	0	0	0	0	0	0	0	0
(Acceptor, Aromatic) 1	0	0	0	0	0	0	0	0	0	0	0	0	0	0	0	0	0	0	0	0	0
(Acceptor, Donor) 2	0	0	0	0	0	0	0	0	+1	0	0	0	0	0	0	0	0	0	0	0	0
(Posinoizable, Posionizable) 20	0	0	0	0	0	0	0	0	0	0	0	0	0	0	0	0	0	0	0	0	0

Fig. 5. LigityScore1D Feature Matrix Generation. A protein-PIP set and a ligand-PIP set are extracted from a PL complex. From each PIP combination taken from the PIP pool, the family pair, and their discrete distance are used to update the binning count in the feature matrix.

is that since the protein structure is essential for SBVS, considering also the protein PIPs in the feature generation process strengthens our model. The distance between each combination is discretised using 1 Å resolutions. These PIP combinations also represents a particular PIP family set (example Acceptor-Donor). Each PIP family pair represents a different row in the feature matrix. Therefore the PIP-family pair is used to index the row of the feature matrix, whilst the discretised distance is used to index the column of the PIP. These coordinates in the feature matrix are then used to increment the bin count of that location. This process is illustrated in Fig. 5. In Fig. 5, an *Acceptor* ligand-PIP is selected, whilst a Donor protein-PIP is selected from the protein-PIP set. A distance of 3.7 Å is discretised to bin 4. In this dummy example the Acceptor-Donor family pair represents row 1 Fig. 5. Therefore in this example location (1, 4) is incremented by 1. If the discrete distance exceeds the allowed max distance the PIP combination is discarded. The feature matrix is initialised to all 0's. All the possible combinations are iterated so that each PIP pair distance increments the bin position in the feature matrix space.

The rules in Table 1 allow six possible PIP families. This corresponds to a total of 21 possible family-family combinations when selecting two families from six with

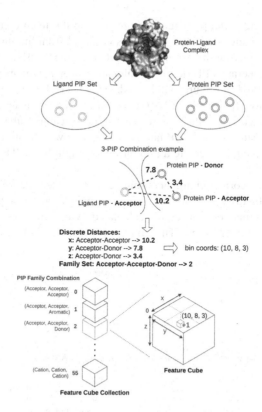

Fig. 6. LigityScore3D *Feature Cube Collection* Generation. A protein-PIP set and a ligand-PIP set are extracted from a protein-ligand complex. From each 3-PIP combination taken from the PIP pool, the family-set, and their discrete distances are used to update the binning count in the Feature Cube. A Feature Cube is built for every available family-set. Reproduced from Azzopardi and Ebejer (2021) [2].

replacement. A total of 21 possible discrete locations are available when considering a maximum distance of 20 Å, with a 1 Å resolution. Therefore each feature matrix has a size of (21×21). Each PIP family combination corresponds to a row vector that represents the discrete distribution from a single distance of the 2-PIP combination, and hence the name LigityScore1D was chosen for this representation.

LigityScore3D. The method used in LigityScore3D is similar to LigityScore1D but is more complex as it considers a combinations of 3-PIPs, choosing one PIP from the ligand-PIP set and two PIPs from the protein-PIP set and vice-versa. The 3-PIP combination creates a triangular structure amongst the PIPs as shown in Fig. 6 and generates a set of three inter-PIP distances (3D). The three distances are discretised as is done in LigityScore1D approach to extract a binning coordinate in 3D space. The voxel, or bin at this location, is incremented by one. In this case the 3-PIP family combination represents a unique feature cube. Taking three out of six families with replacement creates a total of 56 possible 3-family set combinations. The unique family set combination is used to index the particular feature cube in the feature cube collection to update the binning count using the coordinates obtained from the three inter-PIP discrete distances. Considering the example in Fig. 6, one ligand PIP and two protein are considered. These generate a PIP-family combination of *Acceptor-Acceptor-Donor*, so the *Acceptor-Acceptor-Donor* cube will be updated at the $(10, 8, 3)$ voxel location. The process is repeated for all possible PIP combinations. Considering a maximum distance of 20 Å in each dimension with 20 Å resolution, each feature cube has a dimension of $21 \times 21 \times 21$. Since each 3-PIP family set has its own feature cube, 56 features cubes are stacked together to create a protein-ligand LigityScore3D representation of size $1176 \times 21 \times 21$.

To ensure that the correct binning coordinates are selected the 3-PIP combinations are ordered by the first two family names so that a unique family sequence is created. Additionally the binning coordinated are calculated by ordering both the family-pairs and their distance at the same time. This concept is illustrated in Fig. 7.

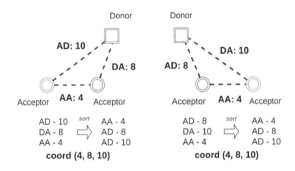

Fig. 7. LigityScore3D 3-PIP binning coordinates. In order to extract the correct binning coordinates, both the families pairs and their corresponding distances are used to sort the distance. This ensures that the same binning coordinates are used for the same structure. Although the structure are a mirror of each other, they still update the same binning coordinate $(4, 8, 10)$.

4.3   CNN Architecture

The architecture used for LigityScore is a deep convolutional neural network with a single regression output neuron used for prediction of binding affinity. The CNN architecture used for both LigityScore1D and LigityScore3D are illustrated in Fig. 8 and 9 which highlight the dimensions at each layer. The model automatically extracts patterns from the protein-ligand representation and encodes these patterns in the weights of the model. The patterns extracted should differentiate the spatial information between different complexes captured from the PIP interactions. A python package "sbvscnn" was developed to configure and build the CNN network. The package provides a dynamic way to construct different CNN architectures using a number of input parameters such as the number on convolution layers, maxpooling, normalisation, dropout at each layer, and the number of the fully connected layers and their dimensions.

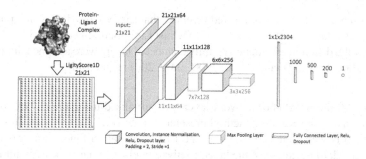

Fig. 8. CNN Architecture for LigityScore1D. The feature representation is directly input to the network with 4 convolutional layers with instance normalisation, RELU activation, and spatial dropout applied in each layer. The output of the last convolution layers is flattened to input to a fully connected network with 3 hidden layers. The output is a single neuron predicting the binding affinity.

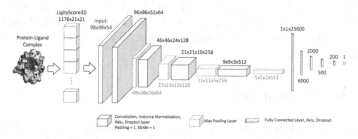

Fig. 9. CNN Architecture for LigityScore3D. The input is reshaped to $(98 \times 98 \times 54)$. Four convolutional layers are used with instance normalisation, RELU activation, and spatial dropout. The output of the last convolution layers is flattened to feed a fully connected network with 4 hidden layers. The output is a single neuron predicting the binding affinity. Reproduced from Azzopardi and Ebejer (2021) [2].

Network. The input for LigityScore1D is (21×21), whilst the input for LigtyScore3D is $(98 \times 98 \times 54)$. These normalised inputs are treated as 2D and 3D tensors respectively, and our approach considers them as to a greyscale and colour image respectively. This analogy allowed us to explore and use image processing techniques to optimise the scoring function model. Data augmentation using rotations of the *"image"*, and normalisation at the convolution layers [39] are techniques used in image processing and are also used in our experiments to verify if they can improve the prediction of the LigityScore scoring function.

The network consists of two components namely the convolutional block, and the fully connected block. The convolutional layers shown in Fig. 8 and 9 are randomly initialised and processed using the PyTorch *conv2D* module. A convolutional kernel size of 5×5 is used, with a padding of two in order to keep the layer output size the same. Each convolution layer includes instance normalisation, RELU activation, and spatial dropout components, followed by a maxpooling layer with a patch of two to reduce the dimensions by half. The output of the last convolution layers is flattened to be used as input to four fully connected layers so that LigityScore1D has an input to the fully connected layers of size ($3 \times 3 \times 256$) whilst LigityScore3D is ($5 \times 5 \times 2 \times 512$). To cater for the difference in inputs the fully connected layers were assigned dimensions of (2000, 1000, 500, 200) and (6000, 2000, 1000, 200) respectively.

Training. All the weights of network layers are initialised using the random uniform distribution using the Kaiming method presented in He *et al.* (2015) [12]. This initialising method is well suited for use with the RELU activation function as this method keeps the standard deviation of the layer's activation close to one. Correctly initialising weights keep the network stable during training preventing the output of the activation layers from exploding or vanishing.

Stochastic gradient descent with the Adam optimisation [16] is used with default parameters for momentum scheduling ($\beta_1 = 0.99$, $\beta_2 = 0.999$) to train the network with a learning rate of 10^{-5}. Adam optimisation was also used by Jiménez *et al.* (2018) [14] and Stepniewska-Dziubinska *et al.* (2017) [36]. Various batch sizes were used for training ranging from mini-batch sizes of 5 to 25. The datasets are shuffled and split into mini-batch is order to speed up the training process. Various experiments were carried for hyperparameter tuning.

5   Results and Evaluation

Several experiments were performed to find the best performing CNN architecture and LigityScore data representation starting from a baseline model. A similar test execution was followed for both 2016 and 2018 PDBbind datasets. The first series of experiments were done to search for the best CNN hyperparameters. Different mini-batch sizes (5, 10, 15, and 25) and kernel size of 3×3 were tested however these did not show any significant improvement.

The LigityScore representations extracted from each protein-ligand complex were each transposed four or eight times so as to artificially augment the training data by four or eight times. This increased the training time and also the input size from 21×21 to 37×37 in order to avoid *clipping* any values at the edges. This type of artificial data augmentation did not improve the model performance as the CNN's equivariant feature extraction process is independent of the features' spatial position. Lipinsky's rule of five based filtering for drug likeliness, also did not impact the performance of the model. Increasing the dropout at the fully connected layers, and increasing the regularisation factor in the ADAM optimizer also did not show improvements in results. For this reason these parameters were not changed from the baseline in other experiments.

Rotations of the LigityScore representation were added for data augmentation during training. Rotations increased the training time, as four or eight different rotated LigityScore representations were trained at each epoch for each protein-ligand complex. Rotations increased the input size from

Normalisation techniques such as *BatchNorm* [13] and *InstanceNorm* [39] proved to be effective in optimising the model efficiency. Training convergence was improved from 140 epoch (70 min) to only 40 epochs (20 min). Although the normalisation techniques did not improve the prediction ability of the model, they were still used throughout the rest of the experiments due to significant increase in efficiency. InstanceNorm showed slightly better convergence times and R results on validation. Therefore, it was used as the preferred choice in further experiments.

After several changes in the CNN parameters that did not improve the prediction performance, a different strategy was adopted to focus on changes to the model representation. It seemed that with the baseline data representation no further learning was possible, and thus a different data representation was required. A considerable improvement in prediction performance was achieved when different PIP threshold factors greater than one were applied to the values listed in Table 1. A higher PIP threshold factor implies that pharmacophoric *hotspots* that are further apart are considered during the LigityScore PIP generation. Figure 10 shows the validation Pearson correlation coefficient (R) performance as the PIP threshold factor is incremented from the baseline 1.0 to 1.6 for LigityScore3D. The PIP threshold factor of 1.6 (purple line graph) reaches a validation Pearson correlation coefficient (R) close to 0.72 recording an improvement of around 30% from the baseline (blue line). The PIP threshold factor of 1.6 clearly outperforms the baseline and the other models in terms of R for the validation set.

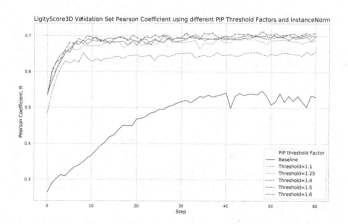

Fig. 10. Validation Set Performance using different PIP thresholds and InstanceNorm. The Pearson correlation coefficient (R) performance increases considerably over the baseline as the PIP threshold increases. LigityScore3D achieves similar results for threshold factors of 1.4, 1.5, and 1.6.

Other tests to change the data representation included i) testing a larger area of interest around the binding site (from 20 Å to 30 Å), and ii) changing the discretisation resolution to 0.5 Å, also did not show improvements in results and were not considered for further experiments. Apart from InstanceNorm and higher PIP generation threshold factors, spatial dropout was found to be effective to increase the generalisation of the model and hence its performance. Further tests were done on the CNN architecture to change the depth of the convolution layers and the number of channels used in each

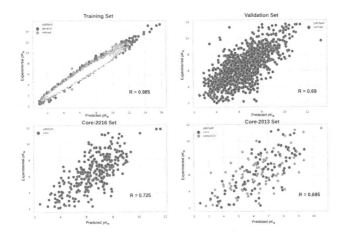

Fig. 11. Experiment Vs Predicted Binding Affinity in pK_a (negative log of disassociation constant, IC50, and inhibition constant) for best LigityScore1D (v2016) model. The top left plots illustrates the optimal predication rate for the training set. The top right represented the validation set taken from the refined set. The bottom plot are the core set v2016 (left), and the core set v2013 (right).

Table 2. Performance of LigityScore1D when trained with PDBbind v2016 and v2018, and LigityScore3D trained with PDBbind v2016, showing average and standard deviation for 10 tests using different validations sets taken from the refined set. LigityScore3D has the better overall performance for Core2013 and Core2016 test sets. Reproduced from Azzopardi and Ebejer (2021) [2].

Set	RMSE (±sd)	MAE (±sd)	SD (±sd)	R(±sd)
LigityScore1D (v2016)				
Training	0.406 (0.151)	0.323 (0.118)	0.393 (0.157)	0.974 (0.027)
Validation	1.438 (0.038)	1.144 (0.031)	1.432 (0.032)	0.698 (0.020)
Core2016	1.556 (0.039)	1.234 (0.031)	1.555 (0.038)	0.699 (0.018)
Core2013	1.861 (0.076)	1.485 (0.051)	1.701 (0.042)	0.657 (0.021)
LigityScore1D (v2018)				
Training	0.964 (0.295)	0.764 (0.237)	0.947 (0.287)	0.845 (0.076)
Validation	1.447 (0.037)	1.158 (0.033)	1.436 (0.029)	0.684 (0.017)
Core2016	1.516 (0.066)	1.223 (0.058)	1.461 (0.038)	0.741 (0.016)
Core2013	1.831 (0.072)	1.472 (0.064)	1.743 (0.054)	0.635 (0.028)
LigityScore3D (v2016)				
Training	0.621 (0.077)	0.490 (0.059)	0.531 (0.116)	0.957 (0.021)
Validation	1.479 (0.020)	1.182 (0.013)	1.435 (0.021)	0.692 (0.009)
Core2016	1.509 (0.034)	1.224 (0.031)	1.497 (0.034)	**0.725 (0.015)**
Core2013	1.676 (0.050)	1.335 (0.040)	1.583 (0.044)	**0.713 (0.019)**

layer. Convolution layers were increased to 4, 5, 6, or 8 in separate experiments, whilst layers with 32 channels were also introduced. Finally, the VGG16 [35] architecture

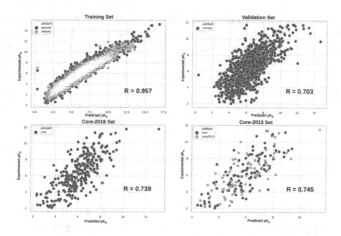

Fig. 12. Experiment vs Predicted Binding Affinity in pK_a (negative log of disassociation constant, IC50, and inhibition constant) for best LigityScore3D (v2016) model. The top left plots illustrates the optimal predication rate for the training set. The top right represented the validation set taken from the refined set. The bottom plot are the core set v2016 (left), and the core set v2013 (right).

was also tested, modified to include less pooling layers due to a smaller input, and to include spatial dropout. These deeper convolution layers, that need more training resources, showed negligible improvement which are easily attributed to changes in the model due to random initialisation across parameters of the model, and also difference in training or validation sets.

LigityScore1D achieved best results when using InstanceNorm at the convolution layers, a PIP threshold factor of 1.4, and spatial dropout of 0.1 and obtained an R of 0.725 for CASF-2016 and 0.695 for CASF-2013 test sets. The 0.1 spatial dropout was applied after the second convolution layers (middle layer with 128 channels) similar to the usage described in Tompson *et al.* (2015). The scatter plots showing the predicted versus experimental binding affinity are highlighted in Fig. 11 for training, validation, and test sets.

The same testing approach was taken for LigityScore3D, and similar to LigityScore1D, the best results were achieved with a PIP threshold factor of 1.4, InstanceNorm, and a spatial dropout probability of 0.2 on all the convolution layers. The predicted Pearson correlation coefficient (R) for LigityScore3D is of 0.745 and 0.739 for the Core-2013 and Core-2016 tests respectively. The scatter plots showing the predicted versus experimental binding affinity are highlighted in Fig. 12. LigityScore3D's additional scoring power results comes at the expense of a more complex network. It has 94M learnable parameters whilst the best model for LigityScore1D has only 3.9M parameters. LigityScore1D training takes 0.54 min per epoch whilst LigityScore3D takes 2.73 min per epoch. This represents a 24 times increase in learnable parameters, and five fold training time.

The LigityScore3D model was also tested using the Conv3d PyTorch module. The Conv3d module allows training of our model using a 4D tensor of dimension

Table 3. LigityScore evaluation on the **CASF-2013** Scoring Power benchmark ranked using the Pearson Correlation Coefficient, R. Our results are in bold achieving 5th and 8th placings from the scoring functions listed in the benchmark, as well as other literature marked with (*) where authors also used the CASF-2013 benchmark for evaluation. Entries without an (*) are taken directly from Li *et al.* (2014a) – only the top 10 are included. Reproduced from Azzopardi and Ebejer (2021) [2].

Scoring function	Rank	SD	R
AGL* [28]	1	1.45	0.792
LearningLigand* NNScore+RDkit [5]	2	–	0.786
OnionNet* [42]	3	1.45	0.782
EIC-Score* [29]	4	–	0.774
PLEC-nn* [40]	4	1.43	0.774
LigityScore3D	**5**	**1.58**	**0.713**
Pafnucy* [36]	6	1.61	0.700
DeepBindRG* [41]	7	–	0.639
LigityScore1D	**8**	**1.74**	**0.635**
X-Score	9	1.77	0.622
X-ScoreHS	10	1.77	0.620
X-ScoreHM	11	1.78	0.614
X-ScoreHP	12	1.79	0.607
dSAS	13	1.79	0.606
ChemScore@SYBYL	14	1.82	0.592
ChemPLP@GOLD	15	1.84	0.579
PLP1@DS	16	1.86	0.568
PLP2@DS	17	1.87	0.558
GScore@SYBYL	18	1.87	0.558

* other literature using CASF-2013 benchmark

$1 \times 54 \times 98 \times 98$, which is essentially the LigityScore3D representation with one input channel. The previous experiments used the Conv2d PyTorch module using a 3D tensor of size $54 \times 98 \times 98$. Experiments that utilised the Conv3D module using a combination of parameters showed an increase in performance. Although these models do achieve relatively good results, they do no outperform the previously reported results. The Conv3d module further increases the complexity of the model as it requires additional training parameters. The Conv3D module increased the learnable parameters by 42% and the training time by approximately 13 times.

The mean and standard deviation of 10 tests of the best performing models were taken, to remove any bias that might be caused from testing using a single holdout validation set. Table 2 summarises these results for LigityScore1D trained using PBD-bind v2016 and PDBbind v2018, and for LigityScore3D using PDBbind v2016. LigityScore3D shows a significant performance improvement for the Core-2013 model with an average Pearson correlation coefficient (R) of 0.713 that is well above the 0.657 and 0.635 achieved for LigityScore1D trained on PDBbind v2016 and PDBbind v2018

Table 4. LigityScore evaluation on the **CASF-2016** Scoring Power benchmark ranked using the Pearson Correlation Coefficient, R. Our results are in bold achieving **7**[th] and **8**[th] placings from the scoring functions listed in the benchmark, as well as other literature marked with (*) where authors also use the CASF-2016 benchmark. Entries without an (*) are taken directly from Su *et al.* (2018) – only the top 10 are included. Reproduced from Azzopardi and Ebejer (2021) [2].

Scoring function	Rank	SD	R
AGL* [28]	1	–	0.830
EIC-Score* [29]	2	–	0.826
LearningLigand NNScore+RDkit [5]	2	–	0.826
K_{deep}* [14]	3	–	0.820
PLEC-nn* [40]	4	1.26	0.817
OnionNet* [42]	5	1.26	0.816
ΔVinaRF20	5	1.26	0.816
Pafnucy* [36]	6	1.37	0.780
LigityScore1D	**7**	**1.46**	**0.741**
LigityScore3D	**8**	**1.50**	**0.725**
X-Score	9	1.69	0.631
X-ScoreHS	10	1.69	0.629
ΔSAS	11	1.70	0.625
X-ScoreHP	12	1.70	0.621
ASP@GOLD	13	1.71	0.617
ChemPLP@GOLD	14	1.72	0.614
X-ScoreHM	15	1.73	0.609
Autodock Vina	16	1.73	0.604
DrugScore2018	17	1.74	0.602

other literature using CASF-2016 benchmark

respectively. On the other hand the results for Core-2016 for LigityScore3D shows comparable performance to the LigityScore1D (PDBbind v2018) models with only 0.01 difference in R. Due to the similarity in results obtained for both CASF-2013 and CASF-2016, LigityScore3D is chosen as the best performing model with R of 0.725 and 0.713. The additional scoring power of approximately 10% for CASF-2013 comes at the expense of a more complex network.

The ranking of LigityScore for the scoring power in CASF-2013 and CASF-2016 are presented in Tables 3 and 4. Apart from the scoring function evaluated directly in CASF, Tables 3 and 4 include other scoring functions, marked with an asterix (*), that represent results reported in literature (in individual publications) that also utilise the CASF benchmarks. Tables 3 and 4 thus provide, to the best of our knowledge, a comprehensive list of the scoring functions developed in recent years to date, that compare and rank the different scoring functions available. LigityScore3D achieved 5th place in the CASF-2013 benchmark with an average Rof 0.713, and exceeds the reported CASF-2013 score for Pafnucy. On the CASF-2016 benchmark, LigityScore models achieve the 7th and 8th places.

6 Conclusion and Discussion

Classical scoring functions are built using expert chemical knowledge, however they still have serious limitations such as having linear based models, imposed functional form, and their inability to learn from new data. Conventional ML methods address some of these limitations, however ML based scoring functions still rely on a degree of feature engineering that requires expert knowledge to preprocess the data. This, in turn, led to the introduction of deep learning methods, and we have thus developed the LigityScore CNN-based scoring function for binding affinity prediction.

In this study, we have hypothesised that pharmacophoric interactions across different feature types contain key information to suitably represent the protein-ligand structure and their binding properties. This hypothesis was extended so that this representation would be suitable to train a CNN model as a scoring function for binding affinity prediction. A key aspect of this representation is that it is built without using expert drug design knowledge, but rather utilise a more *simplistic* representation that is passed to the CNN to automatically extract the underlying complex representations. These CNN feature maps can then be used to distinguish the relationship between the protein and the bound ligand and estimate their affinity using a regression type output. To this effect we have developed the LigityScore representations that are extracted directly from the 3D structure of both the protein and ligand using pharmocophoric features inspired by the Ligity method [8]. The pharmacophoric features across both the protein and ligand are used to extract pharmacophoric interaction points (PIPs) that need to conform to specific family types and distance thresholds so as to capture only the stronger interactions between the protein's and ligand's pharmacophoric feature. LigityScore1D uses a *single* distance between the protein PIP and the ligand PIP, hence the name LigityScore1D. Each distance for each PIP pair combination is discretised to increment binning counters for its corresponding pharmacophoric family-pair vector. The different pharmacophoric family pair combinations are grouped to construct a matrix representation of the complex. The other representation, LigityScore3D, uses a combination of 3-PIPs at a time to extract three different distances from the triangular structure formed by the 3-PIP combination. For the selection of the 3-PIPs combination, the cases where two PIPs are chosen from the protein PIP pool and one from the ligand PIP pool, and vice versa, are both considered. In each combination at least one of the three PIPs must be on the other molecule. This varies from the Ligity method where only combinations of ligand PIPs were considered. These distances are also discretised and are used as binning coordinates in a feature hypercube for each PIP family set. A number of experiments were carried out using a random hyperparameter optimisation technique to outline a suitable CNN model. The best results were achieved when using higher PIP threshold factors to include *non-local* electrostatic interactions, InstanceNorm normalisation, and small spatial dropout at the convolution layers. Various parameters relating the selection of PIPs were tested to seek out the best possible representation of the protein-ligand complex. The data representation component and the CNN architecture, tuned for the representation to provide the best prediction performance, together constitute the LigityScore scoring function.

LigityScore models are evaluated on the latest two CASF benchmarks. The Pearson correlation coefficient (R), and the standard deviation in linear regression are used to compare LigityScore with the benchmark model, and also other models in literature published in recent years. The scoring functions from both the benchmark, and the literature reviewed were compiled in an updated list (Tables 3 and 4) in order to provide a better understanding of LigityScore performance across a comprehensive list of scoring functions. The LigityScore3D has achieved better results than LigityScore1D and showed similar performance for both the CASF-2016 and CASF-2013 benchmarks.

The major contribution for this study is in the presentation of a novel protein-ligand representation for use as a CNN scoring function for binding affinity prediction adapted from Ebejer *et al.* (2019). Representation engineering is required when using CNN for SBVS as the data needs to represent the protein-ligand structure. LigityScore still relies on the automatic feature extraction of CNNs for feature extraction. Since LigityScore is based on distances between pharmacophoric features, it also presents a rotationally invariant representation. Additionally, the method shows relatively good performance that marginally exceed the Pafnucy R performance on the CASF-2013 benchmark by 0.01 on average, using a less computationally complex model that can be trained 16 times faster. The LigityScore models can potentially be used for affinity predictions for novel molecules, and as a scoring function for docking in virtual screening.

Shen *et al.* (2020) have recently used the CASF benchmarks to assess all the power metrics for 14 machine learning-based scoring functions. The authors have stressed the importance of assessing the scoring function in all four powers (scoring, ranking, docking, and screening) of the CASF benchmark for a 360° performance evaluation. Our evaluation of LigityScore focuses on the scoring power aspect such as the work done by Stepniewska-Dziubinska *et al.* (2017), Jiménez *et al.* (2018), and Zheng *et al.* (2019). The additional benchmark powers will be considered for future work.

Although we understand the importance of evaluating the scoring function in all powers, we argue that this view represents a more *traditional* approach to the development of scoring functions. The shift from human expert knowledge to automatic feature extraction is providing researchers with the ability to be more dynamic and efficient in their approach to build scoring functions. This gives the flexibility to adopt and optimise a scoring function for the particular use case (power). We therefore argue that every use case might need a *modified* scoring function ML model optimised for a particular purpose. A particular ML scoring function may not be suited for every use case, and therefore a different model, trained for the particular scoring function scope, might be better. As an example, the screening power as defined by Su *et al.* (2018) [37] would require the scoring function model to differentiate between actives and inactives. However, the models trained with the PDBbind dataset do not include any inactive information. ML models, including DL, use learning by representation to extract the underlying function in the data. Therefore, if the dataset does not include the inactive class it is intuitive that the model might not respond well when presented with inactive information. Due to the lack of experimentally-validated inactives there are no evaluation datasets that include inactive molecules highlighting the need for better and more complete datasets [34]. Therefore it would be difficult to optimise a ML scoring function for virtual screening when such data is not available. One way to workaround this is to use decoys with a manual preset binding affinity set to zero or negative value to indicate its non-binding nature. However this approach is less realistic and would need to be validated. Therefore in this sense such a ML model that is trained with inactives, might be better suited for screening, whilst a model trained on experimental data only, might be better suited for scoring power assessment. An ML scoring function model can be developed to cater for the particular requirements, leveraging on the flexibility they provide to adjust and derive their parameters from the given training data. The LigityScore protein-ligand complex representation is critical for the performance of the scoring function, and future work would definitely need to enhance this representation element by seeking ways to incorporate alternate types of features within LigityScore. In this regard one of the research tasks would be to look into additional pharmacophoric feature families (or types) that could help create an enriched descriptor. Other features such as the spatial distribution count for distances between key atom type combinations could be considered as another dimension to the LigityScore representation. Deep learning resultant models can be seen as a *black box* where the actual features that are important to the model may be difficult to determine. Therefore, future work would apply techniques such as SHAP [25] to determine the critical features used for predictions. Another method would be to exclude certain PIP families from the representation during the processing of the feature generation. Each PIP family combination would be systematically excluded to determine the effect it has on the prediction performance when compared to the baseline model.

Finding a suitable representation of the protein-ligand complex is a major challenge when building a scoring function, and is key for accurate predictions using deep learning techniques. In our work we have successfully found a suitable rotationally invariant representation that to the best of our knowledge was never used for binding affinity prediction, which provides good results and ranked 5th in the CASF-2013 benchmark. Therefore, although our work did not outperform the top scoring function we deem it is still a valid contribution to the area and may be further enhanced in future work, or may also serve as motivation and inspiration for other researchers to seek out alternative methods that increase the effectiveness of scoring functions and virtual screening in general.

We believe a deeper understanding of CNN in the domain of SBVS is still required, and a breakthrough like the work of Krizhevsky *et al.* (2012) in the computer vision domain is still being sought after in this challenging domain. Nonetheless, we also believe that ML and DL techniques will lead the future of the development of scoring functions.

Acknowledgements. We would like to thank the AWS Research Credits Team for supporting our research with AWS credits to develop our models.

References

1. Ain, Q.U., Aleksandrova, A., Roessler, F.D., Ballester, P.J.: Machine-learning scoring functions to improve structure-based binding affinity prediction and virtual screening. Wiley Interdisc. Rev.: Comput. Mol. Sci. **5**(6), 405–424 (2015)
2. Azzopardi, J., Ebejer, J.P.: LigityScore: convolutional neural network for binding-affinity predictions. In: Bioinformatics, pp. 38–49 (2021)

3. Ballester, P.J., Mitchell, J.B.: A machine learning approach to predicting protein-ligand binding affinity with applications to molecular docking. Bioinformatics **26**(9), 1169–1175 (2010)
4. Berman, H., Henrick, K., Nakamura, H.: Announcing the worldwide protein data bank. Nat. Struct. Mol. Biol. **10**(12), 980–980 (2003)
5. Boyles, F., Deane, C.M., Morris, G.M.: Learning from the ligand: using ligand-based features to improve binding affinity prediction. Bioinformatics **36**(3), 758–764 (2020)
6. Ching, T., et al.: Opportunities and obstacles for deep learning in biology and medicine. J. R. Soc. Interface **15**(141), 20170387 (2018)
7. Dunbar Jr., J.B., et al.: CSAR benchmark exercise of 2010: selection of the protein-ligand complexes. J. Chem. Inf. Model. **51**(9), 2036–2046 (2011)
8. Ebejer, J.P., Finn, P.W., Wong, W.K., Deane, C.M., Morris, G.M.: Ligity: a non-superpositional, knowledge-based approach to virtual screening. J. Chem. Inf. Model. **59**(6), 2600–2616 (2019)
9. Goldberg, Y.: A primer on neural network models for natural language processing. J. Artif. Intell. Res. **57**, 345–420 (2016)
10. Goodfellow, I., Bengio, Y., Courville, A.: Deep Learning. MIT Press, Cambridge (2016)
11. Gund, P.: Three-dimensional pharmacophoric pattern searching. In: Hahn, F.E., Kersten, H., Kersten, W., Szybalski, W. (eds.) Progress in Molecular and Subcellular Biology, vol. 5, pp. 117–143. Springer, Heidelberg (1977). https://doi.org/10.1007/978-3-642-66626-1_4
12. He, K., Zhang, X., Ren, S., Sun, J.: Delving deep into rectifiers: surpassing human-level performance on ImageNet classification. In: 2015 IEEE International Conference on Computer Vision (ICCV), pp. 1026–1034 (2015)
13. Ioffe, S., Szegedy, C.: Batch normalization: accelerating deep network training by reducing internal covariate shift. In: Proceedings of the 32nd International Conference on Machine Learning. Proceedings of Machine Learning Research, vol. 37, pp. 448–456. PMLR, Lille, 07–09 July 2015
14. Jiménez, J., Skalic, M., Martinez-Rosell, G., De Fabritiis, G.: K deep: protein-ligand absolute binding affinity prediction via 3D-convolutional neural networks. J. Chem. Inf. Model. **58**(2), 287–296 (2018)
15. Kaggle, M.: Kaggle: Merck molecular activity challenge (2012). https://www.kaggle.com/c/MerckActivity, https://www.kaggle.com/c/MerckActivity. Accessed 8 Feb 2019
16. Kingma, D.P., Ba, J.: Adam: a method for stochastic optimization (2014). arxiv:1412.6980. Comment: Published as a conference paper at the 3rd International Conference for Learning Representations, San Diego, 2015
17. Landrum, G.: RDKit: open-source cheminformatics (2020). https://www.rdkit.org, accessed April, 2020
18. Leach, A.R., Gillet, V.J., Lewis, R.A., Taylor, R.: Three-dimensional pharmacophore methods in drug discovery. J. Med. Chem. **53**(2), 539–558 (2010)
19. LeCun, Y., Bengio, Y., Hinton, G.: Deep learning. Nature **521**(7553), 436–444 (2015)
20. Li, Y., et al.: Comparative assessment of scoring functions on an updated benchmark: 1. Compilation of the test set. J. Chem. Inf. Model. **54**(6), 1700–1716 (2014)
21. Li, Y., et al.: Assessing protein-ligand interaction scoring functions with the CASF-2013 benchmark. Nat. Protoc. **13**(4), 666 (2018)
22. Lipinski, C.A., Lombardo, F., Dominy, B.W., Feeney, P.J.: Experimental and computational approaches to estimate solubility and permeability in drug discovery and development settings. Adv. Drug Deliv. Rev. **23**(1–3), 3–25 (1997)
23. Liu, Z., et al.: Forging the basis for developing protein-ligand interaction scoring functions. Acc. Chem. Res. **50**(2), 302–309 (2017)
24. Liu, Z., Cui, Y., Xiong, Z., Nasiri, A., Zhang, A., Hu, J.: DeepSeqPan, a novel deep convolutional neural network model for pan-specific class i HLA-peptide binding affinity prediction. Sci. Rep. **9**(1), 794 (2019)

25. Lundberg, S.M., Lee, S.I.: A unified approach to interpreting model predictions. In: Advances in Neural Information Processing Systems, vol. 30, pp. 4765–4774. Curran Associates, Inc. (2017)
26. Ma, J., Sheridan, R.P., Liaw, A., Dahl, G.E., Svetnik, V.: Deep neural nets as a method for quantitative structure-activity relationships. J. Chem. Inf. Model. **55**(2), 263–274 (2015)
27. Mysinger, M.M., Carchia, M., Irwin, J.J., Shoichet, B.K.: Directory of useful decoys, enhanced (dud-e): better ligands and decoys for better benchmarking. J. Med. Chem. **55**(14), 6582–6594 (2012)
28. Nguyen, D.D., Wei, G.W.: AGL-score: algebraic graph learning score for protein-ligand binding scoring, ranking, docking, and screening. J. Chem. Inf. Model. **59**(7), 3291–3304 (2019)
29. Nguyen, D.D., Wei, G.W.: DG-GL: differential geometry-based geometric learning of molecular datasets. International journal for numerical methods in biomedical engineering **35**(3), e3179 (2019)
30. Paszke, A., et al.: PyTorch: an imperative style, high-performance deep learning library. In: Advances in Neural Information Processing Systems, vol. 32, pp. 8024–8035. Curran Associates, Inc. (2019)
31. Pérez-Sianes, J., Pérez-Sánchez, H., Díaz, F.: Virtual screening meets deep learning. Curr. Comput. Aided Drug Des. **15**(1), 6–28 (2019)
32. Ragoza, M., Hochuli, J., Idrobo, E., Sunseri, J., Koes, D.R.: Protein-ligand scoring with convolutional neural networks. J. Chem. Inf. Model. **57**(4), 942–957 (2017)
33. Rifaioglu, A.S., Atas, H., Martin, M.J., Cetin-Atalay, R., Atalay, V., Dogan, T.: Recent applications of deep learning and machine intelligence on in silico drug discovery: methods, tools and databases. Brief. Bioinform. **10** (2018)
34. Sieg, J., Flachsenberg, F., Rarey, M.: In need of bias control: evaluating chemical data for machine learning in structure-based virtual screening. J. Chem. Inf. Model. **59**(3), 947–961 (2019)
35. Simonyan, K., Zisserman, A.: Very deep convolutional networks for large-scale image recognition. In: ICLR 2015 (2014)
36. Stepniewska-Dziubinska, M.M., Zielenkiewicz, P., Siedlecki, P.: Pafnucy-a deep neural network for structure-based drug discovery. Stat **1050**, 19 (2017)
37. Su, M., et al.: Comparative assessment of scoring functions: the CASF-2016 update. J. Chem. Inf. Model. **59**(2), 895–913 (2018)
38. Szegedy, C., et al.: Going deeper with convolutions. In: Proceedings of the IEEE Conference on Computer Vision and Pattern Recognition, pp. 1–9 (2015)
39. Ulyanov, D., Vedaldi, A., Lempitsky, V.: Improved texture networks: maximizing quality and diversity in feed-forward stylization and texture synthesis. In: The IEEE Conference on Computer Vision and Pattern Recognition (CVPR). IEEE (2017)
40. Wójcikowski, M., Kukiełka, M., Stepniewska-Dziubinska, M.M., Siedlecki, P.: Development of a protein-ligand extended connectivity (PLEC) fingerprint and its application for binding affinity predictions. Bioinformatics **35**(8), 1334–1341 (2019)
41. Zhang, H., Liao, L., Saravanan, K.M., Yin, P., Wei, Y.: DeepBindRG: a deep learning based method for estimating effective protein-ligand affinity. PeerJ **7**, e7362 (2019)
42. Zheng, L., Fan, J., Mu, Y.: OnionNet: a multiple-layer intermolecular-contact-based convolutional neural network for protein-ligand binding affinity prediction. ACS Omega **4**(14), 15956–15965 (2019)

Chaotic Changes in Fingertip Pulse Waves and Psychological Effects of Reminiscence Therapy Intervention

Eri Shibayama[✉] and Taira Suzuki

Graduate School of International Studies, J.F. Oberin University, Machida, Tokyo 194-0294, Japan
eri.shibayama.psychology@gmail.com

Abstract. Population aging is a problem in developed countries today. Dementia, a general term that covers various disorders leading to disturbances in life caused by a decline in intellectual functions, is a severe health problem in older adults. Reminiscence therapy has been used to prevent dementia and the deterioration of symptoms. There are reports that reminiscence is effective, but no empirical studies using physiological indicators have been conducted yet. Therefore, the present study focused on chaos analysis of fingertip pulse waves, which are correlated with mental and physical health and can be measured simply and non-invasively. The present results indicated an increase in fingertip pulse-wave LLE and a decrease in negative psychological scores only in the retrieval group, indicating that recalling and talking about memories increased fingertip pulse-wave LLE and improved psychological indices, differently from mere vocalization. Since there are few studies that combine reminiscence and physiological indicators, further research is needed.

Keywords: Reminiscence therapy · Chaos · Fingertip pulse waves

1 Introduction

Population aging is a problem in developed countries today. The total population of the world in 2015 was approximately 7,383 million which will reach 10,222.6 million in 2060. The proportion of people aged 65 or older is called the aging rate, globally 8.3% in 2015 and will reach 17.8% in 2060. Aging will further progress in the future [1]. For example, Japan has the highest aging rate in the world, at 28.1% in 2019. Japan has already become a super-aging society [2]. Whereas the total population is decreasing in Japan, the aging rate is increasing and will reach approximately 40% in 2060. It is an urgent issue to deal with the aging problem from various aspects, including medical care and welfare. Dementia, a general term that covers various disorders leading to disturbances in life caused by a decline in intellectual functions, is a severe health problem in older adults. The core symptoms of dementia include memory loss, abstract thinking and judgment disorders, apraxia, agnosia, aphasia, and executive function disorders.

© The Author(s), under exclusive license to Springer Nature Switzerland AG 2022
C. Gehin et al. (Eds.): BIOSTEC 2021, CCIS 1710, pp. 45–60, 2022.
https://doi.org/10.1007/978-3-031-20664-1_3

1.1 Reminiscence Therapy

Reminiscence therapy has been used to prevent dementia and the deterioration of symptoms. It is an interpersonal assistance method, generalized from Butler's concept of the life review [3], which encourages older adults to recollect memories, relieve their death anxiety, and facilitate attaching positive meanings to life, rather than only focusing on negative aspects [4]. Reminiscence therapy is often used for patients with dementia. Talking about nostalgic memories and sharing them with others might stimulate the brain and improve cognitive functions. Tadaka & Kanagawa [5] provided long-term reminiscence therapy to patients with Alzheimer-type dementia and reported a significant improvement in social withdrawal and cognitive functions.

Tadaka et al. [6] reviewed previous reminiscence studies conducted with older adults having dementia and suggested that specific issues in reminiscence therapy's essential efficacy and significance have not been sufficiently identified. Especially, empirical studies on the effects of reminiscence therapy using objective indices are scarce. Developing empirical reminiscence studies is significant in Japan, a super-aging society. However, assessment methods placing heavy burdens on participants are not realistic in such studies because participants are older adults. Therefore, the present study focused on chaos analysis of fingertip pulse waves, which are correlated with mental and physical health and can be measured simply and non-invasively.

1.2 The Chaos of Fingertip Pulse Waves

The keyword "chaos" attracted scientists' attention together with the keywords "Fractals" and "Complex systems" around the end of the 20th century. According to Aihara [7], chaos is "a phenomenon with very complicated, irregular, and unstable behaviors because of the nonlinearity of the system, although the system is following deterministic laws, and it is impossible to predict the future state". Chaos is a "fluctuation of phenomena" often observed in biological, physiological, social, economic, and psychological phenomena, analyzed by "chaos analysis", a nonlinear time series analysis that quantifies the strength of chaos in data. This analysis reconstructs the attractor in the phase space based on the delay time and embedding dimensions to capture the orbital instability in the time-series data, enabling us to geometrically reproduce time-series data and understand the characteristics of the data based on the attractor shape. We can visually evaluate the attractor when the embedding dimensions are less than three. However, it becomes impossible for four dimensions. Therefore, we calculate the Largest Lyapunov Exponent (LLE) to quantify the shape complexity; when time-series data is chaos, LLE values become positive. In other words, LLE indicates the chaotic degree of the time-series data [8].

Many natural and biological phenomena are complex systems that fluctuate with chaos. For example, fingertip pulse waves, which are biosignals that include information about the central nervous system and the autonomic nervous system, are considered chaotic phenomena. Previous studies have indicated that the LLE of the fingertip pulse waves, calculated through chaos analysis, correlated with physical and mental health. Physical and mental health cannot be maintained when a low-level fingertip pulse-wave LLE continues, i.e., when a non-fluctuant condition continues for a long time, which leads to a decline in external adaptability. Previous studies have indicated that the attractor of patients with depression or dementia had low fluctuations and LLE decreased [9]. Yaregani, Rao, Tancer, & Uhde [10] demonstrated that providing selective serotonin reuptake inhibitors (SSRI) to patients with panic disorders decreased excessively high LLE, suggesting that fingertip pulse-wave LLE might be closely correlated with physical and mental health. Moreover, we can easily measure fingertip pulse waves using a fingertip cuff and complete the measurement in only 1–2 min, which is a non-invasive method that places a low physical and mental burden on participants. Conventional objective measurement methods, such as EEG analysis or diagnostic imaging, need high skills and knowledge and are expensive. On the other hand, fingertip pulse waves are effective objective indices, easily measured, and available for a wide range of generations, from children to older adults.

1.3 Purpose

The increasing number of patients with dementia is a severe problem in aging societies. Previous studies have reported positive effects of reminiscence therapy for preventing deterioration of dementia, among others. However, only a few studies have used objective indices. This study empirically examined the effects of reminiscence therapy using chaos analysis of fingertip pulse wave LLE, which are correlated with physical and mental health and can be easily and non-invasively measured.

No studies have correlated reminiscence therapy and chaos analysis of fingertip pulse waves. Therefore, we must examine the effects of memory retrieval used in reminiscence therapy on psychological indices and fingertip pulse-wave LLE. Shibayama and Suzuki [11] reported that the recollection of autobiographical memories increased LLE and resulted in positive effects on cognitive functions. The present study conducted additional experiments and a more detailed examination by considering the sample size. Moreover, we examined whether the ease of recollecting happy memories in childhood might influence the effects of memory retrieval to suggest a more effective implementation and targets of reminiscence therapy.

2 Methods

The experiments were conducted from October to December 2018 to January 2022. We selected male and female participants aged 18–35 years for the current fundamental study on the effects of recalling memories and sharing them with others using words. We excluded three participants with missing data and analyzed the data of 25 participants. They participated in the experiment twice; (1) recalling childhood memories (retrieval group) and (2) vocalizing Japanese syllabary (control group), which was used to control the effects of vocalizing on blood flow (Average age $= 22.76$, SD $= 3.24$).

2.1 Materials

Participants responded to the POMS2 Brief form Japanese Version for Adults [12], a psychological index assessing mood. POMS2 is composed of seven subscales; Anger-Hostility, Confusion-Bewilderment, Depression-Dejection, Fatigue-Inertia, Tension-Anxiety, Vigor-Activity, and Friendliness. Responses to POMS 2 are made using a 5-point scale ranging from 0 (Never) to 4 (Very often). We can evaluate the mood state on the specified time axis based on POMS2 subscale scores and Total Mood Disturbance (TMD) scores, which comprehensively express the negative mood state. The participants were required to respond to how they currently felt.

Participants completed an original check sheet after recalling memories. The check sheet included seven items; "I was happy in my childhood", "I immediately recall happy memories in my childhood", "I immediately recall negative memories in my childhood", "I could talk well in the experiment", "I think the experimenter carefully listened to me", "I could easily talk", and "I enjoyed talking". Participants answered the items using a 10-point Likert scale ranging from 1 (Not at all) to 10 (Very true).

2.2 Equipment

Fingertip pulse waves were measured as a biological index by connecting a cuff sensor to a Lyspect 3.5 computer. We used a laptop computer (NEC, Versa Pro VD-9) and analyzed data using software (Lyspect). We set delay time at 10.0 ms and embedding dimensions (d) at 4, following Sano & Sawada (1985). The time-series data of fingertip pulse waves were sampled at a frequency of 200 Hz.

2.3 Procedures

The Fig. 1 shows the procedure of the experiment. Firstly, we measured participants' fingertip pulse waves at rest for three minutes. Then, the participants responded to POMS2. We instructed the retrieval group as follows; "Please talk about your happiest memory in your childhood and tell me when you finish talking". Simultaneously, we measured the participant's fingertip pulse waves. We listened carefully to participants' talk when they recalled memories and asked questions about the content if they stumbled. We instructed the control group as follows; "Please slowly read aloud the Japanese syllabary written on the paper for three minutes, without considering about your pronunciation or the loudness of your voice. Please restart from the beginning if you reach the end of the syllabary and repeat the reading". Simultaneously, we measured the participant's fingertip pulse waves. After completing the task, we measured the fingertip pulse waves of both groups for three minutes. Only the retrieval group responded to the original check sheet.

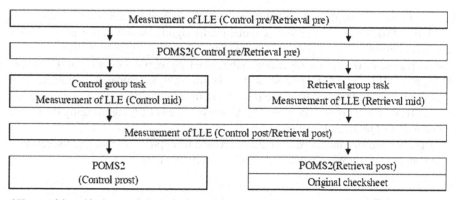

*They participated in the experiment twice.
*The second experiment was conducted after an interval of one or more days.

Fig. 1. The procedure of the experiment.

2.4 Ethical Considerations

Participants were instructed that they could quit the experiment even in the middle for any reasons and that they would incur no disadvantages for not responding, quitting the experiment, or based on the content of their responses. Moreover, they were explained that the data would be stored in a USB memory stick that has been encrypted. They were also told that no individuals would be identified from the data. The participated took part in the experiment after giving their consent to the explanation.

3   Results

We did not limit the recall time to prevent inhibiting retrieval. We deleted the excess data if it exceeded three minutes in matching the length of the control task, which was three minutes long. Firstly, we looked for significant differences between the two groups before the experiment (pre) using a one-way analysis of variance (ANOVA), which indicated no significant differences ($<.05$). Next, we examined the main effects of the group and repetition and the interaction between the group and repetition. The present study omitted descriptions of main effects and described only significant or marginally significant interactions. Subsequently, we tested simple main effects.

3.1   Mean LLE Changes in the Two Groups

Table 1 shows fundamental statistics of mean LLE in the two groups. We conducted 2×3 ANOVA to examine significant differences in mean LLE changes in the two groups, before (pre), during (mid), and after (post) the experiment (Table 2). The results indicated a significant difference between Control mid and Retrieval mid (F (1,49) = 18.38, p < .001, η^2_p = .27), as well as a marginally significant difference and mid-level effect size between Control post and Retrieval post (F (1,49) = 3.55, p = .07, η^2_p = .07). The simple main effect of the repetition in the retrieval group was significant (F(2,48) = 20.21, p < .001, η^2_p = .46). The results of the Holm multiple comparisons indicated that LLE significantly increased from pre to mid and from pre to post in the retrieval group (p < .001, g = 1.25: p = 0.05, g = .41). Moreover, mean LLE significantly decreased at mid and post in the retrieval group (p < .001, g = .84).

The above results indicated that LLE increased from pre to mid only in the retrieval group, and the effect was maintained at post-experiment (Fig. 2).

Table 1. Fundamental statistics of mean LLE in the two groups.

$n = 25$	Mean	SD	SE	95% CI lower	95% CI upper
Control pre	4.68	1.33	0.27	4.13	5.23
Control mid	4.75	1.47	0.29	4.14	5.36
Control post	4.57	1.31	0.26	4.03	5.12
Retrieval pre	4.70	1.40	0.28	4.12	5.28
Retrieval mid	6.39	1.12	0.22	5.93	6.85
Retrieval post	5.25	1.18	0.24	4.77	5.74

Table 2. 2 × 3 ANOVA to examine significant differences in LLE changes in the two groups.

	F	p	η^2_p	Result
Interaction	8.41 (2,98)	<.001	0.15	Control < Retrival
Main effect pre	.01 (1,49)	0.96	.00	Control < Retrival
Main effect mid	18.38 (1,49)	<.001	0.27	
Main effect post	3.55 (1,49)	0.07	0.07	
Simple main effect (control)	.19 (2,48)	0.83	0.01	
Simple main effect(Retrival)	20.21 (2,48)	<.001	0.46	pre < mid (p < .001, g = 1.25) pre < post (p = .05, g = .41) mid > post (p < .001, g = .84)

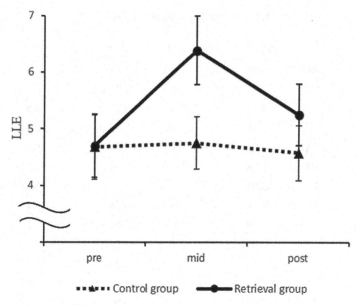

Fig. 2. Mean LLE changes in the two groups.

3.2 Changes in the Psychological Indices of the Two Groups

Table 3 shows POMS2 subscale statistics; Anger-Hostility (AH), Confusion-Bewilderment (CB), Depression- Dejection (DD), Fatigue-Inertia (FI), Tension-Anxiety (TA), Vigor-Activity (VA), and Friendliness (F), and TMD scores. We conducted 2 × 2 ANOVA on changes in the two groups before and after the experiment, with POMS2 subscale scores and TMD scores as dependent variables (Table 4). The results indicated that the simple main effect of repetition in the retrieval group was significant for Confusion-Bewilderment, Depression-Dejection, Fatigue-Inertia, and Tension-Anxiety. The post score was significantly lower than the pre score in the retrieval group ($p < .001$, $\eta^2_p = .48$: $p = .01$, $\eta^2_p = .30$: $p = .00$, $\eta^2_p = .36$: $p < .001$, $\eta^2_p = .43$). Moreover, the TMD score, which comprehensively assesses negative mood states, significantly decreased only in the retrieval group ($p < .001$, $\eta^2_p = .54$). On the other hand, in the control group, the Depression-Dejection, Fatigue-Inertia tended to decrease, and Vigor-Activity decreased.

The above results indicated that recalling memories can decrease negative psychological scores. As for Depression-Dejection, Fatigue-Inertia, the control group also showed a decrease in scores, so it is possible that the effect of vocalization reduced the scores.

Table 3. POMS2 subscale statistics.

n = 25		Mean	SD	SE	95% CI Lower	95% CI Upper
Control pre	AH	5.08	4.74	0.95	3.12	7.04
	CB	7.92	5.20	1.04	5.77	10.07
	DD	6.24	5.64	1.13	3.91	8.57
	FI	8.16	5.43	1.09	5.92	10.40
	TA	7.64	5.19	1.04	5.50	9.78
	VA	10.28	5.18	1.04	8.14	12.42
	F	13.84	5.02	1.00	11.77	15.91
	TMD	24.76	24.18	4.84	14.78	34.74
Control post	AH	4.20	3.30	0.66	2.84	5.56
	CB	7.60	5.71	1.14	5.24	9.96
	DD	5.92	5.75	1.15	3.54	8.30
	FI	7.56	5.12	1.02	5.45	9.67
	TA	7.04	5.08	1.02	4.94	9.14
	VA	9.12	5.09	1.02	7.02	11.22
	F	12.56	5.42	1.08	10.32	14.80
	TMD	23.20	23.49	4.70	13.51	32.89
Retrieval pre	AH	5.28	0.97	0.97	3.27	7.29
	CB	8.40	1.08	1.08	6.18	10.62
	DD	6.56	0.85	0.85	4.80	8.32
	FI	8.44	1.00	1.00	6.38	10.50
	TA	7.84	0.93	0.93	5.93	9.75
	VA	10.56	0.99	0.99	8.52	12.60
	F	14.08	1.25	1.25	11.50	16.66
	TMD	25.96	4.24	4.24	17.21	34.71
Retrieval post	AH	4.32	0.63	0.63	3.02	5.62
	CB	6.52	0.94	0.94	4.58	8.46
	DD	5.48	0.78	0.78	3.88	7.08
	FI	6.72	0.93	0.93	4.79	8.65
	TA	6.28	0.85	0.85	4.52	8.04
	VA	10.64	0.92	0.92	8.74	12.54
	F	13.80	1.14	1.14	11.46	16.14
	TMD	18.68	3.82	3.82	10.79	26.57

Table 4. 2 × 2 ANOVA on changes in the two groups before and after the experiment.

		F	p	η^2_p
AH	Interaction	.04 (1,49)	.85	.00
CB	Interaction	7.68 (1,49)	.01	.14
	Main effect pre	.10 (1,49)	.76	.00
	Main effect post	.51 (1,49)	.47	.01
	Simple main effect (control)	.66 (1,24)	.43	.03
	Simple main effect (retrival)	21.94 (1,24)	<.001	.48
DD	Interaction	3.88 (1,49)	.06	.08
	Main effect pre	.05 (1,49)	.83	.00
	Main effect post	.10 (1,49)	.76	.00
	Simple main effect (control)	2.87 (1,24)	.10	.11
	Simple main effect (retrival)	10.32 (1,24)	.01	.30
FI	Interaction	3.74 (1,49)	.06	.07
	Main effect pre	.04 (1,49)	.85	.00
	Main effect post	.35 (1,49)	.56	.01
	Simple main effect (control)	3.09 (1,24)	.09	.11
	Simple main effect (retrival)	13.55 (1,24)	.00	.36
TA	Interaction	3.29 (1,49)	.08	.06
	Main effect pre	.02 (1,49)	.89	.00
	Main effect post	.32 (1,49)	.58	.01
	Simple main effect (control)	2.51 (1,24)	.12	.10
	Simple main effect (retrival)	17.77 (1,24)	<.001	.43
VA	Interaction	2.87 (1,49)	.10	.06
	Main effect pre	.04 (1,49)	.85	.00
	Main effect post	1.18 (1,49)	.28	.02
	Simple main effect (control)	4.09 (1,24)	.05	.15
	Simple main effect (retrival)	.03 (1,24)	.86	.00
FI	Interaction	2.26 (1,49)	.14	.05
TMD	Interaction	11.92 (1,49)	.00	.20
	Main effect pre	.03 (1,49)	.86	.00
	Main effect post	.54 (1,49)	.47	.01
	Simple main effect (control)	2.75 (1,24)	.11	.10
	Simple main effect (retrival)	28.47 (1,24)	<.001	.54

Table 5. Fundamental statistics of changes in mean LLE and psychological scores.

$n = 25$		*Mean*	*SD*	*SE*	95% CI lower	95% CI upper
Control	LLE mid-pre	0.07	1.67	0.69	−0.62	0.76
	LLE post-pre	−0.11	1.29	0.53	−0.64	0.43
Retrival	LLE mid-pre	1.69	1.60	0.32	1.03	2.35
	LLE post-pre	0.55	0.80	0.16	0.22	0.89
Control post-pre	AH	−0.88	1.95	0.39	−1.68	−0.08
	CB	−0.32	1.93	0.39	−1.12	0.48
	DD	−0.32	0.93	0.19	−0.70	0.06
	FI	−0.60	1.67	0.33	−1.29	0.09
	TA	−0.60	1.85	0.37	−1.37	0.17
	VA	−1.16	2.81	0.56	−2.32	0.00
	F	−1.28	2.16	0.43	−2.17	−0.39
Retrival post-pre	AH	−0.96	2.25	0.45	−1.89	−0.03
	CB	−1.88	1.97	0.39	−2.69	−1.07
	DD	−1.08	1.65	0.33	−1.76	−0.40
	FI	−1.72	2.29	0.46	−2.67	−0.77
	TA	−1.56	1.81	0.36	−2.31	−0.81
	VA	0.08	2.23	0.45	−0.84	1.00
	F	−0.28	2.44	0.49	−1.29	0.73

3.3 Discriminant Analysis

We conducted a discriminant analysis to examine the extent to which each experimental content explained changes in mean LLE and psychological scores with the groups as explained variables (Table 5). We set the degree of change in fingertip pulse-wave LLE as "mid-pre" and "post-pre" and that of psychological scores as "post-pre" and created dummy variables. We assigned "1" to the control group and "2" to the retrieval group. The results of using the degree of change in mean LLE and psychological scores as discriminant variables are as follows. The standardized discriminant function coefficients of mid-pre, Vigor-Activity, Friendliness, and post-pre were large, whereas the amount of change from pre to post in Tension-Anxiety, Fatigue-Inertia, Confusion-Bewilderment, Depression-Dejection, and Anger-Hostility was negative (Table 6). The centroid coefficient of the group was −.84 in the control group and .87 in the retrieval group. The above results indicated that when an increase in LLE from pre to mid or post was larger, the subject was more classified into the retrieval group, and when a decrease in negative psychological scores was smaller, the subject was more classified into the control group. The percentage of correct classifications was 80.4% in total. The above results indicated that the changes in mean LLE and psychological scores could discriminate between recalling memories and vocalizing Japanese syllabary with a high probability, i.e., changes in LLE and psychological scores were significantly different between memory retrieval and mere vocalization.

Table 6. The results of Discriminant analysis.

		Canonical discriminant function coefficients	Standardized discriminant function coefficients
LLE mid-pre		.37	.62
LLE post-pre		.12	.13
post-pre	AH	−.01	−.03
	CB	−.13	−.26
	DD	−.10	−.14
	FI	−.16	−.32
	TA	−.26	−.42
	VA	.16	.42
	F	.17	.39
	Constant number = 0.79		

Eigenvalue = .75 Canonical correlation coefficient = .66 Wilks $\lambda = \chi^2(9) = .57$

Predicted group membership			
	Control group	Retrieval group	Total
Control group	21 (80.8)	5 (19.2)	26
Retrieval group	5 (20.0)	20 (80.0)	25

The percentage of correct classifications was 80.4% in total.

3.4 LLE Changes Depending on the Easiness of Recalling Childhood Memories

Table 7 shows fundamental statistics of the check sheet that participants responded to after recalling memories. We used the items "I immediately recalled happy memories of my childhood" and "I immediately recalled negative memories of my childhood" to examine whether the easiness of recalling happy childhood memories might influence the effect of recalling memories. We used the mean LLE of mid-pre and post-pre to examine the correlation between the above two items' scores and LLE changes.

Table 7. Fundamental statistics of the check sheet that participants responded to after recalling memories.

$n = 25$			*Mean*	*SD*	*SE*	95% CI lower	95% CI upper
"Immediately recalling happy childhood memories"			4.72	2.16	0.43	3.83	5.61
"Immediately recalling negative childhood memories"			5.84	2.13	0.43	4.96	6.72
Happy childhood memories	High	LLE mid-pre	0.05	1.47	0.42	−0.88	0.98
		LLE post-pre	−0.12	1.25	0.36	−0.83	0.59
	Low	LLE mid-pre	0.49	1.95	0.54	−0.68	1.67
		LLE post-pre	0.15	1.27	0.35	−0.62	0.92
Negative childhood memories	High	LLE mid-pre	−0.56	0.83	0.24	−1.09	−0.03
		LLE post-pre	−0.41	1.01	0.29	−1.05	0.23
	Low	LLE mid-pre	1.06	2.00	0.55	−0.15	2.26
		LLE post-pre	0.42	1.35	0.38	−0.40	1.23

The Difference in LLE Changes Depending on the Level of "IMMediately Recalling Happy Childhood Memories"

We classified the participants into two groups based on item score, "I immediately recalled happy memories of my childhood," those higher than the mean (4.72, SD = 2.16) into the high group and those lower than the mean into the low group. Then, we examined the difference in mid-pre and post-pre LLE, which indicated no significant difference between the two groups in either mid-pre or post-pre.

The Difference in LLE Changes Based on the Level of "Immediately Recalling Negative Childhood Memories"

We classified the participants into two groups based on the item for, "I immediately recalled negative memories of my childhood", those higher than the mean (5.84, SD = 1.52) into the high group and those lower than the mean into the low group. Then, we examined differences in mid-pre and post-pre LLE, which indicated a mid-level effect size ($F (1, 23) = 2.70$, $p = .11$, $\eta^2 = .11$), i.e., the post-pre LLE value of the high group was smaller than the low group, and the mid-pre LLE value of the high group was significantly smaller than the low group ($F (1, 23) = 6.23$, $p = .02$, $\eta^2 = .21$).

The above results indicated that an increase in LLE from pre to mid or post was smaller in participants that tend to recall bad childhood memories, i.e., fluctuation of pulse waves caused by memory retrieval was low in such participants.

3.5   Changes in the Attractor

The present study focused on LLE, which quantitatively describes chaos. The results indicated a significant change in the attractor. It is difficult to quantitatively express attractors. Therefore, we report the results of the visual assessment. Figure 3 shows an example of attractor changes in the control group, and Fig. 4 shows that in the retrieval group. Generally, the attractor structure becomes dynamic as LLE increases. The control group's attractor did not significantly change, or the dynamic structure decreased. On the other hand, the retrieval group's attractor structure became more dynamic from pre to mid or post, suggesting that recalling and talking about memories, not only vocalizing syllabary, made the attractor's structure more dynamic. Visual evaluation would also become possible.

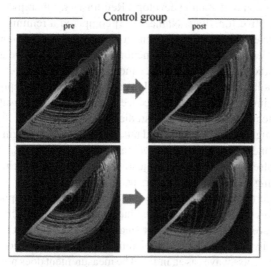

Fig. 3. Attractor changes in the control group.

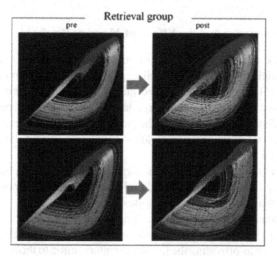

Fig. 4. Attractor changes in the retrieval group.

4 Discussion

The present experiment indicated an increase in fingertip pulse-wave LLE and a decrease in negative psychological scores in the retrieval group, indicating that recalling and talking about memories increased fingertip pulse-wave LLE and improved psychological indices, differently from mere vocalization.

As previously described, fingertip pulse-wave LLE, which is biological data, is closely correlated with mental and physical health. It is reported that low-level LLE continues as depression or dementia develops. Reminiscence therapy might be effective for improving cognitive functions. Namazi [13] compared a reminiscence group talking about a topic relevant to participants and a general tea party group and reported an improvement in older adults' cognitive functions in the reminiscence group. Moreover, Arean et al. [14] indicated that reminiscence therapy was useful for relieving depression in healthy older adults. Watt & Cappeliez [15] also indicated that depressive symptoms were significantly improved by a reminiscence intervention. The results of the present study were consistent with the preceding studies cited above.

These results suggest that recalling and talking about memories might have positive effects on mental and physical health as well as cognitive functions. We might be able to use fingertip pulse-wave LLE as an objective index of reminiscence therapy effect, recalling and sharing memories with others using words.

Measuring fingertip pulse waves is easy and non-invasive, which places a low burden on the mind and the body. Various studies have reported the effects of reminiscence intervention. However, there are only a few studies using physiological indices. It might be possible to easily assess the effects of reminiscence intervention by using chaos analysis of fingertip pulse waves as an index. The measurement does not need specialized skills or knowledge. Therefore, participants themselves or caregivers can easily measure and record the data.

4.1 Childhood Memories and the Effects of Memory Retrieval

The original check sheet and LLE analysis indicated that the increase in LLE was smaller when participants tended to recall negative childhood memories. Tani, Fujiwara, & Kondo [16] reported that the percentage of developing dementia was higher in people with more adverse childhood experiences. We did not ask participants about their adverse childhood experiences, and the participants did not mention their unpleasant memories. Nevertheless, negative childhood memories might have influenced the effects of memory retrieval.

The life review suggested by Butler is partly different from reminiscence therapy, although there is no detailed definition. Reminiscence therapy generally aims at the recreation accompanied by recalling memories, whereas life review is a psychological therapy for individuals, in which they attach meanings to negative aspects of the past and recollect them. The present study results suggest that taking measures suitable for each participant, such as providing the life review intervention to those that tend to recall negative memories, might be essential. We need to examine differences in reminiscence intervention effects based on the type of participants in the future.

4.2 Future Perspectives

The present study set the age range of the participants as 18 to 35 years to examine the effects of memory retrieval on fingertip pulse waves. In the future, we need to provide reminiscence therapy intervention to older adults or older adults with dementia and examine the intervention effects using objective indices based on the present study. Moreover, the present study provided individual-based intervention. However, group-based intervention is usual in reminiscence therapy, in which participants interact with others and communicate. We need to examine correlations between characteristics of group intervention and cognitive functions and fingertip pulse-wave LLE. Empirical studies on reminiscence therapy are still scarce. Future developments using other physiological indices, including fingertip pulse waves, are desirable.

References

1. United Nations: World Population Prospects: The 2017 Revision. United Nations (2017)
2. Japan Cabinet Office: WHITE PAPER Information and Communications in Japan30. https://www8.cao.go.jp/kourei/whitepaper/w-2018/html/zenbun/index.html. Accessed 10 Feb 2022
3. Butler, R.N.: The life review: an interpretation of reminiscence in the aged. Psychiatry **26**, 65–75 (1963)
4. Lewis, C.N., Butler, R.N.: Life-review therapy. Putting memories to work in individual and group psychotherapy. Geriatris **29**, 165–173 (1974)
5. Tadaka, E., Kanagawa, K.: Effects of reminiscence group in elderly people with Alzheimer disease and vascular dementia in a community setting. Geriatr. Gerontol. Int. **7**(2), 167–173 (2007). (in Japanese)
6. Tadaka, E., et al.: Literature review on the significance and effect of reminiscence on the elderly with dementia (in Japanese). J. Jpn. Acad. Gerontol. Nurs. **9**(2), 56–63 (2005). (in Japanese)
7. Aihara, K.: Chaos a completely new wave of creation-. Tokyo, Koudansya, Tokyo (1993)
8. Imanishi, A., Oyama, M.: A new analysis method in physiologcal psychology and psychophysiology: chaos analysis in biologcal signals. J. Humanit. **58**(3), 23–42 (2008)
9. Oyama, M.: Psychology of "fluctuation" for strengthening the mental immune system. Shodensha, Tokyo (2012)
10. Yeragani, V.K., Radhakrishna, R.K.A., Tancer, M., Uhde, T.: Paroxetine decreases respiratory irregularity of linear and nonlinear measures of respiration in patients with panic disorder. Neuro Psychobiol. **49**, 53–57 (2004)
11. Shibayama, E., Suzuki, T.: Chaotic changes in fingertip pulse waves during autobiographical memory retrieval. In: Proceedings of the 14th International Joint Conference on Biomedical Engineering Systems and Technologies, pp. 35–41 (2021). https://doi.org/10.5220/0000145600002865
12. Yokoyama, K.: Profile of Mood States 2nd Edition Japanese Version. Kanekosyobou, Tokyo (2015)
13. Namazi, K.H., Haynes, S.R.: Sensory stimuli reminiscence for patients with Alzheimer's disease. Clin. Gerontol. **14**(4), 29–46 (1994)
14. Arean, P.A., Perri, M.G., Nezu, A.M., Schein, R.L., Christopher, F., Joseph, T.X.: Comparative effectiveness of social-solving therapy and reminiscence therapy as treatments for depression in older adults. J. Consult. Clin. Psychol. **61**, 1003–1010 (1993)

15. Watt, L.M., Cappeliez, P.: Integrative and instrumental reminiscence therapies for depression in older adults: intervention strategies and treatment effectiveness. Aging Ment. Health **4**, 166–177 (2000)
16. Tani, Y., Fujiwara, T., Kondo, K.: Association between adverse childhood experiences and dementia in older Japanese adults. JAMA Netw. Open (2020). https://doi.org/10.1001/jam anetworkopen.2019.20740

Determination of Charge Transfer Resistance from Randles Circuit Spectra Using Elliptical Fitting

Norman Pfeiffer[1]([✉])([iD]), Toni Wachter[1], Jürgen Frickel[2], Hamdi Ben Halima[3], Christian Hofmann[1], Abdelhamid Errachid[3], and Albert Heuberger[1,2]

[1] Fraunhofer IIS, Fraunhofer Insitute for Integrated Circuits IIS,
Am Wolfsmantel 33, 91058 Erlangen, Germany
norman.pfeiffer@iis.fraunhofer.de
[2] Lehrstuhl für Informationstechnik mit dem Schwerpunkt Kommunikationselektronik (LIKE),
Friedrich-Alexander-Universität Erlangen-Nürnberg,
Am Wolfsmantel 33, 91058 Erlangen, Germany
[3] Institut des Sciences Analytiques, Université de Lyon,
5 rue de la Doua, 69100 Villeurbanne, France

Abstract. Physical and chemical phenomena of an electrochemical system can be described by electrochemical impedance spectroscopy (EIS). The spectral response of impedimetric biosensors is often modeled by the Randles circuit, whose parameters can be determined by regression techniques. As one of these parameters, the charge transfer resistance R_{ct} is often used as the sensor response. Regression in the laboratory environment is usually performed using commercial software, which is typically computationally intensive. Therefore, applications of biosensors outside the laboratory require more efficient concepts, especially when miniaturized or portable instrumentations are used. In this work, an approach for geometric elliptical fitting of the graph in the Nyquist diagram is presented and compared with the complex nonlinear least squares (CNLS) regression. The evaluation is based, on the one hand, on artificial spectra and, on the other hand, on real data from a immunologically sensitive field-effect transistor (IMFET) for cortisol measurement in saliva. For simulated noisy data, the average error in computing R_{ct} using the elliptical fit with -2.7% is worse than using the CNLS with 0.024%, but the former required only about $1/225$ of computation time compared to the latter. Applying the elliptic fitting to real data from an IMFET, the determination of R_{ct} showed deviations of only $0.7 \pm 2.7\%$ compared to CNLS. The impact of these variations on a standard addition method (SAM) was demonstrated for quantitative analysis of cortisol concentration. After application-oriented evaluations considering the possible accuracies, the elliptical fitting could prove to be a resource-saving option for the analysis of impedance spectra in mobile applications.

Keywords: Electrochemical impedance spectroscopy · Elliptical fitting · Randles circuit · Least squares fitting · Charge transfer resistance · Complex nonlinear least squares · ImmunoFET · IMFET

© The Author(s), under exclusive license to Springer Nature Switzerland AG 2022
C. Gehin et al. (Eds.): BIOSTEC 2021, CCIS 1710, pp. 61–79, 2022.
https://doi.org/10.1007/978-3-031-20664-1_4

1 Introduction

Electrochemical impedance spectroscopy (EIS) for the analysis and measurement of biosensors is increasingly used in a variety of research areas. Through this powerful measurement technique, several chemical and physical phenomena of an electrochemical system can be observed separately. Thus, electrical properties of the sensor surface and interfacial reaction mechanisms can be characterized [17]. From a medical perspective, EIS has been used in diverse applications. A small selection among these is the diagnosis of heart disease [12], the diagnosis of Alzheimer's disease [25], the detection of bacteria such as Escherichia coli or viruses [16] or the detection of cancer cells [9]. There are various types of impedimetric biosensors, such as aptamer-based, cell-based, enzyme-based or immunosensors [2]. The latter are biosensors that respond to the reaction between immobilized antibodies and corresponding antigens. The advantages of EIS include the realization of label-free measurements, the possibility of miniaturization and low production costs. This results in opportunities for multi-channel architectures or miniaturized, microprocessor-controlled point-of-care testing (POCT) systems [23].

After the impedance spectra are collected, electrical modeling of the biofunctionalized sensor surface is usually performed to interpret the data. For this purpose, equivalent circuit diagrams representing the electrochemical cell are used, which allow to characterize the main electrochemical and physical processes. An example of an equivalent circuit is the Randles circuit, which describes an electrode in contact with an electrolyte. Here, a one-step charge transfer process that involves the diffusion of reactants to the interface is described [3]. When using biosensors, the charge transfer resistance R_{ct} in particular is used as the relevant parameter after fitting the equivalent circuit to the acquired impedance spectrum [20].

In most EIS studies reported in the literature, commercial impedance spectrometers are used to perform measurements. In addition to the hardware, software tools running on laboratory computers are usually provided to allow the impedance spectra to be fit using complex nonlinear least squares (CNLS) [14]. However, manual estimates of R_{ct} are often used as an alternative in the electrochemical domain [24]. This takes advantage of the fact that the Randles circuit typically forms a semicircle in the high-frequency region in the Nyquist diagram. This semicircle is determined by the electrolyte resistance R_s, the double-layer capacitance C_{dl}, and R_{ct}. By geometrically estimating the extrapolated intersections with the real axis, R_{ct} can thus be estimated.

Electrochemical biosensors can be applied to different body fluids such as blood, urine, saliva and sweat [10, 26, 28]. The latter examples, in particular, provide an opportunity for the development of novel non-invasive POCT devices. The advent of mobile and small POCT devices outside a laboratory can lead to new requirements for evaluation electronics. Thus, depending on the application, it may be advantageous to analyze the data directly on the portable measurement electronics to minimize the response time of the system [30], which in turn requires efficient algorithms. This can also be relevant for the design of micro total analysis systems (μTAS), in which, for example, embedded systems with appropriate onboard processing transmit only relevant parameters as the result of the data analysis. Compared to an architecture in which the raw data is sent wirelessly to a computing unit for analysis, embedded evaluation has the advantage of reducing dependence on the overall system architecture and thus minimizing sources of error. For example, alarm systems or real-time diagnostic tools can be designed that do not require (continuous) wireless communications and consequently have a lower risk of malfunction.

An example of biosensors that are potentially suitable for integration into POCT devices or μTAS are biosensitive field-effect transistors (BioFETs) [29]. These sensors are based on ion-sensitive field-effect transistors (ISFET), which are metal-oxide-semiconductor field-effect transistors (MOSFETs) whose gate solid-state conducting electrode has been replaced by an analyte and a counter electrode (CE). In this simplest form, the ISFET is sensitive to pH, but can be made sensitive to various biomolecules by functionalizing the gate insulator. For example, these types of sensors can also be used as immunosensors by using antibodies as bioaffinity elements. In this case, these are called immunological field-effect transistors (IMFETs). The change in the electrostatic charge environment or the charge transfer due to the binding of biomolecules with the sensor surface leads to a change in the gate voltage. BioFETs can also be characterized by an EIS in the subthreshold region. An advantage in this case is that the exponential behavior of the curves of the transconductance versus the gate-source voltage $g_m(V_{GS})$ in subthreshold operation is used for signal amplification [5, 15].

To address this issue, this work proposes an approach that allows an automatic, efficient analysis of impedimetric biosensors to obtain the parameter R_{ct}. Therefore, a geometric fit of an ellipse in the Nyquist plot is used to analyze the impedance spectrum of a Randles circuit. This is intended to increase reproducibility and accuracy compared to manual analysis methods while reducing computation time compared to CNLS.

To analyze the proposed method described above, both elliptical fitting and CNLS were implemented in Python and compared. Some aspects of this work have been recently presented by the authors in the 14th International Conference on Bio-inspired Systems and Signal Processing [22]. This extended version not only considers simulated data to compare the methods, but also uses recorded impedances of cortisol-sensitive IMFETs in human saliva. Thus, not only the behavior with real data can be investigated, but also their influences on the performance of a standard addition method (SAM).

2   Materials and Methods

The following paragraph describes the generation of the simulated data and the implementation of the electrochemical measurements by an IMFET for cortisol sensing. Subsequently, CNLS regression is presented as the state of the art for analyzing EIS data, followed by the ellipse fitting to be investigated.

2.1   Simulation of Electrochemical Impedance Spectroscopy Data

For the studies presented here, the Randles circuit is assumed to be the equivalent circuit of a sensing element as shown in Fig. 2. This equivalent circuit includes the electrolyte resistance R_s, the charge transfer resistance R_{ct}, the double layer capacitance C_{dl} and the Warburg impedance Z_w. The serial connection of R_{ct} and Z_w describes the impedance of Faraday charge exchange characterizing the ion exchange between the electrolyte and the conducting metal electrode [32].

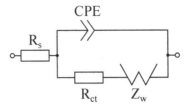

Fig. 1. Equivalent circuit of the Randles circuit used for the simulation of EIS data [22].

Table 1. Applied parameter value range of the Randles circuit to simulate artificial spectra: R_s electrolyte resistance, R_{ct} charge transfer resistance, Q_w prefactor of Warburg impedance Z_w, Q prefactor of CPE, n exponent of CPE [22].

Parameter	Min	Max	Unit
R_s	10^3	10^5	Ω
R_{ct}	10^4	$9 \cdot 10^6$	Ω
Q_w	10^{-8}	10^{-6}	$S \cdot \sqrt{s}$
Q	10^{-11}	10^{-6}	$S \cdot s^n$
n	0.5	1	–

Due to non-ideal conditions such as porous electrodes, the double layer capacitance C_{dl} is replaced by a constant phase element CPE:

$$Z_{CPE}(f) = \frac{1}{Q(i2\pi f)^n} \qquad\qquad n \in [0, 1], \tag{1}$$

with the pre-factor Q and the exponent n. At $n = 1$ the equation of an ideal capacitor is given [27].

Assuming an infinite area of the electrodes leading to unlimited diffusion at the electrode surfaces, Z_w is a special case of CPE with $n = 0.5$, giving a constant phase of $45°$:

$$Z_w(f) = \frac{1}{Q_w \sqrt{(i2\pi f)}}. \tag{2}$$

Thus, finite-length or finite-space Warburg impedances are not considered for simplification. The parameter limits of the simulations were chosen to generate typical and analyzable spectra. For this purpose, the Warburg impedance should not interfere too much with the effects of R_{ct} and C_{dl} in the high-frequency range, which accordingly means that the typical semicircle in the Nyquist plot is still recognizable. The chosen value ranges are shown in Table 1.

To obtain a logarithmic distribution of randomly simulated spectra, each parameter β was divided into a factor a and an exponent b such that $\beta = a \cdot 10^b$. Then, a and b were drawn randomly to generate artificial spectra from Randles circuits. Even with the restricted value ranges of the parameters, in some cases the Nyquist plot showed no semicircle, due to the $45°$ line overlaying it. This effect depends on the relative ratios between the parameters. Affected spectra were sorted out by checking whether the phase response shows a minimal level of change.

Each of the 100 spectra was simulated twice, resulting in one version without noise superposition and one with. A Gaussian noise with argument ($\mu = 0$, $\sigma^2 = 1\%$) and phase ($\mu = 0$, $\sigma^2 = 1°$) was chosen.

2.2 Evaluation with Real Data of a Cortisol-Sensitive IMFET

Data obtained from a cortisol-sensitive IMFET were used to apply and to evaluate the developed algorithms. These data were generated by the measurement setup and procedure described below and have already been used to evaluate the IMFET itself [6].

The ISFETs used were developed and produced by the Institute of Micoelectronics of Barcelona (IMB-CNM) of the Spanish National Research Council (CSIC). The microelectronic fabrication process of a 4-channel ISFET with a sensor area of $20 \times 400\,\mu m$ each has already been described elsewhere [31].

Biofunctionalization of the sensor surface was achieved by chemical binding of anti-cortisol monoclonal antibody (mAb-cortisol) to the surface and is intended for application to saliva samples. The fabrication process of the functionalization as well as its responsiveness and specificity have already been published [6] and are not further described here.

The EIS was performed with the potentiostat VMP3 (BioLogic Science Instruments, Seyssinet-Pariset, France). In order to generate a direct current (DC) voltage to apply a drain-source voltage to the IMFET, an additional electrical circuit was developed and a printed circuit board (PCB) was designed. It mainly consists of a low-dropout regulator (LDO) and an impedance converter that require an external supply voltage between 4 and 7 V. For all presented measurements, the power supply unit SNG-24-48W-A (Voltcraft, Wollerau, Switzerland) was utilized. The LDO regulates the power supply voltage to 0.5 V, which is buffered by an impedance converter. The latter is based on the AD8534 with a closed-loop output impedance of $40\,\Omega$ and an output current up to 250 mA. Its output voltage (0.5 V) serves as drain-source voltage of the IMFET at its operating point. Figure 2 shows the connection of the developed circuit and the potentiostat. During the measurement process, the VMP3 applies an AC sinus voltage of 75 mV between 10 kHz and 10 Hz to the CE. The potentiostat is keeping the potential between the Ag/AgCl reference electrode (RE) and source of the IMFET at 0 V, which will operate the IMFET in the subthreshold condition. The resulting drain current I_D is measured at the input Ref1. To perform EIS, the sensors were placed in a Faraday cage to minimize electrical and light-sensitive interference. After incubation of the IMFET with the analyte for 30 min at room temperature ($20 \pm 2°C$), the measurement was performed in 7 mL phosphate buffer solution (PBS).

This measurement setup was used to quantify cortisol concentrations in real saliva samples by the SAM. Therefore, the sample is measured without and with standards of different concentrations. Linear regression can then be used to determine the concentration of the biomarker in the original sample. A detailed description of the manufacturing process of the standard solutions has already been described elsewhere [6]. For the evaluation of the SAM, normalized resistances $R_{ct,norm}$ were calculated using the

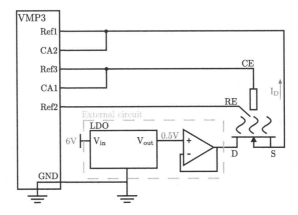

Fig. 2. Electrical setup of the performed measurements. Both ground potentials of the external circuit and the potentiostat BioLogic VMP3 are short circuited. The low-dropout regulator (LDO) has a output voltage of 0.5 V, that is buffered by an impedance converter and functions as drain-source voltage of the IMFET. The parameter to be measured is the drain current I_D. A platinum counter electrode (CE) and a silver-silverchlorde Ag/AgCl reference electrode (RE) are used. The designations of the inputs of the VMP3 correspond to those of the manual.

charge transfer resistance of the samples $R_{ct,S}$ and that of the reference measurement in mAb-cortisol solution ($10\,\mu g/mL$ in PBS) $R_{ct,Ref}$:

$$R_{ct,norm} = \frac{R_{ct,S} - R_{ct,Ref}}{R_{ct,Ref}} = \frac{\Delta R_{ct}}{R_{ct,Ref}}. \tag{3}$$

The measured saliva sample was taken from a healthy person (female, 39 years). For this purpose, a synthetic swab (Salivette®, Sarstedt, Germany) was moved in the oral cavity by the subject for 2 min. Subsequently, saliva was collected by centrifuging the swab at 7000 rpm for 5 min at 4 °C. The saliva sample was divided into two aliquots. Aliquot A contained the saliva as such, aliquot B was spiked with $7.5\,ng/ml$ cortisol. Both aliquots were diluted by a factor of 20.0. The data generated by this measurement setup has already been used to evaluate the described IMFETs [6] and are used to investigate the algorithms presented here.

2.3 Complex Nonlinear Least-Squares Regression

To determine R_{ct}, all parameters $B = (\beta_1, \beta_2, ..., \beta_n) \in \mathbb{R}^n$ of the equivalent circuit are determined using the least squares (LS) method on the measured values z_{acq}. Thus, the residuals r_m between the values of the model curve z_{mod} and the acquired data z_{acq} are minimized with respect to the measurement frequency f_m:

$$r_m(B) = z_{acq}(f_m) - z_{mod}(B, f_m) \tag{4}$$

Accordingly, the sum of error squares R over all frequencies $f_m = (f_1, f_2, ..., f_M) \in \mathbb{R}^M$ is described by

$$R(B) = \frac{1}{2} \sum_{m=1}^{M} r_m(B)^2. \tag{5}$$

Parameters B that minimize the sum of squared residuals are to be determined:

$$R_{min} = \min_{B \in \mathbb{R}^M} \frac{1}{2} \sum_{m=1}^{M} r_m(B)^2 \tag{6}$$

The solution approach to be chosen for this minimization problem depends on the nature of the model function [19]. Since the application described here is a nonlinear optimization problem, the Gauss-Newton method was chosen. This numerical approach can be used to solve nonlinear minimization problems using the LS method. For this purpose, the nonlinear cost function R is linearized in order to subsequently optimize it using LS. The linearization is achieved by the first order Taylor expansion. Using the Jacobi matrix $J = \nabla r_m(B^{(k)})^T$, a linearization for the residual r_m with parameters $B^{(k)} \in \mathbb{R}^N$ at iteration step k gives

$$\tilde{r}_m(B, B^{(k)}) = r_m(B^{(k)}) + \nabla r_m(B^{(k)})^T(B - B^{(k)}). \tag{7}$$

Accordingly, the minimization problem is:

$$\begin{aligned} B^{(k+1)} &= \min_{B \in \mathbb{R}^M} \sum_{m=1}^{M} \tilde{r}_m(B, B^{(k)})^2 \\ &= B^{(k)} - ((J|_{B^{(k)}} \cdot (J|_{B^{(k)}})^T)^{-1}(J|_{B^{(k)}}) \cdot R(B^{(k)}) \end{aligned} \tag{8}$$

This iterates until the result converges [7]. In order to ensure minimization and to guarantee handling of a singular matrix JJ^T, the Gauss-Newton iteration step can be optimized assuming $\alpha(k) \geq 0$ to:

$$B^{(k+1)} = B^{(k)} - \alpha^{(k)}((J|_{B^{(k)}}) \cdot (J|_{B^{(k)}})^T + \Delta^{(k)})^{-1}(J|_{B^{(k)}}) \cdot R(B^{(k)}) \tag{9}$$

Here $\Delta^{(k)}$ is chosen so that $(J|_{B^{(k)}}) \cdot (J|_{B^{(k)}})^T + \Delta^{(k)}$ is positive definite. Choosing $\Delta^{(k)}$ as a positive multiple of the unit matrix $\Delta^{(k)} = \lambda^k I, \lambda \geq 0$ leads to the Levenberg-Marquardt algorithm (LMA) [7]. In this work, the LMA is applied to determine the component values of the Randles circuit as shown in Fig. 1.

The Jacobi matrix is determined in the regression by numerical differentiation. It should be noted that the parameters of the equivalent circuit have strong differences in size due to the use of capacitors and resistors. Thus, it results that the existing differences in the magnitude of the parameter values have an unbalanced influence on the numerical differentiation. Additionally, the different sizes of the parameters can cause further problems during the regression with the LMA. The step size is adjusted for each parameter within an iteration by estimating the error between the measured value and the calculated value and evaluating the influence of changing a single parameter. In the present case, however, a small step size for a resistor may have only an insignificant influence on the calculated impedance value, while the same step size for a capacitor may be very significant.

These previously described influences can be counteracted in particular by normalizing the parameter values [21]. Therefore, in the present work, a normalization of the parameter values and a standardization of the impedance spectra were applied [22].

To realize the former, each parameter β of the equivalent circuit is normalized to a uniform range of values by first dividing it into a factor γ and an exponent ϵ:

$$\beta = \gamma \cdot 10^{\epsilon} \tag{10}$$

The number of parameters is consequently doubled. In the next step, the obtained parameters $\theta = \gamma$ or ϵ are scaled to the range of values $W \in [t_1, t_2]$ and are subsequently applied to the regression:

$$\theta_{scaled} = t_1 + \frac{\theta - \min(\theta)}{\max(\theta) - \min(\theta)} \cdot (t_2 - t_1) \tag{11}$$

The standardization is applied to the acquired impedances z_{acq} and the calculated impedances z_{cal} separately to real and imaginary part. Thus, in cases where the semicircle experiences a strong compression in the imaginary axis or there is a dominant Warburg impedance, the real and imaginary parts have the same influence on the calculated error. Using the mean $\bar{z}$ and the standard deviation σ, the z-score is applied:

$$z_{standard} = \frac{z - \bar{z}}{\sigma} \tag{12}$$

Here $\bar{z}$ and σ calculated from z_{acq} are also applied to z_{cal}. The z-score was chosen because it is better at handling outliers than a min-max normalization, which is especially important for real measured spectra.

The result of the LMA depends strongly on the used start parameters, since unfavorable start parameters may result in finding only local optima. Typically, start parameters are determined empirically and manually, which, however, should be automated and reproducible in the context of the research presented here. In general, the start parameters should be chosen to be close to the actual parameter sizes. Due to the wide value ranges for the individual parameters, it is therefore not possible to make a general, fixed preselection for all simulations. Therefore, the pre-fit method was used to estimate appropriate start parameters for the LMA [4]. The combined application of normalization of parameter values, standardization of impedances and pre-fit could already achieve a success rate of 97.75% for the fitting of simulated data of a Randles circuit [21].

For the pre-fit, a CNLS is performed with a circuit corresponding to a series connection of two RC elements (R_m, C_m for m = 1, 2) and a series resistor R_0 (see Fig. 3) before performing the actual analysis of the Randles circuit. The obtained results can then be used as start parameters for the actual CNLS with the Randles circuit. For this purpose, the components of the pre-fit must be assigned to the components of the Randles circuit, for which the time constants $\tau_m = R_m C_m$ of the determined RC elements are sorted by size in ascending order.

Considering that τ for diffusion is much larger than that of a charge exchange, an assignment of the RC elements to the Randles circuit can be made. Here it is evident that R_s is given by the series resistance R_0. The remaining components are assigned based on their ordinal number (m = 1 for CPE, R_{ct} and m = 2 for Z_w) according to the time constants sorted by size. Consequently, the smaller time constant derived from the pre-fit is assigned to the CPE. Accordingly, the capacitor value C_1 is used as the

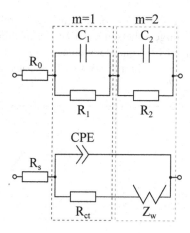

Fig. 3. Mapping between the components of the equivalent circuit of the pre-fit (top) with those of the Randles circuit (bottom) using the time constant τ_m [22].

initial value for Q (see Eq. 1). Since there is no equivalent for the exponent of the CPE by the RC network, it is always set to n = 0.75. Furthermore, R_1 is assigned to R_{ct} as well as C_2 to Q_w (see Eq. 2). An example illustration of the result obtained from the pre-fit is shown in Fig. 4.

For all investigations presented later in this paper, a CNLS without pre-fit is carried out first, whose start parameters are the logarithmic means of the value ranges. If the fit is unsuccessful, the same is done with an anterior pre-fit.

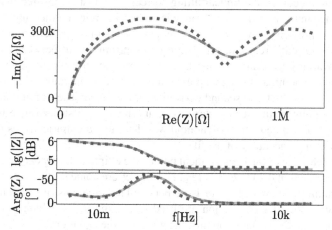

Fig. 4. Example Nyquist and Bode plots of a simulated impedance spectrum (green) with the result of the pre-fit (blue) and the resulting output of the CNLS (red) [22]. (Color figure online)

2.4 Elliptical Fitting

For the sole determination of the parameter R_{ct}, a geometric approach based on an elliptical fit in the Nyquist plot was applied [22]. For this approach it is assumed that the influence of the Warburg impedance is only significant at relatively low frequencies. The elliptical fitting hereby targets the semicircle which is created in the Nyquist plot in the higher frequency range by the parallel connection $R_{ct}||CPE$, as shown in Fig. 5. This semicircle may be shifted on the real axis by the series resistor R_s and may also be compressed by CPE [18,27].

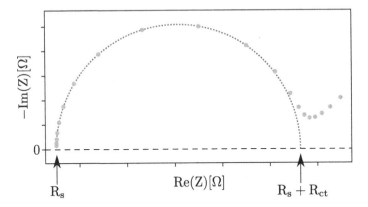

Fig. 5. Nyquist plot of a simulated impedance spectrum of a Randles circuit (red) with the corresponding fitted ellipse (blue). The zero crossing of the semicircle near the origin of coordinates represents R_s, the zero crossing in the low frequency region describes $R_s + R_{ct}$ [22]. (Color figure online)

To perform a geometric elliptical fitting correctly, it must be ensured that the Warburg impedance in the low-frequency range is not used as relevant measurement points. Accordingly, a pre-selection of the measurement points must be performed, selecting only those of the semicircle. For this purpose, the turning point between the semicircle and the Warburg impedance is used, which represents the cut-off point. To detect this characteristic point, a 5th degree polynomial is fitted to the impedance curve in the Nyquist plot, whose first and second derivatives are derived. The turning point results from the zero point of the second derivative, at which the first derivative is positive. The choice of the degree of the polynomial was determined empirically, as this avoids overfitting with high accuracy of the fit.

After the selection of the measurement points, the elliptical fitting can be performed, as already described in detail elsewhere [11]. Ellipses are conic sections on a plane that does not contain the apex or base or is perpendicular to the axis of rotation. Sections perpendicular to the axis of rotation are used to obtain circles, which is therefore a special case of an ellipse. Based on this, the general cone equation :

$$F(a, x) = ax^2 + bxy + cy^2 + dx + ey + f = 0 \qquad (13)$$

is applied for the fit, where $a = \begin{bmatrix} a\ b\ c\ d\ e\ f \end{bmatrix}^T$ and $x = \begin{bmatrix} x^2\ xy\ y^2\ x\ y\ 1 \end{bmatrix}^T$. Since no rotation of the ellipse is to be expected in the present case, b = 0 applies.

The algebraic distance $F(a, x)$ to be minimized is defined as the distance of a point (x, y) from the intersection $F(a, x) = 0$. Here also trivial solutions like $a = 0$ exist, which have to be avoided by additional conditions on the solution. Therefore the eigenvalue problem can be solved, for which a quadratic condition matrix C is set up:

$$D^T D a = \lambda C a \tag{14}$$

$D = \begin{bmatrix} x_1 & x_2 & \dots & x_n \end{bmatrix}^T$ represents the design matrix [8]. Because of C the vector a should describe an ellipse. This can be achieved by a negative discriminant $b^2 - 4ac$, which is difficult to solve in general. However, this application leaves the freedom to scale the parameters arbitrarily. Thus, the equality condition $4ac - b^2 = 1$ can be obtained [11], from which follows

$$a^T C a = 1 \tag{15}$$

where

$$C = \begin{bmatrix} 0 & 0 & 2 & 0 & 0 & 0 \\ 0 & -1 & 0 & 0 & 0 & 0 \\ 2 & 0 & 0 & 0 & 0 & 0 \\ 0 & 0 & 0 & 0 & 0 & 0 \\ 0 & 0 & 0 & 0 & 0 & 0 \\ 0 & 0 & 0 & 0 & 0 & 0 \end{bmatrix}. \tag{16}$$

By calculating the eigenvectors of Eq. 14, the minimization problem can now be solved. Assuming a pair of eigenvalue and eigenvector (λ_i, u_i) satisfies the system of equations, $(\lambda_i, \mu u_i)$ also does for any value of μ. Based on Eq. 15, a μ can now be found for which applies:

$$\mu_i^2 u_i^T C u_i = 1 \tag{17}$$

It follows that

$$\mu_i = \sqrt{\frac{1}{u_i^T C u_i}}. \tag{18}$$

The ellipse parameters for solving the optimization problem (Eq. 15) are thus given by

$$\hat{a}_i = \mu_i u_i. \tag{19}$$

3   Results

To evaluate the elliptical fitting, it is applied to simulated spectra from Randles circuits as well as to real data from an IMFET for the detection of cortisol. The results are compared with those of CNLS.

3.1   Simulated Data

The simulated impedance spectra were analyzed by both algorithms, so that at least R_{ct} can be extracted from each of the approaches. An example dataset with superimposed noise and the corresponding fits is shown in Fig. 6.

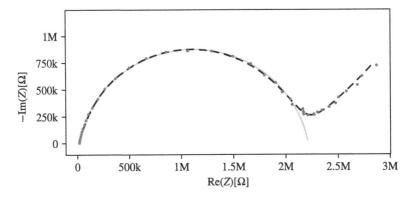

Fig. 6. Blue: one of the 100 simulated spectra with noise superimposed ($R_s = 1.72 \cdot 10^4$, $R_{ct} = 2.10 \cdot 10^6$, $Q_w = 2.83 \cdot 10^{-7}$, $Q = 3.13 \cdot 10^{-10}$, n = 0.88); black: fit of CNLS; red: elliptical fitting. In this example, CNLS achieved an error for determining R_{ct} of -0.05%, elliptical fitting achieved 0.26% [22]. (Color figure online)

The calculated values of R_{ct} derived with both approaches were compared with the values used to simulate the data sets. For this purpose, both the noisy and the raw data are examined. To avoid falsification of the evaluation by outliers, simulated spectra that could not be fitted by any of the presented approaches were discarded for further investigation. In order to compare performance, the required computation times for each fitting procedure are also measured. All approaches are implemented in the Python programming language and were run on an 1.90 GHz Intel® Core™ i7-8650U processor with 16 GB RAM.

A summary of all results is shown in Table 2. Here, the relative error E_R represents the difference between the calculated value $R_{ct,c}$ and the true value $R_{ct,t}$, with respect to $R_{ct,t}$. The linear relationship $R_{ct,c} = mR_{ct,t} + b$ with the slope m and the intercept b were determined which is exemplified in Fig. 7 for the noisy impedance spectra. Here, the coefficient of determination R^2 was also determined. N_d is the number of discarded spectra. For CNLS, the pre-fit must be used as an additional step for 33 spectra (raw spectra) or 31 spectra (noisy spectra).

Table 2. Results for CNLS and the elliptic fitting (EF) using raw ($CNLS_r$, EF_r) and noisy signals ($CNLS_n$, EF_n). Investigated parameters are: mean relative error E_R, slope m, intercept b, coefficient of determination R^2, number of discarded spectra N_d and mean computation time t_{cal} [22].

	E_R [%]	m	b [Ω]	R^2	N_d	t_{cal} [s]
$CNLS_r$	$1.5 \cdot 10^{-6} \pm 1.5 \cdot 10^{-5}$	1.00000	$1.2 \cdot 10^{-3}$	1.00000	1	$4.6 \cdot 10^{-1}$
EF_r	-2.7 ± 4.2	1.01027	$5.6 \cdot 10^3$	0.99957	2	$2.0 \cdot 10^{-3}$
$CNLS_n$	$2.4 \cdot 10^{-2} \pm 4.6 \cdot 10^{-1}$	0.99934	$5.3 \cdot 10^2$	0.99997	0	$4.5 \cdot 10^{-1}$
EF_n	-2.7 ± 4.3	1.00965	$5.6 \cdot 10^3$	0.99950	2	$2.0 \cdot 10^{-3}$

To measure the computation time, all necessary steps of the approaches were considered. This includes e.g. pre-selection of the measuring points, normalization or the

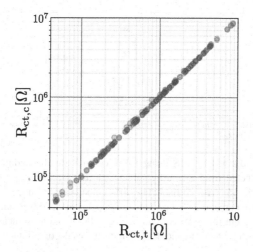

Fig. 7. Linear relationship between the calculated values $R_{ct,c}$ and the true values of the simulated impedance spectra $R_{ct,t}$. Red: CNLS, blue: elliptical fitting [22]. (Color figure online)

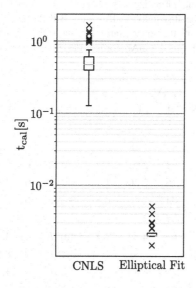

Fig. 8. Boxplots of the computation times for CNLS and the elliptical fit examining 100 simulated spectra without noise [22].

fitting of a polynomial. The obtained computation times are shown exemplarily as a boxplot in Fig. 8 for the spectra without noise superimposition.

3.2 Measured Real Data

To validate the approaches with real data, cortisol-sensitive IMFETs were used for saliva samples with EIS (see Sect. 2.2). Figure 9 shows all measurements that were

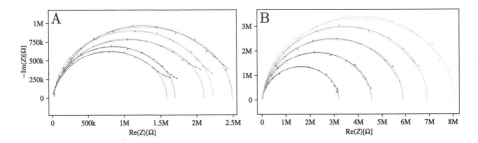

Fig. 9. Nyquist plots obtained by EIS using IMFETs with standard addition method (SAM). Aliquot A: saliva collected from a healthy subject; aliquot B: saliva collected from a healthy subject and spiked with 7.5 $^{ng}/_{mL}$ cortisol. The different standard solutions in PBS are indicated by color (green: 0.0 $^{ng}/_{mL}$, red: 0.2 $^{ng}/_{mL}$, cyan: 0.4 $^{ng}/_{mL}$, purple: 0.6 $^{ng}/_{mL}$, orange: 1.0 $^{ng}/_{mL}$). References (blue) represent the mAb-cortisol baseline. Points indicate measured samples, solid lines the results of CNLS with pre-fit and dashed lines the results of elliptical fitting. (Color figure online)

Table 3. Results from analyses of the impedance spectra generated by the IMFETs using CNLS and elliptic fitting (EF). R_{ct} and normalized resistance $R_{ct,norm}$ (see Eq. 3) are examined. Aliquot A is saliva collected from a healthy individual. Aliquot B is the same saliva sample spiked with 7.5 $^{ng}/_{mL}$ cortisol. C represents the concentrations of the standard solutions in PBS. The reference measurement Ref represents the mAb-cortisol baseline. The relative error between CNLS and EF is given as E_R.

	C [$^{ng}/_{mL}$]	R_{ct} [MΩ]			$R_{ct,norm}$		
		CNLS	EF	E_R [%]	CNLS	EF	E_R [%]
Aliquot A	Ref	1.52	1.57	+3.3	–	–	–
	0.0	1.63	1.68	+3.1	$7.24E-02$	$7.01E-02$	+3.3
	0.2	1.98	2.08	+5.1	$3.03E-01$	$3.25E-01$	−6.8
	0.4	2.16	2.20	+1.9	$4.21E-01$	$4.01E-01$	+4.9
	0.6	2.44	2.46	+0.8	$6.05E-01$	$5.67E-01$	+6.8
Aliquot B	Ref	3.27	3.16	−3.4	–	–	–
	0.0	4.60	4.52	−1.7	$4.07E-01$	$4.30E-01$	−5.5
	0.2	5.93	5.85	−1.3	$8.13E-01$	$8.51E-01$	−4.4
	0.4	6.70	6.85	+2.2	$1.05E+00$	$1.17E+00$	−10.2
	1.0	8.22	8.00	−2.7	$1.51E+00$	$1.53E+00$	−1.2

recorded as part of the SAMs for both aliquots. CNLS and the elliptic fitting were used to determine R_{ct}. In contrast to the studies with simulated data, for measurements with biosensors the true value of R_{ct} is not known. Thus, only the error of the elliptical fitting with respect to CNLS can be determined. CNLS is therefore assumed to be the gold standard for the determination accuracy of R_{ct} in this case. The average error E_R obtained by the elliptical fitting over 10 analyzed impedance spectra for R_{ct} is $0.7 \pm 2.7\%$. A detailed list of results is shown in Table 3.

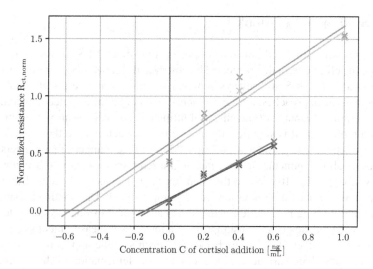

Fig. 10. Standard addition diagram of the measurements with aliquot A (dark) and B (light colors) and respective application of CNLS (red) and elliptical fitting (blue). Aliquot A is a saliva sample from a healthy subject, Aliquot B the same saliva sample spiked with $7.5\,\mathrm{ng/mL}$ cortisol. X-axis scaling includes the dilution factor of 20.0. The cortisol concentration in aliquot A resulted in 2.2 (CNLS) and $2.7\,\mathrm{ng/mL}$ (elliptical fitting), in aliquot B in 10.2 (CNLS) and $11.3\,\mathrm{ng/mL}$ (elliptical fitting), respectively. (Color figure online)

To perform the SAM, the normalized resistances $R_{ct,norm}$ were calculated using the reference measurements according to Eq. 3. Due to normalization, the relative error of the elliptical fitting with respect to CNLS has deteriorated to $-1.6 \pm 6.1\%$ by error propagation. The results of the SAM for both aliquots using CNLS and elliptical fitting are shown in Fig. 10. Linear regression for aliquot A resulted in $R_{ct,norm} = 0.8586C + 0.0928$ ($R^2 = 0.9859$) for CNLS and $R_{ct,norm} = 0.7834C + 0.1057$ ($R^2 = 0.9566$) for elliptical fitting. Based on linear regression, the absolute value of the cortisol concentration of the original sample is obtained from the intercept with the x-axis multiplied by the dilution factor (here: 20.0). Consequently, a cortisol concentration of 2.2 (CNLS) and $2.7\,\mathrm{ng/mL}$ (elliptical fitting) could be determined for aliquot A, respectively. Aliquot B, i.e., the same saliva sample spiked with $7.5\,\mathrm{ng/mL}$, resulted in a linear relationship of $R_{ct,norm} = 1.0408C + 0.5294$ ($R^2 = 0.9460$) (CNLS) and $R_{ct,norm} = 1.0296C + 0.5834$ ($R^2 = 0.9032$) (elliptical fit). The concentrations determined in this case were 10.2 for CNLS and $11.3\,\mathrm{ng/mL}$ using elliptical fitting. Consequently, an average error of $0.8\,\mathrm{ng/mL}$ occurs in the analysis of both aliquots by the elliptical fitting versus CNLS. The concentration difference of both aliquots, which is theoretically $7.5\,\mathrm{ng/mL}$, could be determined to 8.0 (CNLS) and $8.6\,\mathrm{ng/mL}$ (elliptical fitting) by the described procedure. This results in an error of 7.5% between the methods.

4   Discussion and Outlook

Investigations with simulated impedance spectra show that CNLS has low errors and is better than the elliptic fit in this respect. The observed differences become smaller using noisy spectra, but CNLS still always achieves the more accurate results. For further comparison of the approaches, artifact influences should be investigated and compared.

However, the advantage of the elliptical fitting can be made clear by measuring the computation times, as it is significantly more efficient (factor $1/225$) than CNLS. Here, it must be noted that the normalization almost doubled the number of parameters, since the values of all components of the equivalent circuit are divided into a factor a and an exponent b (see Eq. 10). While this step improves the success rate and minimizes the error, it also makes the regression more complex [21]. The obtained results suggest that elliptic fitting is suitable for implementation on embedded systems due to its performance. Thus, the power consumption of a low-power measurement system could be optimized. However, it must be checked for each specific application whether the accuracies achieved are sufficient. For an efficient implementation of this approach on embedded systems, the algorithm may need to be further adapted depending on the hardware to minimize power consumption and optimize accuracies.

Both approaches achieve a very high success rate in fitting and have to discard only very few simulated spectra. It should be noted that the pre-fit is a strong improvement for CNLS, because otherwise 33% would not be fitable. For the elliptical fit, on the other hand, only 2 of the 100 spectra could not be fitted, despite the significantly lower computation time. In general, it is also noticeable for CNLS that the success rate is improved by the superimposed noise, although otherwise strong susceptibilities to noise are described [14]. The elliptical fitting should be further optimized so that success rate can be improved. One possibility for this is that impedance spectra, where Z_w already dominates near the imaginary minimum of the semicircle, are treated differently. For such spectra, due to the fitting of the polynomial and the detection of a turning point, the preselection of the measurement points could be erroneous. Depending on the application, current and future approaches of preselection must also be evaluated with different types of the Warburg impedance (finite length, finite space).

The simulated impedance spectra investigated here cover a wide range of values of the individual parameters of the equivalent circuit. The approaches presented thus allow generic modeling for a wide range of applications. However, as soon as these are to be transferred to a real application scenario, they should be adapted to achieve better results. For example, narrow value ranges may obviate the need for pre-fit or normalization. In case the equivalent circuit of the sensor technology under investigation has a C_{dl} instead of the CPE, one parameter is omitted for CNLS and also the elliptical fitting could be transferred to a circular fitting.

Measurements with IMFETs showed that the application of the elliptical fit is also possible on real data. Here, the determined values of R_{ct} by the elliptical fit differ from CNLS by an average of $0.7 \pm 2.7\%$. For the investigated use case of measuring cortisol in saliva as an indication of cardiac disease, elliptical fitting may nevertheless be a promising approach for future μTAS, considering the cortisol concentration variations that have been published [13]. When measuring real biosensors, the actual values of the parameters in the equivalent circuit are of course not known, thus CNLS had to be used as a reference. It must be noted that errors caused by the application of CNLS can influence the result of the elliptical fitting accordingly. A possible approach for further evaluation would be to physically simulate the equivalent circuit including the Warburg impedance by means of an RC network. Thus, this could be measured by an impedance spectroscope with the actual values known.

In principle, CPE does not cause any compression of the semicircle, even if it appears so when exclusively considering the fourth quadrant of the Nyquist plot. CPE rather causes a rotation of the circle around the zero point. Further research should therefore be conducted to compare the fitting of a circle with the presented method, particularly in terms of accuracy, efficiency and success rate. Related approaches have already been described for the analysis of bioimpedances [1].

Acknowledgements. This research was funded by EU H2020 research and innovation program entitled KardiaTool with grant N⁰ 768686.

References

1. Ayllon, D., Seoane, F., Gil-Pita, R.: Cole equation and parameter estimation from electrical bioimpedance spectroscopy measurements - a comparative study. In: Annual International Conference of the IEEE Engineering in Medicine and Biology Society. IEEE Engineering in Medicine and Biology Society. Annual International Conference 2009, pp. 3779–3782 (2009). https://doi.org/10.1109/IEMBS.2009.5334494
2. Bahadır, E.B., Sezgintürk, M.K.: A review on impedimetric biosensors. Artif. Cells Nanomed. Biotechnol. **44**(1), 248–262 (2016). https://doi.org/10.3109/21691401.2014.942456
3. Barsoukov, E., Macdonald, J.R.: Impedance Spectroscopy: Theory, Experiment, and Applications. Wiley, Hoboken (2005). https://doi.org/10.1002/0471716243
4. Barsukov, Y., Macdonald, J.R.: Electrochemical impedance spectroscopy, pp. 1–17. American Cancer Society (2012). https://doi.org/10.1002/0471266965.com124
5. Bausells, J., et al.: On the impedance spectroscopy of field-effect biosensors. Electrochem. Sci. Adv. (2021). https://doi.org/10.1002/elsa.202100138
6. Ben Halima, H., et al.: Immuno field-effect transistor (immunoFET) for detection of salivary cortisol using potentiometric and impedance spectroscopy for monitoring heart failure. Talanta 123802 (2022). Manuscript submitted for publication
7. Bertsekas, D.P.: Nonlinear Programming, Second Edition (1999)
8. Bookstein, F.L.: Fitting conic sections to scattered data. Comput. Graphics Image Process. **9**(1), 56–71 (1979). https://doi.org/10.1016/0146-664X(79)90082-0
9. Chowdhury, A.D., Ganganboina, A.B., Park, E.Y., Doong, R.A.: Impedimetric biosensor for detection of cancer cells employing carbohydrate targeting ability of Concanavalin A. Biosens. Bioelectron. **122**, 95–103 (2018). https://doi.org/10.1016/j.bios.2018.08.039
10. Dang, W., Manjakkal, L., Navaraj, W.T., Lorenzelli, L., Vinciguerra, V., Dahiya, R.: Stretchable wireless system for sweat pH monitoring. Biosens. Bioelectron. **107**, 192–202 (2018). https://doi.org/10.1016/j.bios.2018.02.025
11. Fitzgibbon, A., Pilu, M., Fisher, R.B.: Direct least square fitting of ellipses. IEEE Trans. Pattern Anal. Mach. Intell. **21**(5), 476–480 (1999). https://doi.org/10.1109/34.765658
12. Halima, H.B., et al.: A novel cortisol biosensor based on the capacitive structure of hafnium oxide: application for heart failure monitoring. In: 20th International Conference on Solid-State Sensors, Actuators and Microsystems and Eurosensors, pp. 1067–1070 (2019). https://doi.org/10.1109/TRANSDUCERS.2019.8808561

13. Hammer, F., et al.: High evening salivary cortisol is an independent predictor of increased mortality risk in patients with systolic heart failure. Int. J. Cardiol. **203**, 69–73 (2016). https://doi.org/10.1016/j.ijcard.2015.10.084

14. Kauffman, G.B.: Electrochemical impedance spectroscopy. By Mark E. Orazem and Bernard Tribollet. Angewandte Chemie International Edition (2009). https://doi.org/10.1002/anie.200805564

15. Kharitonov, A.B., Wasserman, J., Katz, E., Willner, I.: The use of impedance spectroscopy for the characterization of protein-modified ISFET devices: application of the method for the analysis of biorecognition processes. J. Phys. Chem. B **105**(19), 4205–4213 (2001). https://doi.org/10.1021/jp0045383

16. Leva-Bueno, J., Peyman, S.A., Millner, P.A.: A review on impedimetric immunosensors for pathogen and biomarker detection. Med. Microbiol. Immunol. **209**, 343–362 (2020). https://doi.org/10.1007/s00430-020-00668-0

17. Macdonald, D.D.: Some advantages and pitfalls of electrochemical impedance spectroscopy. Corrosion **46**(3), 229–242 (1990). https://doi.org/10.5006/1.3585096

18. Orazem, M.E., Tribollet, B.: Electrochemical Impedance Spectroscopy. Wiley (2008). https://doi.org/10.1002/9780470381588

19. Papageorgiou, M., Leibold, M., Buss, M., Papageorgiou, M., Leibold, M., Buss, M.: Methode der kleinsten Quadrate. In: Optimierung (2015). https://doi.org/10.1007/978-3-662-46936-1_6

20. Pejcic, B., De Marco, R.: Impedance spectroscopy: over 35 years of electrochemical sensor optimization. Electrochim. Acta **51**(28), 6217–6229 (2006). https://doi.org/10.1016/j.electacta.2006.04.025

21. Pfeiffer, N., Jechow, M., Wachter, T., Hofmann, C., Errachid, A., Heuberger, A.: Impact of normalization, standardization and pre-fit on the success rate of fitting in electrochemical impedance spectroscopy. Curr. Dir. Biomed. Eng. **7**(2), 492–495 (2021). https://doi.org/10.1515/cdbme-2021-2125

22. Pfeiffer, N., Wachter, T., Frickel, J., Hofmann, C., Errachid, A., Heuberger, A.: Elliptical fitting as an alternative approach to complex nonlinear least squares regression for modeling electrochemical impedance spectroscopy. In: Proceedings of the 14th International Joint Conference on Biomedical Engineering Systems and Technologies, pp. 42–49. SCITEPRESS - Science and Technology Publications (2021). https://doi.org/10.5220/0010231600420049

23. Prodromidis, M.I.: Impedimetric immunosensors—a review. Electrochim. Acta **55**(14), 4227–4233 (2010). https://doi.org/10.1016/j.electacta.2009.01.081

24. Randviir, E.P., Banks, C.E.: Electrochemical impedance spectroscopy: an overview of bioanalytical applications. Anal. Methods **5**(5), 1098–1115 (2013). https://doi.org/10.1039/c3ay26476a

25. Rushworth, J.V., Ahmed, A., Griffiths, H.H., Pollock, N.M., Hooper, N.M., Millner, P.A.: A label-free electrical impedimetric biosensor for the specific detection of Alzheimer's amyloid-beta oligomers. Biosens. Bioelectron. **56**, 83–90 (2014). https://doi.org/10.1016/j.bios.2013.12.036

26. Sgobbi, L.F., Razzino, C.A., Machado, S.A.: A disposable electrochemical sensor for simultaneous detection of sulfamethoxazole and trimethoprim antibiotics in urine based on multi-walled nanotubes decorated with Prussian blue nanocubes modified screen-printed electrode. Electrochim. Acta **191**, 1010–1017 (2016). https://doi.org/10.1016/j.electacta.2015.11.151

27. Shoar Abouzari, M.R., Berkemeier, F., Schmitz, G., Wilmer, D.: On the physical interpretation of constant phase elements. Solid State Ion. **180**(14–16), 922–927 (2009). https://doi.org/10.1016/j.ssi.2009.04.002

28. Sun, A., Venkatesh, A.G., Hall, D.A.: A multi-technique reconfigurable electrochemical biosensor: enabling personal health monitoring in mobile devices. IEEE Trans. Biomed. Circuits Syst. **10**(5), 945–954 (2016). https://doi.org/10.1109/TBCAS.2016.2586504
29. Sung, D., Koo, J.: A review of BioFET's basic principles and materials for biomedical applications. Biomed. Eng. Lett. **11**(2), 85–96 (2021). https://doi.org/10.1007/s13534-021-00187-8
30. Tu, J., Torrente-Rodríguez, R.M., Wang, M., Gao, W.: The era of digital health: a review of portable and wearable affinity biosensors. Adv. Func. Mater. **30**(29), 1906713 (2020). https://doi.org/10.1002/adfm.201906713
31. Vozgirdaite, D., et al.: Development of an immunofet for analysis of tumour necrosis factor-α in artificial saliva: application for heart failure monitoring. Chemosensors **9**(2), 26 (2021). https://doi.org/10.3390/chemosensors9020026
32. Yuan, X.Z., Song, C., Wang, H., Zhang, J.: Electrochemical impedance spectroscopy in PEM fuel cells. Springer, London (2010). https://doi.org/10.1007/978-1-84882-846-9

Towards Segmentation and Labelling of Motion Data in Manufacturing Scenarios

António Santos[1]([✉]) [iD], João Rodrigues[1,3] [iD], Duarte Folgado[1,2] [iD], Sara Santos[2], Carlos Fujão[3], and Hugo Gamboa[1,2] [iD]

[1] Laboratório de Instrumentação, Engenharia Biomédica e Física da Radiação (LIBPhys-UNL), Departamento de Física, Faculdade de Ciências e Tecnologia, FCT, Universidade Nova de Lisboa, 2829-516 Caparica, Portugal
`alm.santos@campus.fct.unl.pt`, `jmd.rodrigues@fct.unl.pt`
[2] Associação Fraunhofer Portugal Research, Rua Alfredo Allen 455/461, 4200-135 Porto, Portugal
`{duarte.folgado,sara.santos,hugo.gamboa}@fraunhofer.pt`
[3] Volkswagen Autoeuropa, Quinta da Marquesa, 2954-024 Quinta do Anjo, Portugal

Abstract. There is a significant interest to evaluate the occupational exposure that manufacturing operators are subjected throughout the working day. The objective evaluation of occupational exposure with direct measurements and the need for automatic annotation of relevant events arose. The current work proposes the use of a self similarity matrix (SSM) as a tool to flag events that may be of importance to be analyzed by ergonomic teams. This way, data directly retrieved from the work environment will be summarized and segmented into sub-sequences of interest over a multi-timescale approach. The process occurs under 3 timescale levels: Active working periods, working cycles, and in-cycle activities. The novelty function was used to segment non-active and active working periods with an F1-score of 95%. while the similarity function was used to correctly segment 98% of working cycle with a duration error of 6.12%. In addition, this method was extended into examples of multi time scale segmentation with the intent of providing a summary of a time series as well as support in data labeling tasks, by means of a query-by-example process to detect all subsequences.

Keywords: Self-similarity matrix · Time series · Industry · Musculoskeletal disorders · Inertial · Segmentation · Summarization · Unsupervised · Labeling

1 Introduction

1.1 Work Related Disorders and Risk Evaluation

Musculoskeletal disorders are a broad variety of health conditions that affect the locomotor system. These are usually described by pain and a reduction of people's mobility, with some of the more common conditions including osteoarthritis,

C. Gehin et al. (Eds.): BIOSTEC 2021, CCIS 1710, pp. 80–101, 2022.
https://doi.org/10.1007/978-3-031-20664-1_5

back and neck pain, fractures associated with bone fragility, injuries and systemic inflammatory conditions such as rheumatoid arthritis.

The burden of impaired musculoskeletal health can be very deteriorating for individual human lives. Pain and disability lead to the inability of performing daily life activities, precluding an active participation in social activities and possibly limiting the work performance of the population. [6,7] Furthermore these may also promote various physical and mental comorbidities. [8–10]

The present work will target work-related musculoskeletal disorders (WMSDs) i.e. MSDs which are induced or aggravated by work and the circumstances of its performance. [11] Workspaces can be pointed out as a significant contributor to MSDs [12], with the added advantage of being also a controlled environment that can be adapted towards health policies concentrated on primary prevention. To project a proper intervention for the work-space it is very important to firs evaluate each separate job-environment relationship. It's not effective to design a "one-fits-all" system for different work settings as it requires specific adaptations designed by trained ergonomist specialists.

In this sense, there have been developed several systems to assess the level of occupational exposure in each workplace. These techniques fall mostly into three main categories, which differ from each other depending on the type of data acquisition method used: (1) Self-report from workers, a protocol that enables workers to individually provide the data about their personal work experience. This can be achieved through the use of questionnaires, diaries, personal interviews or checklist surveys so that they might be further evaluated by experts; (2) Observational methods, which consists on the visual surveillance of the work routine by trained experts, where, conventionally, their metrics are then provided by pre-designed ergonomic risk assessment sheets; (3) Direct Measurements, that propose the use of new technologies to retrieve more precise/accurate information from the work environment. This is made through the usage of sensors usually attached to specific subjects performing work routines.

It has been proven, overall, that an ergonomic assessment of the work environment can indeed reduce the prevalence of MSDs by helping to identify possible risk factors, and in the interest of this work we'll argue that there are also advantages in a transition towards more direct measurement techniques. As a more objective form of describing the interaction between workers and the workplace doesn't suffer from any variability dependent on the worker or specialist observer, as the "Self-reporting" and "Observational" methodologies do.

However, despite direct measurements affording a more objective representation of the reality, it still has limitations regarding greater costs associated with its implementations and the narrow success on a practical environment. Being mostly used successfully under controlled simulated laboratories. Another important concern is its interpretability with the analysis of motion sensors being complex and requiring specific insights to retrieve relevant knowledge.

1.2 Motivation

The current information era, in conjunction with technological developments, is promoting a shift in the way industries manage and perform their work. With the inclusion of sensing devices, dashboards and machine learning algorithms, many tasks can be better evaluated with direct quantitative measures. This can be made for machines to prevent breakdowns and optimize their performance, but can also be used for humans, namely their occupational health, to prevent work-related disorders. The prevention of work-related disorders implies a specialized intervention to perform changes in the workplace, the worker's training process and/or other organizational strategies. The process of deciding a need for intervention implies a previous risk evaluation of the worker's routines. The direct measures from inertial sensors provide relevant information for a more objective and personalized risk assessment [1]. However, before the actual ergonomic risk evaluation, a considerable number of steps in preparing the data are needed. Data preparation is an important part of any analysis or task that requires further deployment in supervised methods, namely the time-consumingtime consuming segmentation and labelling process. This is an impediment that has become extensively common in various types of industries and social sectors, stalling sometimes further development. As the rate of information that we acquire from the world tends to increase there is a greater need for processes that can automaticaly retrieve useful knowledge from that data, as people don't have that same capacity.

Tools capable of segmenting time series to support and ease the labelling process of motion and posture data are highly valued, since it is a sensitive and time-consuming process, but highly necessary for the risk analysis and the deployment of semi-supervised and supervised methods [2]. In this case, motion data in real scenarios are even more complex since it is highly rich and diverse in behaviors. For instance, although cyclic and repetitive activities performed in industrial scenarios are mostly consistent from cycle to cycle, perfect conditions cannot be met all the time. Eventually, the working process can inadvertently be stopped or delayed. In addition, ergonomic risk assessment methods have to analyze each working cycle, which means that a previous segmentation of each one of these instances has to be made. Sub-activities that make the sequence of actions comprehended in the working cycle can also be sub-segmented for further recognition and association with risk measures. For instance, the *ergonomist* might have an interest in understanding which actions from the working cycle have a significant association with a high or low risk measure, to adapt the working station with intervention strategies that could help prevent future disorders. Another relevant analysis is the study of changes in the working behavior over time, since by segmenting the working cycle and its sub-activities, we can compare them over time and perform higher level associations (e.g. how the worker adjusted his behavior over the morning and afternoon periods).

This work studies the hypothesis of using the *Self-Similarity Matrix* (SSM), already applied for audio information retrieval [4], for segmentation and assisted labeling of time series from inertial motion and postural data of workers in an assembly line of an automotive industry. Several results are provided showing the ability of using this method for segmentation tasks, and examples with exploratory results are given to extend the segmentation power of the method for multi time-scale segmentation, summarization and assisted labeling. The contributions are towards having an unsupervised tool to perform time series segmentation in multiple and hierarchical time scales that can further be applied for time series summarization and/or personalized labelling-by-example in occupational health datasets.

To provide an illustrative example to the reader of our intent, we show a multi-scale segmentation of an electrocardiogram (ECG) signal with the proposed method in Fig. 1.

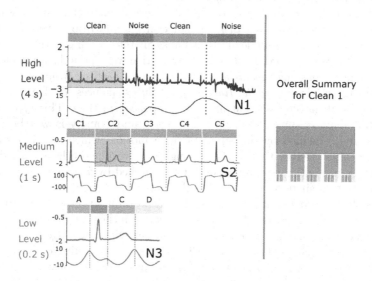

Fig. 1. Example of a multi time scale segmentation of a simple ECG signal with noise. The signal is from the Physionet [5]. Each row of signals indicates a smaller timescale, zooming-in a specific sub-segment of the previous segmentation. On the right, an example of how we could summarize the first portion of the signal with this type of segmentation.

Figure 1 shows three levels of segmentation from higher to lower time scale. The first is segmented by the novelty function (N1) with a time scale of $4\,s$, which peaks separate clean ECG from noise. The segments of interest can then be segmented into ECG cycles by the valleys of the similarity function (S2), calculated with a time scale of 1 s. Finally, inside each cycle, the most significant sub-segments are each of the P, T waves and QRS complex, segmented by the novelty function (N3) with a time scale of $0.2\,s$. This example is illustrative of the goal we want to reach with this work towards a tool that can perform a meaningful multi time-scale segmentation that contributes to transform the data into a summary and that can be used to assist the analyst in performing labelling of the segments identified.

1.3   Towards Occupational Data Segmentation

This work proposes the usage of the *SSM* created by a feature-based representation of the time series from the worker's motion while performing tasks. From this representation, we will present visual evidence of its usage for the identification of events with ergonomic significance and summarize the working activity. The summarization process is performed by segmenting the data into sub-sequences of interest in a multi-timescale approach, as defined below.

1. **Active working periods** *(higher time scale)*: *Active and non-active segments* indicate sub-sequences of the time series where the worker was performing the cyclic working tasks or not doing them, respectively (e.g.: stop on the working line that leads to a pause in the working activity). In this work, transitions between active and non-active work periods are made, with the intent in focusing (*zoom-in*) our attention to each *working cycle*;
2. **Working cycles** *(middle time scale)*: Sub-sequences of highly similar sequences of movements that are being repeated in time. This type of segmentation pre-assumes that the time series under analysis will be mostly (or entirely) defined by the repetition of a motion, which are the examples of tasks analyzed in this work. Having each working-cycle identified, *sub-activities* inside the working cycle can be searched by focusing (*zoom-in*) our attention to a single working-cycle sub-sequence;
3. **In-cycle activities** (lower time scale): A working cycle is structured in a sequence of *sub-activities*. The transition between these might be related with a significant change in the worker's motion behavior or change in posture. In this context, what will be intended is to divide the working cycle into more primitive segments and understand if the segmentation is consistent over each of the analyzed cycles.

In addition to the several levels of segmentation, we will also provide an example in how a labelling process can be performed with the same *SSM* by means of a *query-by-example*. This methodology will be exemplified to identify instant repetitions of a given pre-specified time series' sub-sequence of the user's interest. For example, if the analyst wants to understand the contribution of a specific segment of the working cycle for the occupational risk, this sub-sequence could be used as a query to search all the other equal segments. Moreover, current risk evaluations of occupational exposure are made with the assistance of video. Such query-by-example methods could be integrated into a video system that let's the analyst select an interval of the video that corresponds to a specific part of a working cycle, and the algorithm segments the remaining other similar segments. This would increase the speed of analysis and/or labeling process.

The segmentation process proposed will rely in the detection of significant events in multiple time-scales. These events are the instants in time that segment any of the aforementioned sub-sequences (1, 2 and 3). This work provides additional content to previous experiments [3] by (a) improving the detection performance of *events 1* with the usage of the *novelty function*, (b) extend the event detection process to a multi time-scale approach by segmenting sub-activities of interest inside a working cycle, and (c) discussing how this method can be used as a tool to support labelling of time series.

This document is organized by first (1) discussing related work, then (2) explaining the data we used, (3) describe the proposed methodology, (4) and (5) demonstrate illustrative examples in occupational inertial data, while discussing these findings and (6) provide final thoughts regarding this work.

2   Related Work

Processes of computer analysis under acquisitions retrieved from a real work environment have already been proven to be very useful in the design of evaluation tools to facilitate ergonomic studies. Under the work of [13], by firstly calculating the orientation of anatomical joints, it was possible to design an adjusted ergonomic risk score. This had the final objective of automatically assessing the operator risk exposure during the work on an assembly line.

In the context of summarizing a work period acquisition by segmenting it into smaller motion segments, the work of [14, 15] has analysed multidimensional angular joint motion time series with each motion segment being represented by dynamic model approximations. The segmentation methodology was based on univariate active forgetting segmentation methods, with a two-step recursive least square algorithm predicting change points in the dynamic behavior of the system. The motion data segments are then represented by parameters derivative from a dynamic model fit, which as the advantage of the features being insensitive to small-time variations, very common in this type of data, and allows for a comparison based on a "kinetic energy-like" measure.

Meanwhile [16], in the process of summarizing human motion, temporally segmented the repetitive human motions, much like we also propose to do. This work used a time series representation of the joint angle of the subjects. This motion data was then converted into a generic full-body kinematic model, by using an unscented Kalman filter, and then retrieved kinematic features by performing a primary frequency analysis to the transformed data. The data was then segmented by based on the zero crossing of these retrieved features, followed by an adaptive k-means clustering to identify which segments are repetitions of each other.

[17] proposed the use of a mask-based Neural Network (NN) capable of extracting desired patterns of interest from a large time series database, without the requirement of a predefined template. Validated under electrocardiogram and human motion signals, this work was an algorithm proposal that could automatically detect specific patterns in biosignals.

The use of an SSM applied on the analysis of human motion, more specifically human motion at work, is still a subject with a short exploration in the literature. However, this work will make the case that it might be a useful tool adapted to this concern.

Notwithstanding, there has been some works on this subject, with [18] discussing in much detail a method that relies on a neighborhood graph to partition the dataset into 1) distinct activities and 2) motion primitives according to a self-similar structures. Alternatively, we can also see the matrix profile algorithm [19], an well established algorithm for an optimized processing of time series, which by focusing on the similarity join problem can additionally compute the answer to the time series motif and discord problem. A matrix profile is in a short summery a "time serie", whose values are the euclidean distance between a subsequence and its nearest neighbor. Under this work, its also proven the validity of this methodology to analyse human motion data.

The use of SSM is a well explored tool for the a rapid analysis of music data. The reason why this type of database is especially fit for this analysis is that it is (1) recurrent in nature, (2) complex enough in nature than other types of processing of the raw data would be demanding enough that converting to a similarity matrix isn't as demanding in comparison. Fortunately, these characteristics also apply to our case. We are using inertial data in time series format, retrieved from various Inertial sensors attached to the subjects' body, which is a complex type of data. Besides, it is recurrent in nature, because the tasks being analysed are cyclic. Therefore, the proposed method is highly inspired by the same method used in audio signals analysis for audio thumbnailing or summarization [20].

3   Dataset Description

3.1   Population

The inertial data available to develop this methodology was acquired in the context of validating an inertial measuring system that would guarantee access to direct measures in occupational industrial environments. This system was previously used to deliver an ergonomic risk assessment based on the angular information retrieved by the raw data of these sensors [1].

The population in which the system was tested is described in this work [1]. The in-field data used was acquired in an industrial environment from an automotive assembly plant. More specifically, the subjects were working in assembly tasks and the data was acquired while the subjects were performing the tasks of a specific workstation. The dataset includes six participants, each monitored while working at two different workstations. In this scenario, each workstation has a specific set of tasks that have to be performed by the worker. These tasks are repeated throughout the working period, being divided into working cycles.

3.2   Instruments and Setup

An inertial measurement unit (IMU) is an electronic device composed internally by three 3-axial sensors: accelerometer (Acc), gyroscope (Gyro) and magnetometer (Mag). When attached to strategic points of the human body, it allows to register that object's specific force, angular momentum, and position, simultaneously. Combined, these provide much information about the movement and posture of the subject.

In this study data from the dominant upper limb of the subjects was measured. The system comprehends a set of four 9-DoF IMUs. These were attached on the upper dominant limb of the subjects, namely:

- **IMU 1** posterior side of the hand
- **IMU 2** posterior side of the forearm (wrist)
- **IMU 3** posterior side of the arm (elbow)
- **IMU** 4 thorax area

All devices were attached so that the Y-axis was aligned upwards. Figure 2 shows how the sensors were placed on the subjects.

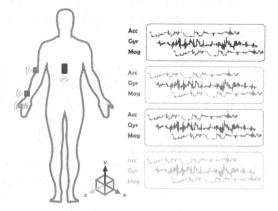

Fig. 2. Schematic of the placement of Inertial sensors, used for the dataset acquisition protocol. Based on [1] and [3]

The signals available for analysis are the 3-axis accelerometer, gyroscope and magnetometer of all IMUs used, collected with a sampling rate 100 Hz. The raw data has all the events described in the ??, namely (1) active working periods intercalated with non-active working periods; (2) working cycles and (3) sub-activity segments. For the ground-truth position of these events, all signals were annotated by means of video-records of the acquisition sessions.

4   Methods

The following section describes the proposed methodologies to detect the various events of interest for the segmentation process. It will, as such, be structured as follows:

1. SSM construction
2. Similarity function
3. Novelty function
4. Sub-sequence search-by-example,

with the first point describing how the *SSM* is structured such that all the remaining strategies are capable of finding relevant event types presented in Sect. 1.

4.1 SSM Construction

Pre-Processing. Before any analysis, the data has to be prepared. This includes tasks such as synchronizing and filtering. The synchronization tends to be an essential process, as the framework usually involves several sensor devices that can have divergent internal clocks. The filtering process is also a fundamental step. In this case, a second-order low pass Butterworth filter 40 Hz was used on the inertial data. The choice of this cut frequency was because experimental studies [21] have already proved that human motion and posture could be well represented by a frequency up 20 Hz.

Feature Retrieval. After all the sensor dimensions have been pre-processed, a new representation of the dataset is made by applying a moving window function, which retrieves a set of predefined features of the temporal, statistical and spectral domain. Extracting relevant features is of great importance to have a rich characterization of the morphology of each signal [22].

This process has the result of turning a multivariate time series with n dimensions and m data points, into a multivariate time series with $n \times f$ feature dimensions and $< m$ number of data points. This is a process of feature retrieval which doesn't necessarily reduces the volume of data, but instead tries to reduce its complexity into simpler components that describe the shape of the data.

This entire process will, of course, be parameterized by the windows length ($Wind_{len}$) and an overlapping fraction ($Overlap_{frac}$). Both $Wind_{len}$, $Overlap_{frac}$ have a large influence on the results, as they define the time scale at which features are extracted and consequently will also define the time resolution of the *SSM*. This means that an adjustment of these parameters changes the time dimension of the events which are gonna be highlighted. In other words, a larger $Wind_{len}$ will result in highlighting similarities between longer sub-sequences of the set of time series, while a shorter $Wind_{len}$ will have the inverse effect. Most studies in the field of human activity recognition consider the use of 1 to 10 s time length windows. [23] However, despite this being a good starting value in an ergonomic analysis, it is required to consider events along the multiple time scales, and without any previous information, there cannot be made any assumptions.

SSM Calculation. An *SSM* is a graphical representation of the similarity between each data sample (or window) and all the remaining samples (or windows) in the rest of a time series. This allows to highlight similar and (dis)similar structures, that can be patterns or dynamic behaviors of the signal.

Obtained the previously described feature matrix

$$F = (x_1, \ldots, x_n)_{(n \in \mathbb{N})},$$

where each coordinate x is also described by a vector of dimensions ($m \in \mathbb{N}$). Then the *SSM*, used for this work, will have a size $n \times n$, with each of its position being defined by

$$SSM(i,j) = s(x_i, x_j)$$

where $s(x_i, x_j)$ is a distance measure, which takes into account the vector points $x_i, x_j \in X$, both of length m and returns a real value, which represents a score of how closely similar are these two point coordinates.

As such, to build an *SSM*, it is necessary to define the distance function s, with the literature on the subject pointing usually to three options: cosine of the angles, euclidean distance and Kullback Leibler distance. This work chose to use the first distance function. To calculate it, the feature representation signal F positions were normalized. Then, the distance function could be described by the simple inner product between two vectors

$$s(x_i, x_j) = \langle x_i, x_j \rangle,$$

which means that the *SSM* can be calculated by the dot product of F and its transposed [25].

$$SSM = X^T X$$

4.2 Similarity Function

A similarity function S_f is a univariate time serie where each value represents how different is a specific time instant when compared with the remaining time series.

Given the *SSM*, built as described in the previous section, the similarity function S_f can be calculated by the sum throughout one of the axes of the *SSM*.

$$S_f(t) = \sum_{i=0}^{n} SSM_{ti},$$

with n being the length of the SSM. Due to the property of symmetry of the *SSM*, this operation can either be applied over the lines or the columns of the matrix, with the final result being the same S_f. This will then be smoothed to facilitate the following processing stages.

In a previous work, it was used to search for highly dissimilar sub-sequences of the signal [3]. In this context, this method was mostly successful in identifying sub-sequences corresponding to periods of non active work. Therefore, by using a simple minimal threshold, it was possible to identify these sub-sequences and remove them from the signal. In addition, the similarity function is useful for the segmentation of periodic events, as is exemplified in Fig. 1. As the dataset being observed is only composed by working cycles, periodically repeated along time, the S_f will approximate to a sinusoidal function. Then, the valleys of S_f will indicate the time instances where there is a transition between the working cycles, which also can be identified by a simple valley detection operation.

4.3   Novelty Function

The Novelty function N_f is also a univariate time serie calculated from the processing of the *SSM*. However, N_f intends to instead provide information on how much the data within a neighborhood distance to the left of that point is different from the data within a neighborhood distance to its right. Being especially relevant in the detection of change points.

When the signal displays a significant change between two states of motion, the corresponding *SSM* will display two distinct blocks along the main diagonal. As such, the novelty function N_f can be calculated by making a *checkerboard* kernel convolution centered along the main diagonal. This kernel in its simplest form can be described as the sum between a kernel that measures coherence and anti-coherence on either side of the center point. In other words, the first component presented in the following equation highlights when the two regions are homogeneous or coherent within each other. Meanwhile, the second component will be highlighted whenever these two regions are also similar within each other. As this last component is negative, the opposite will be expected [25].

$$K_{Box} = \begin{bmatrix} 0 & 1 \\ 1 & 0 \end{bmatrix} - \begin{bmatrix} 1 & 0 \\ 0 & 1 \end{bmatrix} = \begin{bmatrix} -1 & 1 \\ 1 & -1 \end{bmatrix}$$

The resulting novelty function N_f is expected to have higher values of intensity whenever it is in the middle of two different blocks [25]. The *checkboard* kernels' dimension will be defined by $(M \times M$, where $M = 2L+1$, for $L \in \mathbb{N}$. The central column and central row coordinates of the kernel K_{Box} will have the values of 0, followed by four planes which will either be 1 or -1 according to the same pattern as previously seen. For example, if L=2, then [25]

$$K_{Box} = \begin{bmatrix} -1 & -1 & 0 & 1 & 1 \\ -1 & -1 & 0 & 1 & 1 \\ 0 & 0 & 0 & 0 & 0 \\ 1 & 1 & 0 & -1 & -1 \\ 1 & 1 & 0 & -1 & -1 \end{bmatrix}$$

The final kernel is then the result of further smoothing by a radially symmetric Gaussian function $(\phi(s,t))$ and normalization (dividing by the sum of all absolute values of the kernel) [25].

$$K_{checkerboard}(k,l) = \frac{\phi(s,t) \cdot K_{Gauss}(k,l)}{\sum_{k,l \in [-L,L]} | K_{Gauss}(k,l) |}$$

The detection of change points is one of the most commonly used techniques in event detection, as by definition they search time instances that display a significant change in the properties of the signal. This work intends to take advantage of this algorithm to also structure the time series into different non overlapping states. In occupational context, we'll use this to separate between *active* and *non-active periods*, and also to divide the work cycles into a sequence of *sub-activities*.

4.4   Sub-sequences Searched-by-example

Another aspect of occupational risk evaluation in industrial scenarios is to compare the occupational risk of sub-segments of the working cycle during the working period. This strategy supports professionals in identifying specific sequences
of sub-activities that occur in-cycle, and search them over the entire set of working cycles for comparative purposes. In addition, if in need of labeling the data,
this method can be quite fruitful as it searches for the exact sub-sequence match
in the matrix. In addition, this process does not match the shape but rather
the sub-diagonal of the matrix, that is, being the sub-diagonal one cycle, we are
matching the exact portion of the cycle being used as an example.

The search procedure is made with an example that is a sub-sequence of
interest in the signal. The search procedure works by sliding the selected example
along the *SSM*. The distance, D, between the example and the segments it slides
over is calculated as the sum of absolute differences:

$$D(x) = \sum_{x=0}^{x=M} \sqrt{(SSM(x) - SSM_t)^2} \tag{1}$$

where $SSM(x)$ is the segment of the *SSM* over which the example, SSM_t, slides
at moment x, starting from 0 to the size of the *SSM*, M. The resulting function
has valleys at the instants where the example matches.

4.5   Illustrative Example

Figure 3 shows an *SSM* representation of the set of inertial signals acquired
while a worker was performing 2 different workstations (A and C). The *SSM*
also shows an interruption in the working line (B). With this illustration, we
can highlight which structures are mainly present in the *SSM*, namely blocks
and parallel sub-diagonals. The first indicates transitions between homogeneous
blocks and can be detected by the novelty function. The second indicates presence of periodicity or cyclic behavior, which can be detected with the similarity
function. In the next section, these functions will be used in examples of signals
from the manufacturing scenario to provide evidence of applying this methodology to perform the segmentation of time series and possible applicability in
summarization and labeling.

The methods explained in this section are deeply inspired by the work from
Meinard Müller in the context of information retrieval from audio records [4,
24]. We performed the *SSM* calculation and novelty searched by means of the
available *libfmp* python library [20, 25, 26].

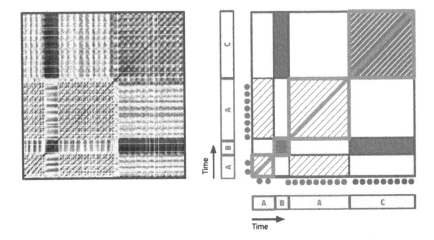

Fig. 3. At the left is the SSM designed from the signals acquired while an operator was performing 2 different workstations. At the right is a simplification of the original SSM, with highlights on the main structures present (Blocks and Diagonals). *A* being workstation 1 and *C* workstation2. *B* is the interruption in the working line. [3]

5   Results and Discussion

The following section delivers the results obtained by applying the aforementioned methodologies to demonstrate the validity of the proposed objectives. As presented as an introductory simple example in Fig. 1, we can use the novelty function to segment homogeneous sub-sequences of the time series, and the similarity function to identify periodic segments. With this in mind, we will now demonstrate the application to more complex scenarios, such as motion data in industrial settings, for time series segmentation, summarization and labeling.

The proposed method is applied in real motion data from an industrial setting to perform the (1) detection of active working periods and (2) segmentation of working cycles. In addition, it provides examples to use these methods to perform a multi timescale analysis and summarization of the data, as well as how this can support a labeling process.

5.1   Active Working Periods Segmentation

In order to detect the transition between *active* and *non-active work* we used the novelty function N_f. This function will display peaks in sections where there is a transition between coherent blocks. To identify these transitions we applied a smoothing and peak detection technique to the N_f.

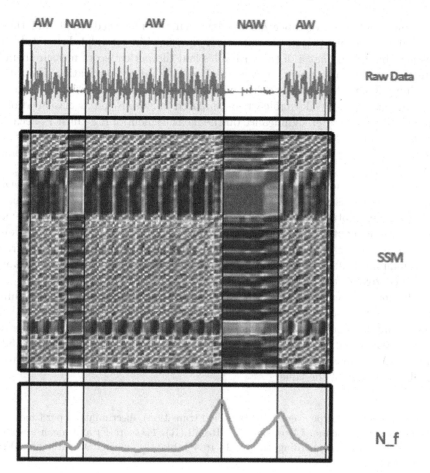

Fig. 4. Schematic of active working period detection, by means of a novelty function. Each image represents a peak detection process. From the top to the bottom, the first step represents the x coordinate of the hand accelerometer during the (Opr4 Wkst1) acquisition. The following images represent the respective SSM and N_f, as labeled. The *active* and *non active* work periods are accordingly represented with the acronyms of AW and NAW at the top of the image [3]

Considering the example provided by Fig. 4. This signal can visibly highlight the time instances where the *SSM* transitions from high valued, squared, and homogeneous blocks, which represent periods of *non-active work*, to blocks with several parallel sub-diagonals, equally spaced, which represent the periods of *active work*.

The measurements of the algorithm's performance are summarized in Table 1. This analysis was made to understand how close were the events identified by the algorithm to the manually annotated labels. For this, we used Precision, Recall and the F_n-score (with the TP annotations having a tolerance of 50s), and how much time distance existed between the identified event and those labelled annotations (Mean absolute error measured in seconds). From Table 1, it is possible to see that 4 of the 7 samples had the perfect score measurements, detecting every single intended event without any false classification. From the remaining 3 samples, the false classifications were all False Positives, which, in this context, are more affordable when compared to False Negative classifications. There is given a greater significance on the measurement of R against P, because a presence of FP could be noticed in a further analysis of the results, as, after all, the motivation of this work is to serve as a support for the analysis of ergonomic data.

Moreover, the identified FP events just tended to divide the *non active work* states into various sub-states. Something understandable as there might be a more complex motion description within these time instances, which wasn't considered for the context of this work. However, this is a manageable error, as long as there is still a clear segmentation between the *active work* time periods from the remaining time series, the segmentation of the *non-active work* is irrelevant for the context of this problem.

The increase in the MAE value is associated with the several smoothing processes applied over the methodology, that distanced the events from their ground annotations. However, when considering that the *active work* period tended to be about 1169.11 s and even the smaller states tended to be of 128.52s. These MAE values (within 8.38–11.87 s), although significant, correspond to a small percentage of the time.

Table 1. Results of type event 1 (work period transition), discriminated per time serie samples. Measurements of Precision (P), Recall (R), F_n-score(F) and mean absolute error(MAE), of each according sample. In this Table, O_{pr} means Operator and W_{kst} is Workstation.

TS sample	P	R	F	MAE (s)
Opr 1 Wkst1	0,78	1	0,88	11,87
Opr1 Wkst2	1	1	1	34,77
Opr2 Wkst1&2	0,86	1	0,92	10,17
Opr3 Wkst1	0,80	1	0,89	3,21
Opr4 Wkst1	1	1	1	8,83
Opr5 Wkst1	1	1	1	8,54
Opr5 Wkst2	1	1	1	8,38

Overall, this process was successful without the necessity of a very intense search, and by performing a simple manual selection of the parameters, most events were able to be detected.

5.2   Working Cycles Segmentation

Much like the work on [3] the best methodology for the segmentation between cycles is the retrieval of the S_f followed by a smoothing and valley detection operation of this signal.

Considering the example provided in Fig. 5, we can see that the similarity function will consistently segment the dataset into positions very close to the annotated ones. Despite usually having a minor delay, the events tend to maintain that delay constantly across the entire time series. The reasoning for this is because the algorithm is unsupervised, it does not have a reference of where the cycle has the "real" start. As such the algorithm will take into consideration the beginning of the data as a reference, which might not be the same precise instant when the operator starts the work cycle. This does not make the detection necessarily incorrect, as long as the following cycles are also segmented in the same transition point, it can be considered a work cycle motif. This consideration means that the assessment will insist more on the question of the consistency of the detections made rather than on how close they are to the labeled positions.

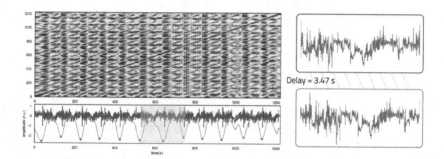

Fig. 5. Schematic of active working period detection, by means of a novelty function. Each image represents a peak detection process. From the top to the bottom, the first step represents the x coordinate of the hand accelerometer during the (Opr4 Wkst1) acquisition. The following images represent the respective SSM and N_f, as labeled. The *active* and *non active* work periods are accordingly represented with the acronyms of AW and NAW at the top of the image [3]

As such, the following metrics will insist on two points: 1) Number of cycles detected 2) consistency of duration of the detected cycles. The last point is described by the mean absolute error between the duration of the ground truth segmentation cycles and the algorithms' segmentation cycles, described by DE (Duration). In the work of 2 the results of the proposed algorithm were also compared with a more well established technique proven to work in similar problems, the Matrix Profile.

Overall, the measures considered for this analysis demonstrate the ability to identify working cycles with good accuracy. Almost all the work cycles of interest were detected, as, within the 157 ground annotation cycles, 154 cycles

Table 2. Detected cycles and duration errors of the working period's event detection. These were made under an occupational context, with the results being separated according with two different methodologies. The SSM is the technique based on the analysis of the similarity function S_f. In this Table, O_{pr} means Operator and W_{kst} is Workstation.

Signal	SSM	
	Detected cycles	Duration error
Opr1 Wkst1	11/11	3.26 s (3.04%)
Opr1 Wkst2	14/15	16.97 s (15.83%)
Opr2 Wkst1	14/14	6.45 s (6.40%)
Opr2 Wkst2	11/11	8.48 s (8.62%)
Opr3 Wkst1	16/16	12.35 s (11.79%)
Opr3 Wkst2	13/13	8.81 s (8.25%)
Opr4 Wkst1	14/14	1.05 s (0.4%)
Opr4 Wkst2	11/11	3.42 s (3.32%)
Opr5 Wkst1	12/12	2.83 s (2.85%)
Opr5 Wkst2	10/11	3.47 s (3.45%)
Opr6 Wkst1	14/15	3.79 s (3.74%)
Opr6 Wkst2	14/15	5.79 s (5.73%)
Total	154/157	6.12%

were detected. The duration error was mostly good with an average value of 6.12% of the working cycle, but still significantly high in some cases (2 and 5). When compared with the MP, the results are comparable. To be clear, we are not trying to say if our algorithm is better or worse than the MP, but simply to have a standard measure of reference to compare with.

5.3   Towards Multi Time-Scale Segmentation

In the two previous sections, we highlighted the ability to perform the segmentation of time series based on novelty, while also being able to segment subsequences of cyclic nature. Now, we intended to extend the usage of the SSM to show how it could be used in an iterative segmentation over multiple timescales, successively over smaller previously segmented sub-sequences. Considering the previously detection of AW as the *high level*, and the segmented working cycles as the *middle level*, this next section devotes its attention to analyse in-cycle detection.

Considering the scenario of occupational health, we are dealing with a multidimensional dataset with some variability in the worker's motion, which means that each working cycle might be relatively different. Still, the sequence of in-cycle activities are the same, with small variations. Using the novelty function with a smaller time scale, we segmented several working cycles of one subject to present as an exploratory example of a lower-scale segmentation. The *SSM* was calculated for each previously segmented working cycle, with a time scale of 2.5 s. In Fig. 6, we present the corresponding novelty functions for 3 working cycles (*C1, C2 and C3*), highlighting their peaks as the segmentation instants.

Firstly, the image shows us that the inertial signals are mostly consistent over working cycles. There are small variations, but the significant changes occur in the same sequence. As the novelty function highlights instants where a change is significant, we expected its peaks to be related to a significant change in the posture/motion of the worker.

In a first inspection, we can see that the peaks of the novelty functions for all cycles match a significant change in the group of inertial signals from which the *SSM* was built. Matching the peaks with a video inspection, we were able to associate the changes with what happened in the video. The caption of Fig. 6 indicates the list of activities. In general, these changes are related to a transition between homogeneous blocks of posture/motion, that is, sub-activities that have a certain pattern and are shifted to another sub-activity by a change of motion/posture. For instance, block *C* indicates a quick motion to a new position to perform a set of tasks with *tool1*. There are also obvious symmetric behaviors that are segmented, such as *I, J and K*, where the subject positions *piece1 (I)*, works on a static posture *(J)* and unfits *piece1*. These actions are well separated in all exemplified cycles.

These are still very preliminary results in a first exploratory experiment on motion data, but we believe that this method, already used in audio thumb-nailling (*technically summarization*), is worth exploring in other types of data for the problematic of time series segmentation and summarization. In addition, we also show that this method is worth exploring in a multi time-scale segmentation process, with simple ECG data (from Fig. 1), but also in more complex data, such as motion and posture.

The importance of summarizing the data is in the way we can then represent the signal in a higher levelled representation. As an example, Fig. 6.*right* shows the length of each sub-activity segmented for each cycle. This type of visual summary gives the analyst a quicker form of getting feedback from the data. Besides, if integrated into an interactive platform, it can provide valuable interactive power.

5.4   Labeling with Query-by-example

Finally, the last scenario focuses on demonstrating the possibility of performing labeling by querying an example along the *SSM*. Figure 7 exemplifies a case where we are trying to label 3 different segments from a working cycle. The segments are highlighted as *A, B and C*. Applying the distance measure across the signal results in the signals $D_A, D_B and D_C$. These distances show how well the valleys (minimal distance) indicate the match with the example. Performing

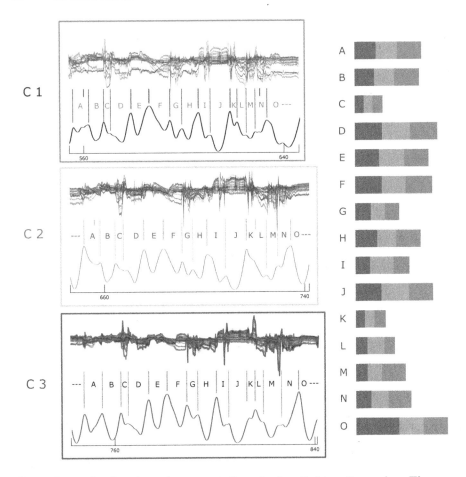

Fig. 6. Example of an in-cycle segmentation of sub-activities of a worker. There are 3 cycles (*C1, C2 and C3*. For each, the corresponding set of inertial signals and the resulting novelty function are presented. The list of activities are labelled from A to O, as follows: A - stretching arms to the top and slowly pulling an object; B - adjusting the object to be fixed on the car; C - picking tool1 and using it on the side of the car; D - moving to the front of the car and use tool1; E - move back to the side and leave tool1; F - perform inverse sub-activity of A; G - walk away from the car; H - walk back to the front of the car; I - Fit piece1 on the car; J - use tool2; K - unfit piece1 from the car; L - walks away from the car; M - drops tools and pieces; N - moves back to the initial position; O - waits for the next cycle.

the match along the sub-diagonals of the *SSM*, it is not *distracted* by similar shapes, but rather by the exact moment the pattern occurs in the working cycle. This method can be used assigned with a label, to semi-automatically label segments of a working cycle, such as *A, B and C*.

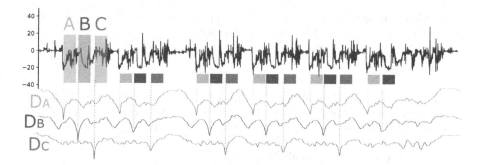

Fig. 7. Query-by-example on the *SSM*. Segments A, B and C are used as examples by being selected on the *SSM* columns. The resulting distance functions $(D_A, D_B$ and $D_C)$ show the ability of this method to find the starting point. The signal is only illustrative, as all the signals available were used to build the *SSM*.

6   Conclusions

One of the objectives of this work was to demonstrate the relevance of retrieving events through the usage of an unsupervised method, for posterior ergonomic analysis. In this sense, the methods were able to structure the time series under different levels of abstraction. Firstly, by detecting the sub-sequences of actual active work movement, then by segmenting the various work cycles, and in the end, by summarizing the work cycle into smaller primitive structures, different from each other. Then it also provided a tool to further detect new instances of an user-defined query.

This methodology shows promise in doing so, as when the events of "Active Working Periods Segmentation" and "Working Cycles Segmentation" were compared with manually labelled annotations they were proven to be mostly all detected. Moreover, when calculating the error duration between the events detected and the annotation these were noticed to be rather short and of little variation. On the other hand, the remaining events were proven by comparison to provide useful and valid information about the work period motion. The most significant utility provided by this algorithm is the automation of processes related to the identification of periods of relevance, segmentation of the signal, and further identification of periodic regions. Moreover, the proposed analysis by means of the *SSM* seems to be a promising approach with the potential to be expanded upon.

The empirical results reported herein should be considered in light of some limitations. The process of feature retrieval is especially time demanding, and the construction of entire *SSMs* for each time series might become too demanding for the storage capabilities. These were concerns that were not noticeable for the dimension of the provided data, which described a short work period extension, but it might become too demanding for acquisitions of entire days. These are points should be further investigated in future research works.

Acknowledgements. This work was partly supported by Fundação para a Ciência e Tecnologia, and Ph.D. grant PD/BDE/142816/2018.

References

1. Santos, S., Folgado, D., Rodrigues, J., Mollaei, N., Fujão, C., Gamboa, H.: Exploring inertial sensor fusion methods for direct ergonomic assessments. In: Ye, X., et al. (eds) Biomedical Engineering Systems and Technologies, BIOSTEC 2020. Communications in Computer and Information Science, vol. 1400. Springer, Cham (2021). https://doi.org/10.1007/978-3-030-72379-8_14
2. Roh, Y., Heo, G., Whang, S.E.: A survey on data collection for machine learning: a big data - AI integration perspective. IEEE Trans. Knowl. Data Eng. **33**(4), 1328–1347 (2021). https://doi.org/10.1109/TKDE.2019.2946162
3. Santos, A., Rodrigues, J., Folgado, D., Santos, S., Fujão, C., Gamboa, H.: Self-similarity matrix of morphological features for motion data analysis in manufacturing scenarios. In: Proceedings of the 14th International Joint Conference on Biomedical Engineering Systems and Technologies - BIOSIGNALS, ISBN 978-989-758-490-9, ISSN 2184-4305, pp. 80-90 (2021). https://doi.org/10.5220/0010252800800090
4. Paulus, J., Müller, M., Klapuri, A.: Audio-based music structure analysis. In: Proceedings of the 11th International Society for Music Information Retrieval Conference, ISMIR 2010, pp. 625–636 (2010)
5. Heldt, T., Oefinger, M.B., Hoshiyama, M., Mark, R.G.: Circulatory response to passive and active changes in posture. Comput. Cardiol. **30**, 263–266 (2003)
6. Song, J., Chang, R.W., Dunlop, D.D.: Population impact of arthritis on disability in older adults. Arthritis Care Res. **55**(2), 248–255 (2006). https://doi.org/10.1002/art.21842. ISSN 21514658
7. Palazzo, C., Ravaud, J.F., Papelard, A., Ravaud, P., Poiraudeau, S.: The burden of musculoskeletal conditions. PLoS ONE **9**(3), e90633 (2014). https://doi.org/10.1371/journal.pone.0090633. Ed. by A. Chopra, ISSN 1932-6203
8. Dominick, C.H., Blyth, F.M., Nicholas, M.K.: Unpacking the burden: understanding the relationships between chronic pain and comorbidity in the general population. Pain **153**(2), 293–304 (2012). https://doi.org/10.1016/j.pain.2011.09.018. ISSN 03043959
9. Antonopoulou, M.D., Alegakis, A.K., Hadjipavlou, A.G., Lionis, C.D.: Studying the association between musculoskeletal disorders, quality of life and mental health. A primary care pilot study in rural Crete, Greece. BMC Musculoskel. Disord. **10**(1), 1–8 (2009). https://doi.org/10.1186/1471-2474-10-143. ISSN 14712474
10. Kadam, U.T., Jordan, K., Croft, P.R.: Clinical comorbidity in patients with osteoarthritis: a case-control study of general practice consumers in England and Wales (2004). https://doi.org/10.1136/ard.2003.007526
11. Luttmann, A., Jager, M., Griefahn, B., Caffier, G., Liebers, F.: World Health Organization preventing musculoskeletal disorders in the workplace (2003). ISSN 924159053X
12. Pruss-Ustun, A., Corvalan, C.: Preventing Disease Through Healthy Environment: A Global Assessment of the Burden of Disease from Environmental Risks, p. 105. World Health Organization, Geneva (2006)
13. Santos, S., Folgado, D., Rodrigues, J., Mollaei, N., Fujao, C., Gamboa, H.: Explaining the ergonomic assessment of human movement in industrial contexts. In: BIOSIGNALS, pp. 79–88 (2020)

14. Lu, C.M., Ferrier, N.J.: Repetitive motion analysis: segmentation and event classification. IEEE Trans. Pattern Anal. Mach. Intell. **26**(2), 258–263 (2004)
15. Lu, C.M., Ferrier, N.J.: Automated analysis of repetitive joint motion. IEEE Trans. Inf Technol. Biomed. **7**(4), 263–273 (2003)
16. Wang, Q., et al.: Unsupervised temporal segmentation of repetitive human actions based on kinematic modeling and frequency analysis. In: 2015 International Conference on 3D Vision. IEEE (2015)
17. Matias, P., Folgado, D., Gamboa, H., Carreiro, A.: Time series segmentation using neural networks with cross-domain transfer learning. Electronics **10**(15), 1805 (2021). https://doi.org/10.3390/electronics10151805
18. Vögele, A., Krüger, B., Klein, R.: Efficient unsupervised temporal segmentation of human motion. In: Symposium on Computer Animation, pp. 167–176 (2014)
19. Yeh, C.-C.M., et al.: Time series joins, motifs, discords and shapelets: a unifying view that exploits the matrix profile. Data Min. Knowl. Discov. **32**(1), 83–123 (2017). https://doi.org/10.1007/s10618-017-0519-9
20. Müller, et al.: libfmp: a python package for fundamentals of music processing. J. Open Source Softw. **6**(63), 3326 (2021). https://doi.org/10.21105/joss.03326
21. Khusainov, R., et al.: Real-time human ambulation, activity, and physiological monitoring: taxonomy of issues, techniques, applications, challenges and limitations. Sensors **13**(10), 12852–12902 (2013)
22. Rodrigues, J., Belo, D., Gamboa, H.: Noise detection on ECG based on agglomerative clustering of morphological features. Comput. Biol. Med. **87**, 322–334 (2017). https://doi.org/10.1016/j.compbiomed.2017.06.009. ISSN 0010–4825
23. Zheng, X., Wang, M., Ordieres-Meré, J.: Comparison of data preprocessing approaches for applying deep learning to human activity recognition in the context of industry 4.0. Sensors **18**(7), 2146 (2018). https://doi.org/10.3390/s18072146
24. Bello, J.P., Grosche, P., Müller, M., Weiss, R.: Content-based methods for knowledge discovery in music. In: Bader, R. (ed.) Springer Handbook of Systematic Musicology. SH, pp. 823–840. Springer, Heidelberg (2018). https://doi.org/10.1007/978-3-662-55004-5_39
25. Müller, M.: Fundamentals of Music Processing: Using Python and Jupyter Notebooks (2021). https://doi.org/10.1007/978-3-030-69808-9
26. Müller, M.: An educational guide through the FMP notebooks for teaching and learning fundamentals of music processing. Signals **2**(2), 245–285 (2021). https://doi.org/10.3390/signals2020018
27. Reyes-Ortiz, J.-L., Oneto, L., Samà, A., Parra, X., Anguita, D.: Transition-aware human activity recognition using smartphones. Neurocomputing **171**, 754–767 (2016). ISSN 0925–2312

Evaluating the Performance of Diadochokinetic Tests in Characterizing Parkinson's Disease Hypokinetic Dysarthria

Pedro Gómez-Vilda[1]([✉]) [iD], Andrés Gómez-Rodellar[2] [iD], Daniel Palacios-Alonso[3] [iD], and Athanasios Tsanas[2] [iD]

[1] NeuSpeLab, CTB, Universidad Politécnica de Madrid,
28220 Pozuelo de Alarcón, Madrid, Spain
pedro.gomezv@upm.es
[2] Usher Institute, Faculty of Medicine, University of Edinburgh, Edinburgh, UK
{a.gomezrodellar,athanasios.tsanas}@ed.ac.uk
[3] E.T.S. de Ingeniería Informática - Universidad Rey Juan Carlos, Campus de Móstoles,
Tulipán, s/n, 28933 Móstoles, Madrid, Spain
daniel.palacios@urjc.es

Abstract. Hypokinetic Dysarthria (HD) is a hampering speech symptom appearing as a consequence of Parkinson's Disease (PD). HD has been traditionally evaluated using diadochokinetic tests such as the fast repetition of monosyllables as [pa], [ta], and [ka] and multisyllable sequences [pataka] and [pakata] towards assessing speech performance. However, the practical validity of these tests in assessing the speech of a person with PD (PwP) to assess performance degradation and infer PD-related symptoms has not been thoroughly investigated. The aim of the present work is to explore the performance of tests consisting in a monosyllabic repetition [...tatata...] vs a multisyllable one [...pataka...]). The methodology proposed is based on estimating distributions of syllable and inter-syllable interval durations obtained from diadichokinetic tests using Kolmogorov-Smirnov Approximations (KSA), and comparing the resulting distributions by means of Jensen-Shannon Divergence (JSD) to assess the efficiency of both types of tests confronting utterances from Healthy Controls (HC) with the ones from PD participants. The results from the evaluation of 30 gender-balanced participants, 18 PwP and 12 HC, show that the monosyllable test does not appear to differentiate well between the two cohorts, whereas the multisyllable test shows better performance. Although the relatively small sample size suggests findings should be cautiously interpreted, they tentatively underline the need to use the most adequate tests to assess HD diadochokinetic performance.

Keywords: Parkinson's disease · Speech diadochokinetic exercises · Hypokinetic dysarthria

This research received funding from grants TEC2016-77791-C4-4-R (Ministry of Economic Affairs and Competitiveness of Spain), and Teca-Park-MonParLoc FGCSIC-CENIE 0348-CIE-6-E (InterReg Programme). The authors want to thank the Parkinson's Disease association APARKAM and the voluntary participants contributing to this initiative.

C. Gehin et al. (Eds.): BIOSTEC 2021, CCIS 1710, pp. 102–119, 2022.
https://doi.org/10.1007/978-3-031-20664-1_6

1   Introduction

Parkinson's Disease (PD) is a neurodegenerative disorder, second in prevalence to Alzheimer's Disease [1]. Its origin has been traditionally attributed to the lack of dopamine in midbrain [2]. This condition causes dramatic neuromotor deterioration affecting body movement [3]. The early work of Dr. James Parkinson [4] described observable neuromotor alterations in patients of shaking palsy, including speech problems, nowadays known as Hypokinetic Dysarthria (HD). It has since then been consistently reported that PD causes considerable alterations in speech and phonation [5,6]. Speech alterations may be broadly categorized as dysphonia (alterations to the production of voice), dysarthria (alterations in the articulation of speech), dysprosody (alterations in the definition of the fundamental frequency modulation in running speech) and dysfluency (alterations in the rhythm of speech production and in speech freezing). The estimation of acoustic markers caused by HD in PD speech allows speech analysis to become a non-invasive and cost-effective tool to characterize and monitor PD. In fact, there is "compelling evidence to suggest that speech can help quantify not only motor symptoms ... but generalized diverse symptoms in PD" [7]. There has been a substantial body of work aimed to characterize PD induced HD, focusing on diadochokinetic tests to assess its degree of severity. Indicative diadochokinetic tests include the repetition of monosyllables as [pa], [ta], and [ka] and multisyllable sequences as [pataka], [pakata], [badaga] and others. Tests consist of repetitions of the sequences as fast as possible, and this setup has been commonly used in PD speech assessment [8]. The efficiency of these tests as a way of assessing speech production as pathological or normative is yet to be further investigated (for a comprehensive review see [9]). The aim of the present study is to explore if the evaluation of some of these tests testing monosyllable vs. multisyllable repetition may serve as a reliable biomarker to compare the performance of two classical diadochokinetic tests as the repetition of a single syllable [...ta...] where an apical-alveolar gesture is involved, versus the repetition of a multisyllable sequence as [...pataka...] that presents bilabial, apical-alveolar, and dorsal-velar gestures. This study further builds and extends our previous findings [10]. The paper is organized as follows: Sect. 2 describes the participants in the experimental framework, the speech recording conditions used, and the statistical methods used in the study. Section 3 describes the results produced by the statistical analysis of speech recordings. Section 4 focus on analysing and discussing the results. Section 5 summarises the main conclusions and findings derived from the present research.

2   Materials and Methods

Eighteen age- and gender-balanced PD participants were selected from the patient associations of Alcorcón and Leganés (APARKAM). Twelve gender-balanced HC participants were recruited from family and friends. The inclusion conditions for PD and HC participants were non-smoking for the last five years, and not presenting any known laryngeal pathology. On top of that, HC participants were selected for not presenting neurological diagnosis as well. The study was approved by the Ethical Committee of Universidad Politécnica de Madrid (MonParLoc, 18/05/2018). Each participant signed a voluntary participation informed consent. The study was fully aligned with the Declaration of Helsinki. The participants were asked to utter two different tests, the first one consisting in the repetition of the syllable [ta] at the fastest speed possible and as long as they could sustain it, as [...tatata...] (monosyllable repetition). The second test consisted of repeating the sequence [pataka] as fast and as long as possible, as [...pataka...]. These two sequences were selected for being regular and monosyllable (the former one) and for involving three different articulation points (bilabial, apical-alveolar and dorsal-velar, the latter one). These tests are especially well suited for the examination of the speaker's fluency, as they do not have any meaning *per se*. The first one is regular and serves as a reference both for HC and PD participants. The second one invokes the three main articulation points (bilabial, apical-alveolar, dorsal-velar), and it forces the speaker to carry on changes on facial, lingual, velar and jaw neuromuscular activity. The recordings were taken in the speech therapist service room of APARKAM. No soundproofing or any other quality-preserving measures were used, except keeping a silent environment inside the room with access limited to participants and assistants. A phantom-fed wireless Audio Technica cardioid Lavalier microphone was used, attached on the speaker's chest at 15–20 cm from the mouth, and digitized on a Motu Traveller board at 50 kHz with 16 bits of resolution. The data were later downsampled at the signal pre-processing stage to 16 kHz (antialias filtering at 8 kHz was previously used), making it compatible with remote recordings using the protocol defined in MonParLoc [11]. The participants were divided in four data sets for the study: 6 male and 6 female HC participants, and 9 male and 9 female PD participants as shown in Table 1.

An experimental framework has been developed to test the relative effects of HD by means of the extraction of syllable and inter-syllable interval durations estimated from the speech signal produced by the participants. The main features considered are the mean, the standard deviation, and the distributions of the syllable and inter-syllable (silence) interval durations, estimated from histograms using KSA. The methodology used in the study is based on the estimation of the following acoustic signals extracted from speech recordings:

- The energy profile estimated using the Teager-Kaiser Energy Operator (TKEO, [12]).
- The glottal residual from Iterative Adaptive Inverse Filtering (IAIF, [13]).
- The Voiced-Unvoiced Intervals (VUI) using the zero-crossings' function of the glottal residual.

These acoustic signals quantitatively express the quality of phonation, the prosody and the fluency. The TKEO, and the VUI, are defined as

$$E_{TKEO}(n) = s^2(n) - s(n+1)s(n-1) \tag{1}$$

$$F_{VUI}(n) = dim\{z(n)\} \tag{2}$$

where

$$r(n) = \begin{cases} 1 \ \epsilon(n) > 0; \\ 0 \ otherwise \end{cases} \tag{3}$$

$$q(n) = r(n) - r(n-1) \tag{4}$$

Table 1. Summary of participant characteristics. 'Code' refers to MC: male control participants; MP: male PD participants; FC: female control participants; FP: female PD participants; H&Y Hoehn and Yahr PD rating scale; State: medication state (ON: under medication; –: not applicable).

Code	Gender	Age	Condition	State	H&Y	Code	Gender	Age	Condition	State	H&Y
MC1	M	69	HC	–	–	FC1	F	66	HC	–	–
MC2	M	70	HC	–	–	FC2	F	62	HC	–	–
MC3	M	68	HC	–	–	FC3	F	65	HC	–	–
MC4	M	67	HC	–	–	FC4	F	67	HC	–	–
MC5	M	61	HC	–	–	FC5	F	65	HC	–	–
MC6	M	68	HC	–	–	FC6	F	65	HC	–	–
MP1	M	71	PD	ON	2	FP1	F	73	PD	ON	2
MP2	M	69	PD	ON	2	FP2	F	73	PD	ON	2
MP3	M	73	PD	ON	2	FP3	F	66	PD	ON	2
MP4	M	73	PD	ON	2	FP4	F	71	PD	ON	2
MP5	M	73	PD	ON	2	FP5	F	78	PD	ON	2
MP6	M	69	PD	ON	2	FP6	F	70	PD	ON	2
MP7	M	87	PD	ON	2	FP7	F	70	PD	ON	2
MP8	M	72	PD	ON	2	FP8	F	74	PD	ON	2
MP9	M	76	PD	ON	2	FP9	F	69	PD	ON	2

$$z(n) = \begin{cases} q(n); & q(n) \neq 0; \\ 0 & otherwise \end{cases} \tag{5}$$

where $\epsilon(n)$ is the inverse filtering residual from IAIF, and $dim\{z(n)\}$ is the number of non-zero samples in z(n). The TKEO and the VUI may be used to determine the inferior and superior syllable interval limits given as a selection function $G_{VAD}(n)$ as

$$G_{VAD}(n) = E_{TKEO}(n)F_{VUI}(n) \tag{6}$$

$$n_i^{lh} = n; \quad if \quad G_{VAD}(n-1) < \vartheta \quad and \quad G_{VAD}(n) \geq \vartheta \tag{7}$$

$$n_i^{lh} = n; \quad if \quad G_{VAD}(n-1) \geq \vartheta \quad and \quad G_{VAD}(n) < \vartheta \tag{8}$$

to divide the speech signal produced by the diadochokinetic test into syllable (Sy) and inter-syllable (Si) intervals, containing the interval duration of syllable $d_{Sy}(i)$ and inter-syllable segments $d_{Si}(i)$

$$d_{Sy}(i) = n_i^{hl} - n_i^{lh}; \quad \forall d_{Sy}(i) > 20ms \tag{9}$$

$$d_{Si}(i) = n_{i+1}^{lh} - n_i^{hl} \tag{10}$$

The normalized distributions of the syllable and inter-syllable interval durations might be considered good candidates to establish a differentiation strategy between the behaviour of PD and HC participants in information theoretic terms, using Jensen-Shannon's Divergence (JSD) [14].

Assuming two probability density functions (PDF) of syllable and/or inter-syllable intervals being $p_i(x)$ and $p_j(x)$, their JSD would be calculated as

$$D_{JSij}\{p_i(x), p_j(x)\} = D_{KLim}\{p_i(x), p_m(x)\} \tag{11}$$

where

$$p_m(x) = (p_i(x) + p_j(x))/2 \tag{12}$$

based on the Kulback-Leibler Divergence defined as

$$D_{KLij}\{p_i(x), p_j(x)\} = -\int_{\zeta=0}^{\infty} p_i(\zeta) ln[p_i(\zeta)/p_j(\zeta)]d\zeta \tag{13}$$

The features used in the comparisons were the PDFs of syllable and inter-syllable intervals in PD vs. HC participants. The following procedure was used to estimate the JSDs between each sequence PDF with respect to the normative set from HC participants:

– All recordings from each participant were down-sampled to 16 KHz.
– Their TKEO was estimated following expression (1).
– The inverse filtering residual was estimated by a 24-order IAIF [13].
– The VUI was estimated following expressions (2–5).
– The 50-bin normalized histogram of syllable $d_{Sy}(i)$ and inter-syllable segments $d_{Si}(i)$ were evaluated as $p_i(k) = h_{ik}/\Sigma_k h_{ik}$, where h_{ik} is the histogram of feature i, and k is the bin number.
– The PDFs of syllable and inter-syllable sequences were were computed using the two-sided Kolmogorov-Smirnov distribution approach using the implementation by Simard and L'Ecuyer accounting for small numbers [15].
– The JSD from each PDF of the male subset ($p_{MSy}(i)$ and $p_{MSi}(i)$) and from the female subset ($p_{FSy}(i)$ and $p_{FSi}(i)$) to their respective average HC subsets ($p_{\mu Sy}(i)$ and $p_{\mu Si}(i)$), was estimated using expressions (11–13).

3   Results

The speech recordings produced by each participant were segmented into intervals with speech emission (syllables) and with no speech emission (inter-syllables) using the TKEO and VUI indexes. Examples of segmented speech [...pataka...] sequences by female HC and PD participants may be seen in Figs. 1 and 2.

The distributions from the diadochokinetic tests [...tatata...] and [...pataka...] uttered by the female HC and PD participants are shown in Figs. 2 and 3. Syllable: a–b, and e–f). Inter-syllable: c–d, and g–h. The average HC distribution is plotted in thick red on the respective templates.

Complementary descriptions of the fluency sequence of syllables and inter-syllables by the male and female datasets (HC vs PD participants) are given in Tables 2, 3, 4 and 5. The the JSDs have been estimated with respect to the HC subsets. The largest and smallest interval numbers, means, standard deviations, and JSDs for each subset are shown in bold in this table and in Tables 3, 4, and 5.

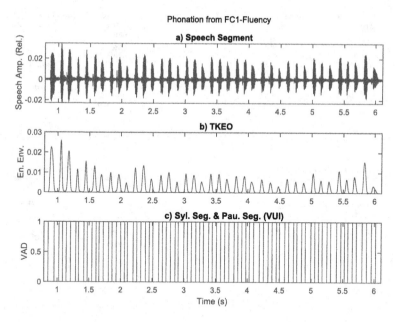

Fig. 1. Segmentation of speech from a female HC participant (FC1): a) Speech utterance; b) TKEO profile; c) Syllable and inter-syllable intervals (VUI).

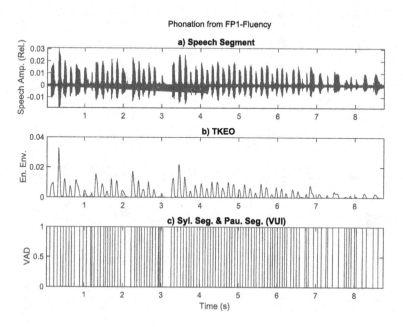

Fig. 2. Similar plot to Fig. 1 for a female PD participant (FP1).

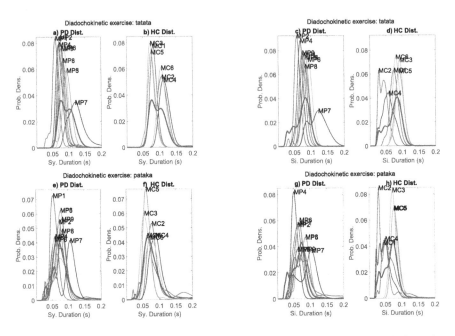

Fig. 3. Distributions of monosyllable (a, b, c, d) and multisyllable (e, f, g, h) intervals for males.

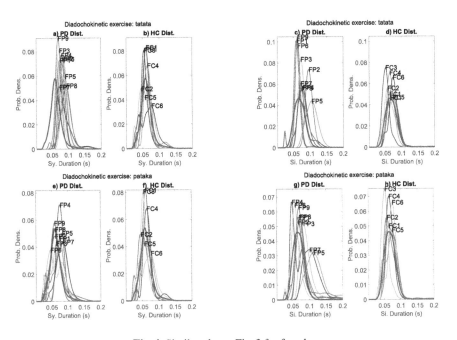

Fig. 4. Similar plot to Fig. 3 for females.

Table 2. Syllable and inter-syllable intervals for monosyllable sequence [...tatata...]. Male dataset.

Syllable intervals							Inter-syllable intervals					
$\mu_{MCSym}=0.096$		$\sigma_{MCSym}=0.013$					$\mu_{MCSim}=0.073$	$\sigma_{MCSim}=0.013$				
Code	Ints	μ_i	$>\mu_{MC}$	σ_i	$>\sigma_{MC}$	JSD	Ints	μ_i	$>\mu_{MC}$	σ_i	$>\sigma_{MC}$	JSD
MP1	38	**0.060**	0	0.012	0	**0.591**	38	0.079	1	0.007	0	0.308
MP2	39	0.076	0	0.008	0	0.412	38	0.059	0	0.007	0	0.523
MP3	**23**	0.093	0	0.012	0	**0.275**	**22**	0.085	1	0.007	0	0.281
MP4	27	0.073	0	0.013	1	0.442	26	0.068	0	0.007	0	0.442
MP5	**23**	0.093	0	0.012	0	**0.275**	**22**	0.085	1	0.007	0	0.281
MP6	39	0.088	0	0.008	0	0.349	38	0.094	1	**0.006**	0	0.396
MP7	33	**0.126**	1	0.028	1	0.374	32	**0.144**	1	**0.096**	1	0.517
MP8	44	0.083	0	0.009	0	0.294	43	0.084	1	0.011	0	0.239
MP9	38	0.080	0	0.010	0	0.362	37	0.074	1	0.008	0	0.351
No. cases			1		2		No. cases		7		1	
MC1	42	0.081	0	**0.007**	0	0.337	41	0.074	1	0.011	0	0.281
MC2	36	0.117	1	**0.036**	1	0.343	35	**0.042**	0	0.012	0	**0.539**
MC3	**54**	0.075	0	0.008	0	0.403	**53**	0.092	1	0.007	0	0.362
MC4	44	0.120	1	0.030	1	0.398	42	0.057	0	0.017	1	0.352
MC5	45	0.076	0	0.009	0	0.373	44	0.091	1	0.009	0	0.317
MC6	36	0.108	1	0.010	0	0.341	35	0.083	1	0.008	0	**0.271**
No. cases			3		2		No. cases		4		1	

Table 3. Syllable and inter-syllable intervals for multisyllable sequence [...pataka...]. Male dataset.

Syllable intervals							Inter-syllable intervals					
$\mu_{MCSyp}=0.079$		$\sigma_{MCSyp}=0.014$					$\mu_{MCSip}=0.066$	$\sigma_{MCSip}=0.013$				
Code	Ints	μ_i	$>\mu_{MC}$	σ_i	$>\sigma_{MC}$	JSD	Ints	μ_i	$>\mu_{MC}$	σ_i	$>\sigma_{MC}$	JSD
MP1	39	**0.056**	0	**0.011**	0	0.401	38	0.065	0	0.012	0	0.234
MP2	46	0.077	0	0.023	1	0.128	45	0.066	1	0.027	1	0.290
MP3	35	0.076	0	0.012	0	0.228	35	0.080	1	0.015	1	0.278
MP4	52	0.066	0	0.016	1	0.145	51	0.054	0	0.009	0	**0.446**
MP5	35	0.076	0	0.012	0	0.226	35	0.080	1	0.015	1	0.280
MP6	59	0.071	0	0.022	1	0.131	58	0.075	1	0.023	1	**0.209**
MP7	**28**	0.091	1	0.028	1	**0.452**	26	**0.091**	1	0.024	1	0.440
MP8	53	0.077	0	0.021	1	0.196	51	0.086	1	0.038	1	0.247
MP9	37	0.080	1	0.016	1	0.215	36	0.076	1	0.023	1	0.192
No. cases			2		6		No. cases		7		7	
MC1	51	0.078	0	0.028	1	**0.097**	50	0.064	0	0.023	1	0.263
MC2	41	**0.099**	1	**0.055**	1	0.219	35	**0.044**	0	0.017	1	0.444
MC3	53	0.061	0	0.013	0	0.300	52	0.073	1	**0.007**	0	0.310
MC4	**74**	0.093	1	0.030	1	0.309	**72**	0.048	0	0.017	1	0.371
MC5	36	0.064	0	0.008	0	0.300	35	0.080	1	0.008	0	0.328
MC6	58	0.079	0	0.016	1	0.144	57	0.088	1	**0.044**	1	0.312
No. cases			2		4		No. cases		3		4	

Table 4. Syllable and inter-syllable intervals for monosyllable sequence [...tatata...]. Female dataset.

Syllable intervals						Inter-syllable intervals					
$\mu_{FCSym}=0.085$		$\sigma_{FCSym}=0.017$				$\mu_{FCSim}=0.077$	$\sigma_{FCSim}=0.016$				
Code	Ints	μ_i	$>\mu_{FC}$	σ_i	$>\sigma_{FC}$	JSD	Ints	μ_i	$>\mu_{FC}$	σ_i	$>\sigma_{FC}$	JSD
FP1	34	0.075	0	0.008	0	0.266	33	**0.060**	0	0.005	0	0.424
FP2	42	0.085	1	0.008	0	**0.126**	41	0.097	1	0.005	0	0.517
FP3	40	0.074	0	0.010	0	0.341	39	0.074	0	0.006	0	0.245
FP4	29	0.082	0	0.016	0	0.191	28	0.079	1	0.011	0	0.160
FP5	30	0.093	1	0.011	0	0.220	29	**0.105**	1	0.015	0	0.495
FP6	45	0.088	1	0.009	0	0.167	44	0.062	0	0.006	0	0.369
FP7	**23**	0.085	1	**0.022**	1	0.186	**22**	0.085	1	**0.053**	1	0.164
FP8	35	0.090	1	0.015	0	0.223	34	0.080	1	0.014	0	**0.141**
FP9	**59**	**0.069**	0	0.006	0	0.444	59	0.064	0	0.007	0	0.363
No. cases		5		1			No. cases		5		1	
FC1	29	0.093	1	0.008	0	0.266	28	0.100	1	**0.004**	0	**0.542**
FC2	30	0.080	0	0.006	0	0.185	29	0.066	0	0.012	0	0.266
FC3	43	0.090	1	0.007	0	0.220	42	0.068	0	0.009	0	0.253
FC4	37	0.078	0	**0.005**	0	0.248	36	0.074	0	0.006	0	0.263
FC5	45	0.073	0	0.008	0	**0.360**	44	0.067	0	0.006	0	0.273
FC6	30	**0.095**	1	0.014	0	0.285	29	0.085	1	0.010	0	0.297
No. cases		3		0			No. cases		2		0	

Table 5. Syllable and inter-syllable intervals for multisyllable sequence [...pataka...]. Female dataset.

Syllable intervals						Inter-syllable intervals					
$\mu_{FCSyp}=0.061$		$\sigma_{FCSyp}=0.016$				$\mu_{FCSip}=0.068$	$\sigma_{FCSip}=0.016$				
Code	Ints	μ_i	$>\mu_{FC}$	σ_i	$>\sigma_{FC}$	JSD	Ints	μ_i	$>\mu_{FC}$	σ_i	$>\sigma_{FC}$	JSD
FP1	53	0.076	1	**0.024**	1	0.316	53	0.085	1	0.037	1	0.197
FP2	73	0.064	1	0.017	1	0.094	72	0.077	1	0.028	1	**0.107**
FP3	39	0.064	1	0.022	1	0.175	38	0.088	1	0.020	1	0.403
FP4	32	0.076	1	**0.008**	0	0.435	31	0.062	1	0.016	0	0.230
FP5	30	**0.082**	1	0.016	0	**0.458**	30	0.119	1	0.032	1	**0.592**
FP6	**78**	0.062	1	0.023	1	0.286	**79**	0.066	0	0.042	1	0.252
FP7	43	**0.082**	1	0.017	1	0.437	43	**0.128**	1	**0.091**	1	0.533
FP8	57	0.064	1	0.017	1	**0.078**	56	0.079	1	0.025	1	0.219
FP9	43	0.059	0	0.013	0	0.082	44	0.087	1	0.045	1	0.214
No. cases		8		6			No. cases		7		8	
FC1	39	0.060	0	**0.008**	0	0.205	38	0.074	1	0.013	0	0.163
FC2	58	**0.053**	0	0.015	0	0.202	58	0.068	1	0.017	1	**0.107**
FC3	49	0.057	0	0.014	0	0.186	49	**0.054**	0	0.014	0	0.400
FC4	**26**	0.068	1	0.017	1	0.211	**25**	0.067	0	**0.010**	0	0.175
FC5	52	0.064	1	0.015	0	0.128	51	0.070	1	0.023	1	0.116
FC6	36	0.067	1	0.023	1	0.261	35	0.074	1	0.012	0	0.234
No. cases		3		2			No. cases		4		2	

The first row from top of each table gives the type of interval segment considered (Syllables or Inter-Syllables) The second row gives the HC subset averages (μ_{MCSym}, μ_{MCSim}, μ_{FCSym}, μ_{FCSim}, μ_{MCSyp}, μ_{MCSip}, μ_{FCSyp}, and μ_{FCSip}) and standard deviations (σ_{MCSym}, σ_{MCSim}, σ_{FCSym}, σ_{FCSim}, σ_{MCSyp}, σ_{MCSip}, σ_{FCSyp}, and σ_{FCSip}). The last sub-index character in the names of means and standard deviations (m or p) specifies the test type, as monosyllable (m) or multisyllable (p).

The third row from left to right gives each participant's code, according to their gender (M: males, F: females), health condition (C: HC, P: PD), and a consecutive number from 1 to 9 (PD) and 1 to 6 (HC); the number of syllable or inter-syllable intervals detected in each sample utterance (ints); the value of the mean interval in seconds for each participant (μ_i); the results of comparing each average duration (μ_i) to the respective control set average shown in the second row (the result of the comparison is 0 if the sequence average is smaller than the subset average, and 1 otherwise); the sequence interval standard deviation (σ_i) in seconds; the result of comparing each sequence standard deviation (σ_i) to the respective control set standard deviation shown in the second row of each table; and the JSD from each PDF of the male subset ($p_{MPSym,p}(i)$ and $p_{MPSim,p}(i)$) and from the female subset ($p_{FPSym,p}(i)$ and $p_{FPSim,p}(i)$) to their respective average HC subsets ($p_{\mu MCSym,p}$, $p_{\mu MCSim,p}$, $p_{\mu FCSym,p}$ and $p_{\mu FCSim,p}$).

Rows 4–12 give the results for each concept listed in the third row for the PD participants. Row 13 gives the number of cases of PD participants exceeding set averages and standard deviations of their respective subsets.

Rows 14–19 give the results for each concept listed in the third row for the HC participants, which are also evaluated to their average means and standard deviations. Row 20 gives the number of cases of HC participants exceeding set averages and standard deviations of their respective subsets.

The emission rates of syllable and inter-syllable segments is also an important participant-specific characteristic reflecting their capability in reproducing monosyllable and multisyllable tests. These are shown in Table 6.

The first row indicates the type of test carried on. The second row gives the participant code (Code), the rate of syllables/10 s (RateSy), the similar tate of inter-syllables/10 s (RateSy), and the difference between RateSy and RateSi for the monosyllable test (Dif), and these scores are repeated in the following three columns for the multisyllable test. The last column (DifMeans) gives the difference between the average multisyllable and monosyllable RateSy and RateSi as $DifMeans = (RateSy_p + RateSi_p)/2 - (RateSy_m + RateSi_m)/2$.

4   Discussion

Figure 1 (a) depicts the speech recording produced by an HC female participant during the emission of [...pataka...]. It shows an initial burst of more energetic emissions (b), to be stabilized to a background leve after 2 s. The rate of syllable and inter-syllable segments seen in (c) is relatively uniform and fast (average syllable duration: 0.062 s, standard deviation: 0.006 s, average inter-syllable duration: 0.073 s, standard deviation: 0.012 s, number of syllables per 10 s: 64.53, number of inter-syllable segments per 10 s: 62.88). The skewness is low in both cases, the kurtosis is below the normal distribution

Table 6. Segment emission rates per 10 s for monosyllable [...tatata...] and multisyllable [...pataka...].

Code	Monosyllable			Multisyllable			DifMeans
	RateSy	RateSi	Dif	RateSy	RateSi	Dif	
MP1	62.33	62.33	0.00	75.88	73.94	1.95	12.58
MP2	68.68	66.92	1.76	61.14	59.81	1.33	−7.33
MP3	52.01	49.75	2.26	57.22	57.22	0.00	6.34
MP4	66.48	64.02	2.46	78.45	76.94	1.51	12.45
MP5	51.82	49.57	2.25	58.21	58.21	0.00	7.51
MP6	53.58	52.21	1.37	66.48	65.35	1.13	13.02
MP7	36.15	35.06	1.10	54.72	50.81	3.91	17.16
MP8	55.46	54.20	1.26	56.92	54.77	2.15	1.01
MP9	63.55	61.87	1.67	63.41	61.70	1.71	−0.16
MC1	63.56	62.05	1.51	67.95	66.61	1.33	4.48
MC2	59.65	57.99	1.66	67.80	57.88	9.92	4.02
MC3	59.33	58.23	1.10	69.27	67.96	1.31	9.83
MC4	56.07	53.52	2.55	70.64	68.73	1.91	14.89
MC5	57.71	56.43	1.28	67.32	65.45	1.87	9.31
MC6	50.21	48.81	1.39	58.65	57.64	1.01	8.64
FP1	64.02	62.14	1.88	62.12	60.97	1.15	−1.54
FP2	50.61	49.41	1.21	67.27	66.34	0.92	16.79
FP3	63.57	61.98	1.59	57.97	56.48	1.49	−5.55
FP4	58.42	56.41	2.01	66.19	64.12	2.07	7.74
FP5	47.53	45.94	1.58	45.16	45.16	0.00	−1.57
FP6	63.87	62.45	1.42	74.54	75.49	−0.96	11.85
FP7	56.26	53.82	2.45	44.51	44.51	0.00	−10.53
FP8	55.56	53.97	1.59	67.46	66.28	1.18	12.11
FP9	69.96	69.96	0.00	60.46	61.87	−1.41	−8.79
FC1	49.91	48.18	1.72	64.58	62.92	1.66	14.71
FC2	66.01	63.81	2.20	79.34	79.34	0.00	14.42
FC3	59.88	58.49	1.39	84.69	84.69	0.00	25.50
FC4	60.48	58.85	1.63	70.09	67.40	2.70	9.08
FC5	69.63	68.08	1.55	72.63	71.23	1.40	3.08
FC6	54.50	52.68	1.82	70.15	68.20	1.95	15.59

one. Figure 1 (a) depicts the speech recording produced by a PD female participant, also corresponding to the utterance of [...pataka...]. It is clearly seen that the energy of syllable emissions (b) is irregular. The rate of syllable and inter-syllable segments in (c) shows clear irregularities (average syllable duration: 0.074 s, standard deviation:

0.016 s, average inter-syllable duration: 0.069 s, standard deviation: 0.015 s, number of syllables per 10 s: 62.12, number of inter-syllable segments per 10 s: 60.95). The skewness is very low for syllables, and rather high for inter-syllables, whereas the kurtosis of syllables is almost normal, and that of inter-syllables is highly leptokurtic. It may be concluded from these simple examinations that the emission of syllables is relatively normal in both tests, although inter-syllable emission appears to be more irregular in participants for the multisyllable test.

The examination of the general results reported in Figs. 3 and 4 allow us to make more general observations. In Fig. 3 (a) and (b) relative to the monosyllable test confronting syllable durations from PD and HC male participants, it may be seen that most of the PD distributions show regular bell-shape patterns below the average, except MP7, but the HC distributions divide within two clusters, a faster one (MC1, MC3 and MC5) and a slower one (MC2, MC4 and MC6). The average reference distribution is clearly bimodal (shown in red). This indicates that most PD participants produced fast and quasi-regular repetitions of [ta], whereas normative ones showed a faster-slower pattern.

Findings are less clear when analyzing inter-syllable intervals (c and d). In this case HC participants showed irregular distributions, whereas PD participants also produced very regular and fast patterns, except MP7 again.

When analyzing the syllable emissions from male HC and PD participants for the syllable test (e and f), the situation reverses, as in this case the emissions from HC participants are more regular and packed together, whereas they are more widespread and irregular when produced by PD participants, especially in the case of MP7.

Inter-syllable emissions in the multisyllable test (g and h) are clearly irregular in the HC group, whereas they are more clustered in PD participants, with the exception of MP7 again.

The results of the same tests from female subsets shown in Fig. 4(a, b) show a rather regular pattern for syllable durations in monosyllable tests, both from the PD and the HC subsets. The situation is more irregular for both PD and HC subsets (c, d) concerning inter-syllable distributions in monosyllable tests. When multisyllable tests are considered (e, f), the PDFs of syllable emissions from HC are more regular than those of PC participants (with the exception of FC6). This seems also to be the case when intersyllable distributions are considered (g, h).

Regarding the results shown in Tables 2, 3, 4 and 5 two important semantic features are the results of comparing each sequence interval averages and standard deviations with respect to the normative subsets. It may be expected that PD participants would produce longer and more disperse syllable and inter-syllable intervals when facing difficulties in repetition as a result of HD. To evaluate this hypothesis, the number of cases fulfilling these conditions for the different tests and participant subsets have been included in the above mentioned tables.

The main observations derived from Tables 2, 3, 4 and 5 are the following:

1. Male subset, monosyllable test, syllable intervals.
   Cases above the HC average: 1/9 (PD), 3/6 (HC).
   Cases above the HC standard deviation: 2/9 (PD), 2/6 (HC).

Observation: PD males produced shorter and less disperse syllable durations than HC males.

2. Male subset, monosyllable test, inter-syllable intervals.
   Cases above the HC average: 7/9 (PD), 4/6 (HC).
   Cases above the HC standard deviation: 1/9 (PD), 1/6 (HC).
   Observation: Both PD and HC males produced shorter and little dispersed inter-syllable durations.

3. Male subset, multisyllable test, syllable intervals.
   Cases above the HC average: 2/9 (PD), 2/6 (HC).
   Cases above the HC standard deviation: 6/9 (PD), 4/6 (HC).
   Observation: Both PD and HC males similar short and disperse syllable durations.

4. Male subset, multisyllable test, inter-syllable intervals.
   Cases above the HC average: 7/9 (PD), 3/6 (HC).
   Cases above the HC standard deviation: 7/9 (PD), 4/6 (HC).
   Observation: PD males produced longer and similar disperse inter-syllable durations than HC males.

5. Female subset, monosyllable test, syllable intervals.
   Cases above the HC average: 5/9 (PD), 3/6 (HC).
   Cases above the HC standard deviation: 1/9 (PD), 0/6 (HC).
   Observation: Both PD and HC females produced similarly short and little disperse syllable durations.

6. Female subset, monosyllable test, inter-syllable intervals.
   Cases above the HC average: 5/9 (PD), 2/6 (HC).
   Cases above the HC standard deviation: 1/9 (PD), 1/6 (HC).
   Observation: PD females produced longer inter-syllables than and HC females, although both subsets produced little dispersed inter-syllable durations.

7. Female subset, multisyllable test, syllable intervals.
   Cases above the HC average: 8/9 (PD), 3/6 (HC).
   Cases above the HC standard deviation: 6/9 (PD), 2/6 (HC).
   Observation: PD females produced longer and more disperse syllable durations than HC females.

8. Female subset, multisyllable test, inter-syllable intervals.
   Cases above the HC average: 7/9 (PD), 4/6 (HC).
   Cases above the HC standard deviation: 8/9 (PD), 2/6 (HC).
   Observation: PD females produced simular although more disperse inter-syllable durations than HC females.

It may be concluded from the above list that the combinations showing stronger differences in μ_i and σ_i between PD and HC subsets are cases 4 (for males) and 7 and 8 (for females).

Another important estimate allowing to establish comparisons between tests and features for male and female subsets are JSDs between each sample (from PD or HC participants) with respect to the HC average JSDs, to determine if a given divergence is to be considered under-normative or over-normative. The main observations in this regard, derived from Tables 2, 3, 4 and 5 are the following:

1. Male subset, monosyllable test, syllable intervals.
   Cases above the HC JSD average: 4/9 (PD), 3/6 (HC).
   Observation: The number of PD to HC JSDs over the HC JSD average is similar.
2. Male subset, monosyllable test, inter-syllable intervals.
   Cases above the HC average: 4/9 (PD), 2/6 (HC).
   Observation: The number of PD to HC JSDs over the HC JSD average is larger.
3. Male subset, multisyllable test, syllable intervals.
   Cases above the HC average: 3/9 (PD), 3/6 (HC).
   Observation: The number of PD to HC JSDs over the HC JSD average is smaller.
4. Male subset, multisyllable test, inter-syllable intervals.
   Cases above the HC average: 2/9 (PD), 2/6 (HC).
   Observation: The number of PD to HC JSDs over the HC JSD average is smaller.
5. Female subset, monosyllable test, syllable intervals.
   Cases above the HC average: 3/9 (PD), 3/6 (HC).
   Observation: The number of PD to HC JSDs over the HC JSD average is smaller.
6. Female subset, monosyllable test, inter-syllable intervals.
   Cases above the HC average: 5/9 (PD), 1/6 (HC).
   Observation: The number of PD to HC JSDs over the HC JSD average is much larger.
7. Female subset, multisyllable test, syllable intervals.
   Cases above the HC average: 5/9 (PD), 4/6 (HC).
   Observation: The number of PD to HC JSDs over the HC JSD average is similar.
8. Female subset, multisyllable test, inter-syllable intervals.
   Cases above the HC average: 7/9 (PD), 2/6 (HC).
   Observation: The number of PD to HC JSDs over the HC JSD average is much larger.

It may be concluded from the results shown in Table 6 that the combinations showing stronger differences between PD and HC subsets are cases 2 (for males) and 6, and 8 (for females).

The examination of the emission rates of syllable and inter-syllable segments given in Table 6 may also provide tentative insights. It may be seen that all the HC controls produce faster emission rates in the multisyllable test than in the monosyllable one (those showing positive DiffMeans), although, counter to expected, some PD participants may produce also faster emission rates in the multisyllable test than in the monosyllable one (7/9 in the male subset, and 4/9 in the female subset). To analyize if these differences had some significance, t-Tests were conducted on the DifMeans from the PD and HC subsets, on the null hypothesis of equal means and different variances. The resulting p-values were 0.619 (male subsets) and 0.025 (female subsets), indicating that differences were not relevant on the male subsets to reject the null hypothesis (no significant differences observed) but were relevant for the female subsets, rejecting the null hypothesis under the limit of 0.05.

Some of these findings may be explained by the relative stability and regularity in syllable and inter-syllable production by PD participants when uttering monosyllable tests, may be related with the effects of repetitive regular cue rates in stabilizing the movements in PD patients [16, 17].

In general, the behavior of the HC male subset is not uniform, as seen in the distributions of syllable and inter-syllable intervals shown in Fig. 3(b, d, f and h). This raises the question if these tests must be conducted under maximum stress or under comfortable conditions. In the first case, the protocols had to be modified to emphasize speech under stress. In turn, the HC female subset in Fig. 4(b, d, f and h) shows a more compact behaviour, thus granting better results in the tests. Another relevant question regarding HC recordings is if HC should be age-matched (showing some co-morbidity behaviour due to aging [18] or if a more normative population (young adults) should be recruited. Regarding the behaviour of the PD datasets in Fig. 3 and 4(a, c, e and g), it may be seen that there is not a common pattern. In general, it may be said that results from inter-syllable distributions (c and g) are more widespread and irregular. However, a certain case as the syllable intervals from the monosyllable test by female participants (Fig. 4a) is a clear example of a rather regular emission cluster. Nevertheless, the inhomogeneity of PD labels is clearly seen in the presence of specific participants showing a stronger degree of HD affection, which is especially present in the case of MP7 and FP5. This observation indicates that although both patients were scored 2 in H&Y, their neuromotor function seems to be more affected than the rest of their respective subsets. Although this may pose specific difficulties in cohort recruiting, it nevertheless shows that distribution estimation is sensitive enough to characterize and differentiate specifically more pathological behaviour from the average background, bringing the methodology into value.

Additional relevant information is provided in Tables 2, 3, 4 and 5, as the number of intervals produced by each speaker, which depends on different factors, respiratory capacity among them. Tables 2, 3, 4 and 5 show the smallest and largest number of intervals in bold. It may be seen that in the male dataset the largest numbers correspond to a member of the HC subset, whereas the smallest comes from the PD subset. This situation is the oposite in the female dataset. Whether this observation is due to pathological or behavioural character is another open question.

Similarly, from the examination of JSDs, it should be expected that the smallest scores should correspond to the HC subsets, and the largest ones to the PD subsets. This expectation is fulfilled by syllable intervals of the male dataset from the multisyllable test only (0.452 and 0.097). In all other cases, either the largest and smallest are within the same PD or HC group, or even reversed (the largest and smallest values of JSD are given in bold over the four tables mentioned).

Analyzing the values of μ_i it should be expected that the largest estimations would correspond to the PD subset, and the shortest to the HC subset, due to bradikinesia. This is fulfilled by the following subsets: syllable intervals, monosyllable test, male subset; inter-syllable intervals, multisyllable test, male subset; syllable intervals, multisyllable test, female subset; and inter-syllable intervals, multisyllable test, female subset.

A symilar analysis on the values of σ_i, assuming that the largest estimations would also correspond to the PD for the same reasons (more widespread activity expected), brings to light that the subsets showing the expected behaviour are: syllable intervals, monosyllable test, female subset (case 5); inter-syllable intervals, monosyllable test, female subset (case 6); inter-syllable intervals, multisyllable test, female subset (case 8).

From the above observations, it seems plausible that normality tests to differentiate PD from HC behaviour might work better with the multisyllable test than with the monosyllable one. Therefore, the best candidate differentiating tests to be checked in a further study would be the syllable intervals from the monosyllable test in the case of males (case 4), and the syllable and inter-syllable intervals from the multisyllable test in the case of females (cases 6 and 7).

It might be inferred from the above that fast purely repetitive tests provide a timely cadence to PD participants which help them in successful fast repetition. On the contrary, mixed-syllable tests require a conscious control of syllable sequence repetition (sequence planning and executing), presenting an added challenge for HC and PD participants, where HC participants seem to utter the multisyllable sequence faster. The added difficulty found in the multisyllable test may be related to executing the neuromotor changes implied in the articulation from bilabial [pa] (orofacial) to apical-alveolar [ta] (lingual) and dorsal-velar [ka] (lingual-pharyngeal), involving quite different neuromuscular systems.

Study Limitations: It seems that the differentiation capability of multisyllabilc diadochokinetic tests is larger than fast purely repetitive tests which may be more easily reproduced by PD patients. Therefore, these tests have to be combined with results from other speech examinations, as phonation [19,20] and articulation [21] to increase differentiation capabilities between pathological an non-pathological behaviour. The main weakness of this study is the limited number of participants suggesting any findings should be cautiously interpreted. Nevertheless, it has exploratory value to initiate a larger scale study. The slightly difference in the age range of HC and PD participants might introduce some bias in the comparisons as well, this fact needing a further study as highlighted in [10,18], although we have relatively well matched ages (with the exception of MP7, well over the average).

5   Conclusions

Repetitive monosyllable and multisyllable tests have been proposed within routine examination protocols of PD HD. Although they may provide important information on a given speaker's competence, their differentiation capability and vulnerability are yet to be explored in depth. The present research allowed to envision some preliminary findings, which are worth of being reviewed:

- The capacity of multisyllable tests to discriminate PD vs HC fast repetition performance appears to be more efficient, compared to monosyllable tests.
- Some PD participants may produce good and regular syllable and inter-syllable monosyllable utterances, and at a faster repetition rate than HC controls. This fact could be explained by the capability of timely regular rhythmics to provide a guided cadence to PD participants which help them in successful fast repetition. The differentiation capability of monosyllable tests may be substantially reduced, and therefore, it should be taken into account in devising examination protocols.
- On the other hand, as PD participants seem to experience more difficulty in uttering multisyllable tests, these tests should be combined with other speech tests in devising examination protocols.

- The average duration of syllable and inter-syllable intervals, and their dispersion measured by the standard deviation seem to be sensitive to HD, and could be used as biomarkers, although a reliable normative database must be granted for comparison, including speech from young adult population, to avoid confounding factors as aging.
- Other reliable biomarkers could be supported by JSDs, under the same premises, relying on multisyllable tests, using inter-syllable PDFs. Again, the need of a well populated normative database is essential.
- The database used in the study is limited in size and variability, as most PD participants are not strongly affected by HD during the ON stage. Therefore, some are competent enough to produce good utterances.
- PD participants were not exhibiting strong HD signs and nevertheless we are putting forward a sufficiently sensitive methodology which appears to have good potential (subject to be validated in larger scale studies), as one of the aims of HD testing is to grant prodromal detection, which depends on the capability of detecting mildly affected PwPs.

The proposed methodology does not require expensive high quality equipment. This is very much aligned with the spirit of the Parkinson's Voice Initiative (PVI), see [17], trying to facilitate low-cost, robust assessment of PD using readily available means.

References

1. De Lau, L.M., Breteler, M.M.: Epidemiology of Parkinson's disease. Lancet Neurol. **5**, 525–535 (2006)
2. Dauer, W., Przedborski, S.: Parkinson's disease: mechanisms and models. Neuron **39**, 889–909 (2003)
3. Duffy, J.R.: Motor Speech Disorders. Elsevier, River Lane, St. Louis (2013)
4. Parkinson, J.: An essay on the shaking palsy. J. Neuropsychiatry Clin. Neurosci. **14**(2), 223–236 (2002). Re-edited from the 1817 monograph by Sherwood, Neely and Jones (London, 1817)
5. Ricciardi, L., et al.: Speech and gait in Parkinson's disease: when rhythm matters. Park. Relat. Disord. **32**, 42–47 (2016)
6. Brabenec, L., Mekyska, J., Galaz, Z., Rektorova, I.: Speech disorders in Parkinson's disease: early diagnostics and effects of medication and brain stimulation. J. Neural Transm. **124**(3), 303–334 (2017)
7. Tsanas, A.: Accurate telemonitoring of Parkinson's disease symptom severity using nonlinear speech signal processing and statistical machine leaning. PhD. Thesis, University of Oxford, UK (2012)
8. Ziegler, W.: Task-related factors in oral motor control: speech and oral diadochokinesis in dysarthria and apraxia of speech. Brain Lang. **80**, 556–575 (2002)
9. Karlsson, F., Schalling, E., Laakso, K., Johansson, K., Hartelius, L.: Assessment of speech impairment in patients with Parkinson's disease from acoustic quantifications of oral diadochokinetic sequences. J. Acoust. Soc. Am. **147**, 839–851 (2020)
10. Gómez, P., Gómez, A., Palacios, D., Tsanas, A.: Performance of monosyllabic vs multisyllabic diadochokinetic exercises in evaluating Parkinson's disease hypokinetic dysarthria from fluency distributions. In: Proceedings of the 14th International Joint Conference on Biomedical Engineering Systems and Technologies (BIOSTEC 2021), vol. 4, pp. 114–123 (2021)

11. Palacios, D., Meléndez, G., López, A., Lázaro, C., Gómez, A., Gómez, P.: MonParLoc: a speech-based system for Parkinson's disease analysis and monitoring. IEEE Access **8**, 188243–188255 (2020). https://doi.org/10.1109/ACCESS.2020.3031646
12. Dimitriadis, D., Potamianos, A., Maragos, P.: A comparison of the squared energy and Teager-Kaiser operators for short-term energy estimation in additive noise. IEEE Trans. Signal Proc. **57**(7), 2569–2581 (2009)
13. Alku, P., et al.: OPENGLOT–an open environment for the evaluation of glottal inverse filtering. Speech Commun. **107**, 38–47 (2019). https://doi.org/10.1016/j.specom.2019.01.005
14. Cover, T.M., Thomas, J.A.: Elements of Information Theory. Wiley, New York (2006)
15. Simard, R., L'Ecuyer, P.: Computing the two-sided Kolmogorov-Smirnov distribution. J. Stat. Softw. **39**(11), 1–18 (2011)
16. Harrison, E.C., Horin, A.P., Earhart, G.M.: Mental singing reduces gait variability more than music listening for healthy older adults and people with Parkinson disease. J. Neurol. Phys. Ther. **43**(2019), 204–211 (2019)
17. Arora, S., Baghai-Rivary, L., Tsanas, A.: Developing a large scale population screening tool for the assessment of Parkinson's disease using telephone-quality voice. J. Acoust. Soc. Am. **145**, 2871–2884 (2019)
18. Gómez, A., Palacios, D., Ferrández, J.M., Mekyska, J., Álvarez, A., Gómez, P.: A methodology to differentiate Parkinson's disease and aging speech based on glottal flow acoustic analysis. Int. J. Neural Syst. **30**, 205558 (2019)
19. Mekyska, J., et al.: Robust and complex approach of pathological speech signal analysis. Neurocomputing **167**, 94–111 (2015). https://doi.org/10.1016/j.neucom.2015.02.085
20. Novotný, M., Dušek, P., Daly, I., Růžička, E., Rusz, J.: Glottal source analysis of voice deficits in newly diagnosed drug-naïve patients with Parkinson's disease: correlation between acoustic speech characteristics and non-speech motor performance. Biomed. Signal Process. Control **57**, 101818 (2020). https://doi.org/10.1016/j.bspc.2019.101818
21. Vásquez, J.C., Orozco, J.R., Bocklet, T., Nöth, E.: Towards an automatic evaluation of the dysarthria level of patients with Parkinson's disease. J. Comm. Disord. **76**, 21–36 (2018). https://doi.org/10.1016/j.jcomdis.2018.08.002

Technology-Based Education and Training System for Nursing Professionals

Conrad Fifelski-von Böhlen[1]([✉])[iD], Anna Brinkmann[1][iD], Sebastian Fudickar[2][iD], Sandra Hellmers[1][iD], and Andreas Hein[1]

[1] Carl von Ossietzky Universität, Ammerländer Heerstraße 114-118, 26129 Oldenburg, Germany
c.fifelski-von.boehlen@uni-oldenburg.de
[2] Institut für Medizinische Informatik, Ratzeburger Allee 160, 23538 Lübeck, Germany

Abstract. Musculoskeletal Disorders (MSD) are one of the most significant health hazards for nurses causing a high rate of sick leave and exit the profession before the retirement age. In this context, physically heavy tasks like lifting patients frequently in awkward stooped or forced postures lead to constant high physical stresses and thus to MSD and physical deterioration. Therefore, in order to reduce physical load, a focus must be placed on the education and training of nurses on ergonomically correct working techniques. At present, technical assistance for the analysis of ergonomic working methods is rarely used in nursing training. In this work, we present a novel sensor system to improve the educational processes in the healthcare profession. The system includes three-dimensional optical sensors, a wearable sensor suit, a ground reaction force plate and surface electromyography to record and analyze nursing tasks. The system is tested and evaluated in a case study with nursing students (n = 13) during a simulated transfer task. The system provided in-depth evaluation of the conducted transfer and increased the feedback quality of an instructor compared to conventional training methods.

Keywords: Nursing education · Ergonomics · Teaching · Optical devices · Feedback · Case studies · Posture

1 Introduction

This article is an extended version of "Evaluating a Multi Depth Camera System to Consolidate Ergonomic Work in the Education of Caregivers" by Fifelski-von Böhlen et al. [1] and is motivated by the upcoming demographic changes and the lack of nurses in western societies. Many absences in this profession are due to musculoskeletal disorders, which can be prevented by improved training of nurses in ergonomically correct work techniques for physically demanding tasks. Therefore, we developed a sophisticated optical sensor system to support nursing education. In addition to the mentioned publication, which focused on the optical system and a dedicated study, we describe in this article further subsystems of

C. Gehin et al. (Eds.): BIOSTEC 2021, CCIS 1710, pp. 120–138, 2022.
https://doi.org/10.1007/978-3-031-20664-1_7

our sensor system for in-depth analyzes of nursing tasks. The system extension enables objective posture and load analysis as well as muscle activity studies to identify incorrect postures and unfavorable loads.

1.1 Demographic Background

Global socio-demographic changes and the estimated shortage of 9 million nurses impact society and healthcare systems tremendously [2,3]. In 2050, the number of people over 80 years is expected to triple from 143 million in 2019 to 426 million [4]. This estimation leads to an increasing number of people requiring health services and an aging nursing workforce [5]. Thus, the imbalance between the provision of health services and the need for these services is steadily increasing, severing the situation in the nursing institutions, which are overbooked even today [6,7].

Musculoskeletal disorders (MSD) are among the most significant health hazards for nurses and are closely associated with a high rate of sick leave and exit the profession before the retirement age [8–10]. Here, low back pain is the most common work-related health problem affecting nurses [11–13]. The risk for MSD and low back pain are mainly caused by repetitive manual patient handling tasks like lifting, holding, or moving large and heavy parts of a patient's weight, and working in asymmetric or flexed postures frequently [11,14].

While musculoskeletal stresses can be significantly reduced by using ergonomic working techniques [15–18] and care aids [15,19], MSD are multifactorial. Biomechanical factors of MSD are targetable by worksite-tailored interventions and rehabilitation programs to potentially reduce functional disabilities and associated absences among nurses that may result from MSD [20]. Specifically, implementing education and training about ergonomic working techniques are essential to avoid harmful postures and actions in manual patient handling tasks to reduce MSD among the nursing workforce [20,21]. However, nursing students and professionals are not routinely educated and trained in ergonomics [22], increasing their risks to experience physical impairments and potential hazards.

1.2 Sensor System Conceptualization

As the demand for training and education of care professionals rises, new concepts, which enhance existing methods, must be implemented beneficially. So far, the education is performed with simulated tasks, where the student performs the nursing tasks in front of the instructor. Afterward, feedback is given, and the performance is evaluated. Recordings are done with standard RGB cameras for revision. As the observation of body postures and the order of movement sequences is necessary for a in-depth feedback by the instructor, questions arise, whether this procedure is suitable or can be enhanced and improved by modern technology. State-of-the-art sensor technology can improve the recordings while keeping the effort low. Because care students are taking different poses during nursing tasks, different view angles and zoom levels may be desirable for the evaluation. As standard imaging lacks these possibilities, using an optical system that provides multiple viewpoints and a three-dimensional data representation would be helpful. Furthermore, additional data by wearable sensors and external sensor systems can enrich an objective evaluation. A tailored solution, where three-dimensional optical data and biomechanical measurements are combined, can significantly improve the previous RGB camera recordings.

In summary, the key element of a sensor system for monitoring nursing actions would consist of a 3D optical imaging system enriched with additional biomechanical sensors for tracking and analyzing body postures, movements and loads. In addition, the data must be presented intuitively to ensure ease of use for care instructors. The technology-based approach with the novel sensor system needs to be tested and evaluated in experimental studies or field trials.

1.3   Related Work

Healthcare systems of western societies are challenged by the lack of nurses and related professionals caused by physical overload. Up to now, current research has focused on detecting and reducing job-related back pain sources by using conventional measures, like real-time auditory feedback or feedback rounds [23] or with sensor- and algorithm-based data evaluation [24, 25]. In particular, depth sensors seem to have broad application fields in the health care sector for body postures or movements analyses [26–28]. In addition to the pure application of sensors, distributed sensor networks can collect additional information about care activities. Jäger et al. have demonstrated this by using different sensors to measure physical load during patient transfers [15]. In addition to the aforementioned depth cameras, multiple sensors of the same type can be used for sensor networks to achieve a higher data density and, thus, a more accurate evaluation. The LiveScan3D by Kowalski et al. for example, is a system that combines the depth images of multiple Kinects V2 depth cameras to scan a human head precisely enough to create 3D printed figurines [29]. This kind of depth camera network can also work for health care applications in simulated nursing tasks [30]. The acquisition of data is only one part of a technology-based evaluation pipeline. Algorithmic approaches and data fusion helps to understand poses and movements [26, 27, 31]. However, multi-sensor networks, which work with different sensor types, are challenging regarding the acquisition, processing, and data representation, especially for non-technical persons. Therefore, an easy and intuitive handling is important.

2   Methods

2.1   The Sensor System

The sensor system used in our case study consists of multiple subsystems. These are an optical system for motion and pose tracking based on multiple depth cameras, a wearable sensor suit, a ground reaction force plate, and a surface electromyograph. The modularity allows using either all sensors or only a subset, depending on the application.

Optical System. For posture and movement analysis, an optical system provides the necessary data. Here, the combination of four Microsoft Kinect v2 depth cameras is used. It is possible to view the scene from indefinitely adjustable view angles in three-dimensional, colored point clouds. Because the point clouds are merely three-dimensional objects, they can be rotated or translated during visualization in real-time or offline. This is beneficial while observing care acts like transfers, due to the possibility to see poses and movements from different perspectives. A depth camera can be occluded by obstacles or humans in the scene. A combination of several depth cameras can compensate the occlusion. Additionally, the point clouds of multiple depth cameras can be combined to a single point cloud. This increases the density of the data and covers scenes from different sides. The depth cameras are situated around the bed and are focusing the center of the bed. All four cameras are installed on tripods at 1.8 m and cover an area of approximately 2 m × 2 m. They tilted towards the ground at 45°. Research by Fankhauser et al. [32] indicates that the best distance from the point of interest to the camera is around 0.8 to 1.2 m. Also, the depth accuracy deteriorates in the corners of the depth image [32]. Therefore, the placement of the cameras needs to follow these findings. Each Kinect v2 is connected to a commercial grade minicomputer with standard Intel i5 Processor of the sixth generation and integrated GPU that runs Windows 10 via USB 3.0. The Kinect v2 Software Development Kit (SDK) only runs on Windows machines. Because the whole room network is ROS-based the minicomputers are communicating to a consumer grade master computer with dedicated Nvidia GTX 1080 GPU and Intel i7 processor of the sixth generation running Ubuntu 16.04 and ROS via private Ethernet connections. A server network PCI card must be installed to handle the traffic. Contrary to standard RGB cameras, the Microsoft Kinect v2 is able of acquiring a depth image alongside with color information. Although it is also possible to obtain other data streams like infrared and a coarse body estimation, we focus on depth and color information. The depth information is obtained at a rate 30 Hz with 512 × 424 pixel, while the color image features 1920 * 1080 Pixel 30 Hz.

The Kinect v2 SDK provides tools to map the color information to the depth image. In short, all color pixels are discarded for regions which are not in the

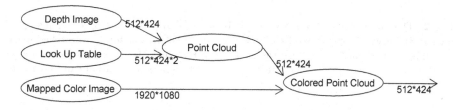

Fig. 1. The generation of the colored point clouds. From the depth image and a look up table, a point cloud is calculated and subsequently colored by a mapped color image [1]. (Color figure online)

depth image. This reduces the resolution of the color image. The depth data must be processed with a static look up table (LUT), internal saved by each camera, in order to calculate point clouds. This is necessary because each Kinect v2 has slightly different lens distortion parameters. The mapped color image stream and the point cloud can be combined to a colored point cloud on the master computer, see Fig. 1. The colored point clouds are displayed for the analysis to the nursing instructor.

Another step that must be done before using the systems is to register the four depth cameras to each other. The 3D registration can be done differently with printed patterns or objects of a unique shape. We use a 15 cm radius Styrofoam sphere. The sphere is placed on at least three different spots in the view of all cameras. This allows calculating the relative position from one camera to another. In the visualization of the four aligned point clouds, the user can adjust the viewpoint. Additionally, we implemented a player that can be used like a standard video player for point clouds, see Fig. 2. Even in the recordings and when the recorded point cloud is paused, it is still possible to change the point of view at any time.

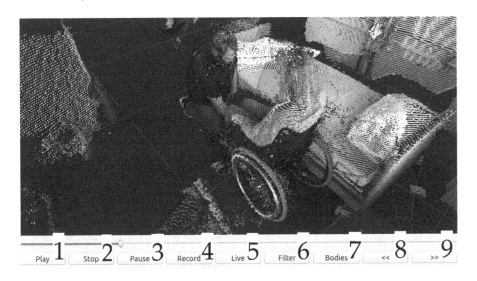

Play 1   Stop 2   Pause 3   Record 4   Live 5   Filter 6   Bodies 7   << 8   >> 9

Fig. 2. The point cloud player window. It is possible to play (1), stop (2), pause (3), rewind(8), forward(9) or record (4) point clouds. The live button (5) switches from recording to live data. To reduce the size of the recorded files it is possible to apply voxel grid and statistical outlier filters (6). The coarse body estimation can be turned on, too (7) [1].

Wearable Sensor Suit. In addition to the optical system, a wearable sensor system was used for body posture analyzes. The sensor suit is a full body motion capture system of Motion Shadow [33]. The system includes 17 motion nodes, which were distributed on the body. A motion node is a measurement unit including a 3D-accelerometer, 3D-gyroscope, and 3D-magnetometer. The sampling rate of each sensor is 100 Hz.

The motion nodes are bilaterally on the feet, lower legs, thighs, hands, forearms, upper arms, shoulders. Additionally, there is a sensor on the head, on the hip and at the back. By distributing the sensors over the entire body, the posture of the back, as well as the movements of the extremities, can be recorded. This allows an analysis of the back torsions and inclinations as well as an evaluation of the leg position.

Ground Reaction Force Sensor. A ground reaction force plate was used for load estimations during the manual patient transfers. Therefore, the force plate was positioned in front of the care bed, see Fig. 2. We used an AMTI AccuPower force plate with a sampling rate of 200 Hz. The force plate measures the vertical forces as well as the forces in mediolateral and anterior-posterior direction. The raw data is filtered by a second-order Butterworth low-pass filter with a cutoff frequency of 20 Hz.

Surface Electromyography. Non-invasive surface electromyography (SEMG) measured the muscle activation behavior during the manual patient transfer tasks. The following knee extensor, knee flexor and hip extensor muscles of the participants' left thigh were equipped with SEMG sensors: vastus medialis (VM, knee extensor), rectus femoris (RF, knee extensor), and biceps femoris (BF, knee flexor and hip extensor). Skin preparation and SEMG electrode placement were done following SENIAM guidelines [34]. Signal recording was done with a device from Biovision (Biovision Inputbox and Dasy-Lab 4.010 software) and amplification (2500 Hz) was done with the use of local amplifiers and an analog-to-digital conversion unit that sent the data to the input box (National Instruments USB-6009, 14-bit) for further processing. The signals were rectified and filtered by root mean square calculation. Then, the signals were labeled according to kinematic and kinetic data.

2.2   Experimental Design

To evaluate our Multi-Kinect-System in the field, audio feedback data is recorded while a nursing instructor uses our system for educating care students. Therefore, we compared a conventional feedback (pure observation without technology) with sensor-enhanced feedback to investigate a measurable effect between both education strategies. The nursing task was a manual patient transfer from a care bed to a wheelchair. In addition, the benefit of the sensor suit, the ground reaction force plate, and surface electromyography as an enriched feedback tool is quantified. All data were synchronized by a trigger signal that involved jumping on the force plate at the start and end of the manual patient handling task.

After conducting the transfer task, the three-dimensional data of the Multi-Kinect-System is presented to the nurse and the nursing instructor. A study organizer is operating the system, following their commands by changing the zoom or the viewpoint and pausing, rewinding, or forwarding the recorded data. Figure 5 depicts the procedure. The nursing instructor articulates which function of the Multi-Kinect-System point cloud player should be used, i.e., what the instructor wants to see. The indirect usage reduces the influence of the usability of the system. The study organizer fulfills these commands on the recording computer. The recordings contain keywords indicating the use of the Multi-Kinect-System. The observed keywords are "stop", "rewind", "forward", "turn view angle" and words with a similar semantic. Furthermore, the time of the feedback rounds is compared, and the criticized aspects are tracked. These aspects are body balance, knee and lunge positioning, back, stand, usage of caretakers movement resources, and the whole movement sequence. The three-dimensional data, which is the foundation for the second feedback by the instructor and the biomechanical measurement, are recorded. Later on, the processed combination of the different sensors helps instructors understand the impact of wrong postures and movements in physically challenging tasks like patient transfers. The resulting data set, which must be analyzed, consists of two audio recordings per study participant. The study organizers are just involved as passive participants [35]. The study is approved by the ethical board of the Carl von Ossietzky University Oldenburg (Drs.EK/2019/004).

Participants. The study participants are nursing students from the nursing school Evangelische Altenpflegeschule e.V. Oldenburg. Although the participants are still in the school courses, they work in nursing homes or similar institutions as caregivers. Some of them are in the courses for further education to obtain a higher qualification in the profession. Therefore, they have a lot of practical experience and are already instructed to use their body and care equipment correctly. Nevertheless, they are making mistakes during the transfer task, too.

Overall, 13 participants have been included in the study and performed the transfer task. The age of the ten women and three men ranges from 18 to 55 years. There are no participants with physical restrictions. The participants enter the study location and are prepared for the transfer task. In addition to the examined Multi-Kinect-System, the sensor suit, the ground reaction force plate, and surface electromyography are used. None of the used sensors are impairing the movement of the participant. Because the participants are differing in height, strength, and expertise, there is not one pattern solution for the conduction of the manual patient transfer task. Nevertheless, the participant should choose the right grips and poses to apply forces according to the nature of the patient's body.

Manual Patient Transfer. The task analyzed in our case study is a manual patient transfer from a care bed to a wheelchair. The patient to be transferred is a 28-year-old woman weighing 63 kg. At the beginning of the task, she is already sitting on the bed's edge and acts like a movement-impaired older adult with abdominal stability while standing. To accomplish the transfer correctly, the participant must use the movement resources of the patient, the care equipment, and the learned knowledge of how to transfer movement impaired people.

Setup. The wheelchair is placed on the right side beside the care bed. Because the force measurement plate elevates the participant 12 cm over the ground, the wheelchair is always elevated on a socket, see Fig. 2. The nursing instructor supervises each transfer by visual inspection, but without the data of the sensor systems at first. This feedback is recorded. Afterward, the same transfer is examined again, but this time with the sensor system. To see the data, the participant and the instructor are gathered around the recording computer. This second feedback round is recorded again. The goal is to find and evaluate the differences between both feedback rounds. The comparison is essential to derive how the sensor system extends the perception of the nursing instructor.

3 Results

As mentioned before, audio data was recorded during the feedback rounds which have been conducted in two conditions: with and without viewing the recordings of the Multi-Kinect-System. In order to assess the quality of both feedback rounds and to compare them, specific characteristics were identified for a quantitative evaluation of the feedback rounds. We chose the following metrics as quantitative indicators:

- the total duration of the feedback rounds,
- frequency of use for specific keywords indicating the use of the Multi-Kinect system,
- and suggested improvements in patient handling.

3.1 Duration of Feedback Rounds

We assume that a higher duration of a feedback round indicates the possible presence of additional information. The feedback rounds with the Multi-Kinect system should therefore last longer than the feedback rounds without, in order to show a possible benefit in the technically supported training. In addition to durations, the information provided in the two feedback rounds is also examined and compared to each other in the following.

Table 1 compares the durations of the analog and digital feedback rounds. The analog feedback rounds are without the Multi-Kinect-System and in the digital feedback round the Multi-Kinect-System was used. Each of the 13 study participants is represented by a three-digit number. The order of the participant numbers in the following graphs and tables do not correspond to the order in which they performed the transfer tasks. The average duration of the analog feedback is 59 s. The average duration of digital feedback is significantly longer with 2 min and 16 s.

Figure 6 shows the differences in the duration of the feedback rounds graphically. Digital feedback that takes more than two minutes longer than analog feedback is marked with an asterisk.

Table 1. Duration of the feedback rounds with (digital) and without (analog) the Multi- Kinect-System [1].

Participant	142	243	424	417	483	107	280	303	350	366	315	437	473
Analog Feedback [min:ss]	0:57	0:43	0:59	0:36	1:00	1:09	1:41	1:29	0:38	1:10	0:38	1:01	0:46
Digital Feedback [min:ss]	4:06	2:58	2:01	2:09	1:55	1:28	2:07	3:37	2:43	1:27	1:07	2:33	1:20

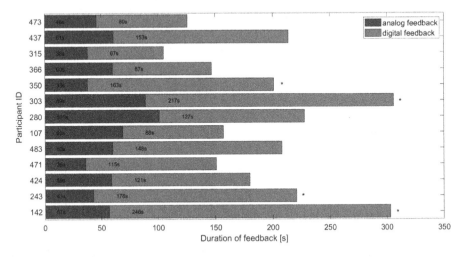

Fig. 3. Duration of the analog and digital feedback rounds. Differences of more than two minutes are marked with an asterisk [1].

3.2   Keywords in Feedback Rounds

An active use of the Multi-Kinect-System indicates a benefit of the system for the feedback rounds, because scenes can be analyzed retrospectively. Therefore, keywords were filtered in the audio recordings to quantify the active use of the system. We found keywords like "stop", "rewind", "forward", "turn view angle" and words with a similar semantic, which can be quantified. Table 2 shows the number of the keywords mentioned in the digital feedback round per study participant. On average, two keywords were mentioned per feedback.

Table 2. Number of keywords used for an active use of the Multi-Kinect-System [1].

Participant	142	243	424	417	483	107	280	303	350	366	315	437	473
Number of keywords	3	3	3	2	1	5	1	1	2	1	1	2	1

3.3   Amount of Criticized Aspects

The overall aim is to train nurses in an ergonomic way of working, taking kinesthetic aspects [36] into account, in order to avoid unfavorable body posture and loads in everyday work. Therefore, it is necessary to compare the improvements and the criticisms mentioned by the nursing instructor in the two feedback rounds. The nursing instructor selected six aspects that are most important for a healthy transfer from the nurses' point of view:

- body balance (BAL)
- knee and lunge positioning (LNG)
- usage and form of the back (BAK)
- stand on the ground (STD)
- usage of the patient's resources (RES)
- movement sequence (MVM)

During the patient transfer, it is important to maintain body balance (BAL) in order to control the patient's weight at all times. To shift the load from the back to the lower extremities, a lunge position with the correct knee angle is recommended (LNG). To avoid lifting with a bent or twisted spine (BAK), the back as well as the neck should be stretched. Overall, inclinations and torsions of the back over 20° should be avoided [37], as most work absences in the nursing field are due to back pain. An appropriate positioning of the feet is also important to ensure a stable stand (STD), since a too narrow stand reduces stability. Patients' movement resources (RES) should be considered to avoid unnecessary strain and to make care more activating. Proper movement patterns and sequences (MVM) should avoid unfavorable postures and movements such as spinal twisting.

The audio is recorded for the analog and digital feedback rounds and the criticized aspects are counted. Table 3 shows the frequencies of the mentioned individual criticisms for each study participant (SP) for both feedback rounds. On average, more aspects were addressed in the digital feedback round than in the analog feedback round. If the number of comments is the same, the cells in the table are highlighted in green; if there are more comments in the digital feedback, the fields are colored in cyan.

Especially the aspects concerning the use and the form of the back (BAK) were addressed significantly more often in the digital feedback round. Seven of the thirteen participants got more feedback in the digital round, five participant got the same number of comments in both rounds and only one participants received more comments in the analog feedback. For study p articipant 107, for example, additional aspects regarding the lunge positioning and one additional aspect regarding the usage of the back were discovered by the nursing instructor in the digital feedback round. This and the higher number of comments in the digital feedback indicates that the usage of the Multi-Kinect-System makes additional aspects visible.

Because the analog feedback was always before the digital feedback, it is more likely, that issues, discussed in the analog feedback, are not mentioned again in the digital feedback round (white cells in Table 3).

Table 3. Number of mentioned improvements and the criticisms in manual patient transfer for both feedback rounds (analog/digital). The same number of aspect for both feedbacks are marked in green. More comments in the digital feedback round are marked in cyan. BAL: body balance, LNG: knee and lunge positioning, BAK: back, STD: stand, RES: usage of patient's resources, MVM: movement sequence, SUM: sum of comments. [1].

Participant	142	243	424	417	483	107	280	303	350	366	315	437	473	SUM
BAL	1/1	0/1	0/1	1/1	1/1	1/1	2/2	0/0	0/0	0/0	0/0	1/1	0/1	7/10
LNG	0/2	0/0	1/0	1/0	0/0	0/1	2/2	1/0	1/0	1/0	0/0	1/1	1/0	9/6
BAK	0/1	0/0	1/1	0/2	0/0	0/1	1/3	1/1	1/2	0/0	0/0	0/1	0/0	4/12
STD	1/2	0/0	0/0	0/0	0/0	0/0	0/1	0/1	0/1	0/0	0/0	0/0	0/0	1/5
RES	1/0	0/2	1/1	1/0	1/1	0/0	0/0	0/0	0/0	0/0	0/1	1/1	0/0	5/6
MVM	1/2	0/1	0/1	0/0	0/0	1/0	0/1	0/0	1/0	1/0	0/0	0/0	0/0	4/5
SUM	4/8	0/4	3/4	3/3	2/2	2/3	5/9	2/2	3/3	2/0	0/1	3/4	1/1	-

3.4   Comparison of Information Content

The pure duration of the feedback alone is no proof of the information content. However, if the feedback duration is taken as an indicator of a more in-depth debriefing and the number of criticized aspects is also taken into account, it can be assumed that the information density is higher when the Multi-Kinect-System is used. The sum of the average criticized aspects is 2.31 for analog feedback and 3.39 for digital feedback. The average analog feedback time is 59 s and 2 min and 16 s for digital feedback. For example, for study participant 142, feedback time increased by 3 min and 9 s between analog feedback and feedback with the Multi-Kinect-System. Dividing the average feedback time by the average number of aspects criticized resulted in a value of 25 s per aspect criticized for analog feedback and 40 s per aspect criticized for digital feedback. This may indicate either that analog feedback requires less time per criticized aspect or that digital feedback is more in-depth due to the possibilities of the Multi-Kinect-System. However, the number of aspects mentioned or criticized should always take precedence over time concerns. In addition, it must be noted that even the passive use of the precedence requires a single-digit number of seconds per participant.

3.5   Feedback by Additional Sensors Systems

In addition to the Multi-Kinect-System, a sensor suit, a ground reaction force plate and SEMG were used to record objective measurements on body posture, mechanical loads and muscle activity.

Using the sensor suit, skeleton models with their joint positions and angles can be extracted. Since special focus is placed on working with a straight back, we automatically calculate the inclinations and torsions of the back. The skeleton model as well as color-coded inclination and torsion angles are visualized in a result report (see Fig. 4). The color-coding is based on the angles ranges for the classification of acceptable, limited acceptable, and unacceptable upper body postures [38]. Limited acceptable angles are marked in yellow (e.g. sagittal inclination angle between 20°-60°), unacceptable angles have red color (sagittal inclination angle >60°, lateral inclination and torsion >20°). Postures with red-marked angles are classified as potentially harmful. Special attention should also be paid to coupled movements (torsion + inclination, sagittal + lateral inclination) since they can be particularly harmful [39].

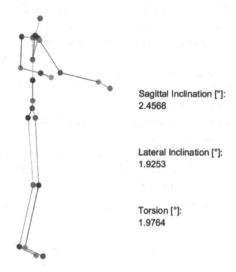

Sagittal Inclination [°]:
2.4568

Lateral Inclination [°]:
1.9253

Torsion [°]:
1.9764

Fig. 4. Skeleton model and corresponding upper body inclination and torsion angles.

Figure 5 shows an example of the analysis of force and sagittal upper body inclination for subject 424. The transfer can be divided into several phases. First, the participant prepares himself and also the patient for the transfer. Then the patient is lifted to an upright position. Next, the patient is turned with small cradle steps so that he or she is standing frontally to the wheelchair. The cradle steps can be recognized in the upper body inclination as well as in the force plate data. Finally, the patient is set into the wheelchair. In phases 'Stand Patient Up' and 'Sit Patient Down', the participant achieves sagittal upper body inclinations of up to 40°. These angles are only limited acceptable and were also noted by the kinesthetic instructor (see Table 3).
This example shows that additional sensors can contribute to training by providing supplementary objective measurements.

In Fig. 5, only sagittal upper body flexion was considered as an example. Flexion in the lateral direction, as well as torsions, are of course also calculated. In addition, the system can also be extended to evaluate the leg position in order to capture further important aspects of ergonomic working. The representation as a skeleton model with objective measurement values can help to reflect retrospectively nursing actions.

In addition to the wearable systems, an optical system is still useful, since the pure use of a sensor suit lacks important contextual information and, for example, the patient is not represented.

The sensor system is extended by using SEMG to record muscle activity data while transferring the patient from bed to wheelchair. Given participant 424, sagittal upper body inclination exceeded an acceptable limit (see Fig. 5 and Table 3) while transferring the patient. Specifically, the phase 'Stand Patient Up' showed the highest sagittal upper body inclination (see Fig. 5) thus requiring further analysis. The nursing teacher instructed the participants to perform the transfer task ergonomically regarding the Kinesthetic care conception [36]. This included working with a straight back while using the leg muscles to lift the patient. Therefore, 424 stood parallel to the patient sitting at the care bed's edge. Then, the participant prepared and shifted the weight through trunk inclination (see Fig. 5) and bent the knee to squat down (see Fig. 7). Here, the upper body is tilted forward (see Fig. 7) and thigh muscle activation is responsible for concentric knee extension as well as eccentrically resisting the flexion of the knee. When lifting the patient to an upright position a combination of different movement patterns occurs, while maintaining stability through adequate muscle activation (see Fig. 6). When rising from the squatting position to lift and stand the patient up, both the VM and RF contract at the same time and BF muscle activity increases (see Fig. 6).

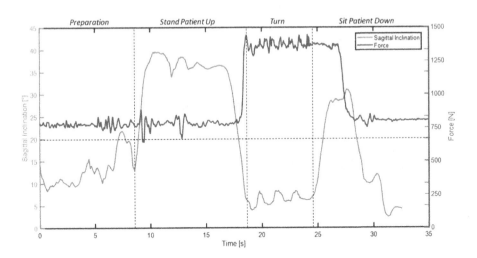

Fig. 5. Sagittal upper body inclination as well as ground reaction force during the transfer from the edge of a bed to a wheelchair for participant 424.

Mean muscle activity of VM, RF and BF of 424 while squatting and lifting the patient are shown in Fig. 7.

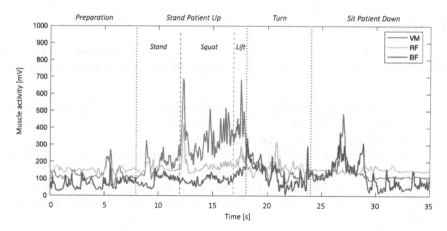

Fig. 6. SEMG data of manual patient transfer from bed to wheelchair for participant 424. The time courses for vastus medialis (VM), rectus femoris (RF) and biceps femoris (BF) muscle activity are shown as a function of the caregiving cycle. The task is divided into four main phases indicated by dashed vertical lines. The phase 'Stand Patient Up' is subdivided into 'Stand', 'Squat' and 'Lift' (see Fig. 7).

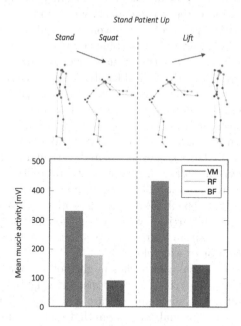

Fig. 7. Mean SEMG data of the subphases 'Squat' and 'Lift' of the manual patient transfer phase 'Stand Patient Up'.

4   Discussion

Considering foreseeable growing demands of care activities, increased effectivity in education of care activities is essential and should address following requirements:

- Increased automation in training of correct executions of care activities (such as patient transfer) can assure a consistent quality of education with decreasing distribution of trainers and students.
- It is critical to minimize the risk of low back pain resulting from falsely executed physically demanding activities, such as patient transfer. Thus an increased level of detail must be achieved in educating caregivers to assure optimal movements and postures for such critical activities of high physical load.

The initially proposed visual system has been generally found to address these requirements. The use of the Multi-Kinect-System resulted in a doubling of the feedback duration time in comparison to the analog feedback. The investigation of the keywords used by the trainers within the digital feedback round clarify that this extension is not a result of lower usability, see Table 3. Instead, it is rather caused by a more detailed feedback, which in some cases included the repeated review of critical postures and movements (cells with green background color) and partly included new aspects (blue color).

We also found that some criticisms which have been discussed in the analog-feedback have been missed in the digital feedback (white color). We assume that this is due to the fact that some aspects that at first glance were considered as critical in the analog feedback were assessed as non-critical in the digital feedback after in-depth analysis.

As we have shown in [40] for the established Ovako Working posture Assessment System (OWAS), the risk of work-related muscular-skeletal disorders can be characterised via visual posture inspection with an sufficient inter-rater (inter-observer) agreement. In detail for 20 raters, an inter-rater reliability of $\kappa = 0.98$ for the arms and $\kappa = 0.85$ (66−97%) for the legs and $\kappa = 0.85$ for the upper body (80−96%). Considering this article, we found that for specific participants it was hard to differentiate correct and erroneous postures based on visual inspection, due to visual occlusion or to wide clothing.

Understanding that visual approaches might not support a complete detection of critical postures, the article at hand also investigated additional sensory to support a semiautomatic screening of care activities. By this sensor-fusion-based approach, we expect to enable a system that semi-automatically can screen the execution and determine relevant phases for detailed investigation.

We indicated the ability of an IMU sensor suite to detect critical body postures. On the basis of the sensor suit data upper body inclinations and torsions can be calculated [37] and body postures can be assessed with regard to their hazardousness. The use of vibrotactile feedback [41] in combination with such sensor suites might even enable online-feedback and thereby help students to directly omit erroneous postures.

The use of non-invasive surface electromyography (SEMG) to record muscle activity during care activities is an additional especially promising system extension due to the following reasons. As the recognition of the muscular load enables the detection of faulty executions via specific peaks in muscular load [17,42], these features represent a reliable indicator for erroneous executions.

Besides, the visualization of the load per muscle can be a suitable visual representation to understand the criticality of incorrect postures and the biomechanical fundamentals of the muscular-skeletal interplay that takes part in such care activities. Thus, in addition to the direct educational benefit to create awareness of the criticality and characteristics of unfavorable or erroneous postures, it might as well enhance the understanding of fundamental biomechanical procedures in the human body, a fact which we want to point out by discussing following example of the study cohort:

For compensating lumbosacral loads in manual patient handling, the use of the leg muscles is essential [18] and advised explicitly by professional associations [43–46]. They recommend squat exercise [43–46] for comprehensive lower limb and spine training. In our study, we analyzed muscle activation behavior of three lower limb muscles (VM, RF, BF). The BF is responsible for hip extension, and the VM and RF for knee extension and hip flexion. Before lifting the patient, VM and RF muscle activation are responsible for concentric knee extension and eccentrically resisting the flexion of the knee [47,48]. The biarticular RF transports moments from the hip to the knee, thereby almost acting as a tendon and redistributing these moments [47,48]. Rising to an upright position through extending the hip by the BF pulls on the RF and extends the knee. In this way, the tendon action of the RF is used [47]. It can be assumed, that an increased activity of RF may lead to sacroiliac pain and may cause lower back disorders [49]. Concerning the mean muscle activation patterns of the lifting performance from our study participant 424, the highest value are found in VM, followed by RF and BF. This type of muscle activation patterns is similar to previous measurements [17] as well as to literature findings [47,48].

To sum up, based on our analysis and the care instructor's feedback, the participant 424 conducted an ergonomic transfer while using the power of the leg muscles but with slightly incorrect ergonomics regarding to upper body posture. This resulted in sagittal upper body inclination angles that were only limited acceptable. Thus, the benefits of the additional IMU and EMG sensors as part of such a training-system are undeniable. However, the reported findings represent only initial results, which clearly have to be confirmed in further studies. Additional studies must be established with more participants and specialized Kinaesthetics [36] trainers. Also the current system is far away from a convenient product to be used in everyday lecturing and, thus, has to be enhanced in terms of usability and - as discussed - automatic detection of relevant phases. It is planned to improve the technical parameters of our Multi-Kinect-System regarding resolution, accuracy and usability with the use of new hard- and software. Additionally, the usage of automatic pose evaluation algorithms [50] is planned to support the instructor's feedback. More in-depth analysis of characteristics of unfavorable poses could also lead to a better understanding why they are common. Furthermore, to integrate our system as an inherent part in the education of nurses, the care instructors need training to use the proposed software on their own, without further help.

Acknowledgements. The study work was carried out at the Evangelische Altenpflegeschule e.V. Oldenburg (Evangelical Nursing School) and was funded by the German Federal Ministry of Education and Research (Project No. 02L14A240). The development of the posture analyses system was funded by the Lower Saxony Ministry of Science and Culture under grant number 11-76251-12-10/19 ZN3491 within the Lower Saxony "Vorab" of the Volkswagen Foundation and supported by the Center for Digital Innovations (ZDIN).

References

1. Fifelski-von Böhlen, C., Brinkmann, A., Fudickar, S., Hellmers, S., Hein, A.: Evaluating a multi depth camera system to consolidate ergonomic work in the education of caregivers. In: Proceedings of the 14th International Joint Conference on Biomedical Engineering Systems and Technologies. HEALTHIN. INSTICC, vol. 5, pp. 39–46. SciTePress (2021)
2. UN World Health Organization (WHO), 2020. State of the world's nursing 2020: investing in education, jobs and leadership. www.who.int. Accessed 10 Feb 2022
3. Hayes, L.J., et al.: Nurse turnover: a literature review-an update. Int. J. Nurs. Stud. **49**(7), 887–905 (2012)
4. United Nations. World Populations Prospects 2019, Volume II: Demographic Profiles. United Nations, New York, US (2019)
5. Haddad, L.M., Annamaraju, P., Toney-Butler, T.J.: Nursing Shortage. StatPearls Publishing LLC, Treasure Island (FL) (2021)
6. Weißert-Horn, M., Meyer, M.D., Jacobs, M., Stern, H., Raske, H.W., Landau, K.: Ergonomisch richtige arbeitsweise beim transfer von schwerstpflegebedürftigen. Zeitschrift für Arbeitswissenschaft **68**(3), 175–184 (2014)
7. Kliner, K., Rennert, D., Richter, M.: Gesundheit und Arbeit - Blickpunkt Gesundheitswesen, vol. 106. BKK, Wolfsburg (2017)
8. Cieza, A., Causey, K., Kamenov, K., Hanson, S., Chatterji, S., Vos, T.: Global estimates of the need for rehabilitation based on the global burden of disease study 2019: a systematic analysis for the global burden of disease study 2019. Lancet **396**, 12 (2020)
9. Koyuncu, N., Karcioglu, Ö.: Musculoskeletal complaints in healthcare personnel in hospital. Medicine **97**, 10 (2018)
10. Hartvigsen, J., et al.: What low back pain is and why we need to pay attention. Lancet **391**, 03 (2018)
11. Gilchrist, A., Pokorná, A.: Prevalence of musculoskeletal low-back pain among registered nurses: results of an online survey. J. Clin. Nurs. **30**, 02 (2021)
12. Jaromi, M., Nemeth, A., Kranicz, J., Laczko, T., Betlehem, J.: Treatment and ergonomics training of work-related lower back pain and body posture problems for nurses. J. Clin. Nurs. **21**, 1776–1784 (2012)
13. Hou, J.Y., Shiao, J.S.: Risk factors for musculoskeletal discomfort in nurses. J. Nurs. Res.: JNR **14**, 228–36 (2006)

14. Chung, Y.C., Hung, C.T., Li, S.F., et al.: Risk of musculoskeletal disorder among Taiwanese nurses cohort: a nationwide population-based study. BMC Musculoskelet Disord **14**, 144 (2013)
15. Jäger, M., et al.: Zentralblatt für Arbeitsmedizin, Arbeitsschutz und Ergonomie **64**(2), 98–112 (2014). https://doi.org/10.1007/s40664-013-0010-4
16. Brinkmann, A.: The aal/care laboratory - a healthcare prevention system for caregivers. Nanomaterials Energy **9**, 27–38 (2020)
17. Brinkmann, A., et al.: Quantification of lower limb and spine muscle activity in manual patient handling - a case study. In: Proceedings of the 18th Annual International Conference on Informatics, Management, and Technology in Healthcare (ICIMTH 2020), pp. 249–252. IOS press (2020)
18. Brinkmann, A.: Relevance of the lower limb in the context of musculoskeletal stress in nursing. Pflegewissenschaft **4**, 229–237 (2021)
19. Rashidi, P., Mihailidis, A.: A survey on ambient-assisted living tools for older adults. IEEE J. Biomed. Health Inf. **17**, 579–90 (2013)
20. Abdollahi, T., et al.: Effect of an ergonomics educational program on musculoskeletal disorders in nursing staff working in the operating room: a quasi-randomized controlled clinical trial. Int. J. Environ. Res. Public Health **17**, 7333 (2020)
21. Garg, A., Kapellusch, J.: Long-term efficacy of an ergonomics program that includes patient-handling devices on reducing musculoskeletal injuries to nursing personnel. Hum. Factors **54**, 608–25 (2012)
22. Tamminen, L., Kimmo, N.: Development of an education scheme for improving perioperative nurses' competence in ergonomics. Work **64**, 1–7 (2019)
23. Doss, R., Robathan, J., Abdel-Malek, D., Holmes, M.W.: Posture coaching and feedback during patient handling in a student nurse population. IISE Trans. Occup. Ergon. Hum. Factors **6**(3–4), 116–127 (2018)
24. Zhao, W.: A privacy-aware kinect-based system for healthcare professionals. In: 2016 IEEE International Conference on Electro Information Technology (EIT), pp. 0205–0210 (2016)
25. Büker, L.C., Zuber, F., Hein, A., Fudickar, S.: Hrdepthnet: depth image-based marker-less tracking of body joints. Sensors **21**(4), 1356 (2021)
26. Lins, C., et al.: Determining cardiopulmonary resuscitation parameters with differential evolution optimization of sinusoidal curves. In: Proceedings of the 11th International Joint Conference on Biomedical Engineering Systems and Technologies, pp. 665–670 (2018)
27. Lins, C., Eckhoff, D., Klausen, A., Hellmers, S., Hein, A., Fudickar, S.: Cardiopulmonary resuscitation quality parameters from motion capture data using differential evolution fitting of sinusoids. Appl. Soft Comput. J. **79**, 300–309 (2019)
28. Clark, R.A., Mentiplay, B.F., Hough, E., Pua, Y.H.: Three-dimensional cameras and skeleton pose tracking for physical function assessment: a review of uses, validity, current developments and kinect alternatives. Gait Posture **68**, 193–200 (2019)
29. Kowalski, M., Naruniec, J., Daniluk, M.: Livescan3d: a fast and inexpensive 3d data acquisition system for multiple kinect v2 sensors. In: 2015 International Conference on 3D Vision, pp. 318–325. IEEE (2015)
30. Fifelski, C., Brinkmann, A., Ortmann, S.M., Isken, M., Hein, A.: Multi depth camera system for 3d data recording for training and education of nurses. In: 2018 International Conference on Computational Science and Computational Intelligence (CSCI), pp. 679–684 (2018)
31. Reichold, J., et al.: Human-machine interaction in care-education. In: Burghardt, M., Wimmer, R., Wolff, C., Womser-Hacker, C., (eds.) Mensch und Computer 2017 - Workshopband, pp. 351–356, Regensburg (2017). Gesellschaft für Informatik e.V

32. Fankhauser, P., Bloesch, M., Rodriguez, D., Kaestner, R., Hutter, M., Siegwart, R.: Kinect v2 for mobile robot navigation: evaluation and modeling. In: 2015 International Conference on Advanced Robotics (ICAR), pp. 388–394. IEEE (2015)
33. Shadow. Motion Workshop, Motion Capture System (2020). https://www.motionshadow.com. Accessed 03 Feb 2022
34. Hermens, H.J., Freriks, B., Merletti, R., Stegemann, D., Block, J., Rau, G.: European recommendations for surface electromyography: results of the seniam project. Roessingh Res. Develop. **8**(2), 13–54 (1999)
35. Musante, K., DeWalt, B.R.: Participant Observation: A Guide for Fieldworkers. Altamira, Lanham (2002)
36. Hatch, F., Maietta, L.K.: Health Development and Human Activity. Urban and Fischer, Munich (2003)
37. Hellmers, S., Brinkmann, A., Böhlen, C., Lau, S., Diekmann, R., Hein, A.: Assessing postures and mechanical loads during patient transfers. In: Proceedings of the 14th International Joint Conference on Biomedical Engineering Systems and Technologies, HEALTHINF, INSTICC, pp. 21–29. SciTePress (2021)
38. Freitag, S., Fincke, I., Dulon, M., Ellegast, R., Nienhaus, A.: Messtechnische analyse von belastenden körperhaltungen bei pflegekräften: eine geriatrische station im vergleich mit anderen krankenhausstationen. ErgoMed **31**, 130–140 (2007)
39. Panjabi, M.M., White, A.A.: Clinical Biomechanics of the Spine. Lippincott, Philadelphia (1990)
40. Lins, C., Fudickar, S., Hein, A.: Owas inter-rater reliability. Appl. Ergon. **93**, 103357 (2021)
41. Lins, C., Fudickar, S.J., Gerka, A., Hein, A.: A wearable vibrotactile interface for unfavorable posture awareness warning. In: Proceedings 4th International Conference on Information and Communication Technologies for Ageing Well and e-Health (ICT4AWE 2018), Funchal/Madeira, Portugal (2018)
42. Brinkmann, A., Fifelski-von Böhlen, C., Hellmers, S., Meyer, O., Diekmann, R., Hein, A.: Physical burden in manual patient handling: Quantification of lower limb EMG muscle activation patterns of healthy individuals lifting different loads ergonomically. In: Proceedings of the 14th International Joint Conference on Biomedical Engineering Systems and Technologies, HEALTHINF, INSTICC, vol. 5, pp. 451–458. SciTePress (2021)
43. Deyo, R.A., Weinstein, J.N.: Low back pain. N. Engl. J. Med. **344**, 363–370 (2001)
44. Ellapen, T.J., Narsigan, S.: Work related musculoskeletal disorders among nurses: systematic review. Ergonomics **4**, S4-03 (2014)
45. Baum, F., Beck, B.B., Fischer, B., et al.: Fischer. Topas r - konzept der bgw für pflege und betreuung. Berufsgenossenschaft Gesundheitsdiens und Wohlfahrtspflege (2012)
46. Kusma, B., Glaesener, J.-J., Brandenburg, S., et al.: Der pflege das kreuz stärken. Trauma Berufskrankheit **17**(4), 244–249 (2015)
47. Roebroeck, M.E., Doorenbosch, C.A.M., Harlaar, J., Jacobs, R., Lankhorst, G.J.: Biomechanics and muscular-activity during sit-to-stand transfer. Clinical Biomechanics (Bristol, Avon) **9**, 235–44 (1994)
48. Schoenfeld, B.: Squatting kinematics and kinetics and their application to exercise performance. J. Strength Conditioning Res. Natl. Strength Conditioning Assoc. **24**, 3497–506 (2010)
49. Hammer, N., et al.: Pelvic belt effects on health outcomes and functional parameters of patients with sacroiliac joint pain. PLoS ONE **10**, 08 (2015)
50. Stoffert, V.: Analyse and einstufung von korperhaltungen bei der arbeit nach der owas-methode. Z. Arbeitswiss. **1**, 31–38 (1985)

Evaluation of Algorithms to Measure a Psychophysical Threshold Using Digital Applications

Silvia Bonfanti and Angelo Gargantini(✉)

Department of Management, Information and Production Engineering,
University of Bergamo, Bergamo, Italy
{silvia.bonfanti,angelo.gargantini}@unibg.it

Abstract. The use of digital applications like in mobile phone or on the web to perform psychophysical measurements led to the introduction of algorithms to guide the users in test execution. In this paper we show four algorithms, two already well known: STRICTN and PEST, and a two that we propose: PESTN and BESTN. All the algorithms aim at estimating the level of a psychophysical capability by performing a sequence of simple tests; starting from initial level N, the test is executed until the target level is reached. They differ in the choice of the next steps in the sequences and the stopping condition. We have simulated the application of the algorithms and we have compared them by answering a set of research questions. Finally, we provide guidelines to choose the best algorithm based on the test goal. We found that while STRICTN provides optimal results, it requires the largest number of steps, and this may hinder its use; PESTN can overcome these limits without compromising the final results.

1 Introduction

The use of computers and digital applications to perform psychophysical measurements has given rise to several automatic procedures to be applied. The objective of these procedures is to determine as rapidly and precisely as possible the value of a psychophysical variable.

In the paper, we focus on estimating psychophysical thresholds by providing a sequence of simple tasks to the patients. Following the classification of methodological for psychophysical evaluation proposed in [12], we can consider three parameters: the task of an observer to judge, stimulus arrangement, and statistical measure. Based on the proposed classification, the set of algorithms taken into account for the comparison fall into the following groups. Regarding the task, we assume that the observer's task is the *classification* of some type. The observer, once a stimulus has been presented, has to judge if some attribute or aspect is present or absent or to classify the stimulus. Regarding the stimuli to be presented, we assume that are *fixed*, i.e. they do not vary during the time they are being observed[1]. Usually, of course, they are varied between observations.

---

[1] This assumption could be relaxed provided that the classification of the stimulus is meaningful.

© The Author(s), under exclusive license to Springer Nature Switzerland AG 2022
C. Gehin et al. (Eds.): BIOSTEC 2021, CCIS 1710, pp. 139–157, 2022.
https://doi.org/10.1007/978-3-031-20664-1_8

Regarding the measure of stimulus, we assume that a level is associated with every observation and this level is used to estimate the psychophysical threshold. Furthermore, in our case study, we assume that the psychophysical of the user could be null as a result of missing capability by the user and the test should discover that.

Before the introduction of digital technologies, psychophysical measurements were made by using simple devices or printed paper cards and the observer had to judge the responses. The observer guided the test procedure that could be partially fixed based on test execution. Nowadays, tests are becoming more computerized, partially automatized and the observer may have only partial control during the test execution. The test execution and the estimation of the psychophysical threshold are decided by an algorithm that should correctly diagnose the level of the measured parameter, by minimizing the number of false positive/negative.

The advantages are that the observer cannot interfere with the testing process and the results can be objectively validated. However, there is the risk that the algorithms are not precise or they are not as efficient as the observer would be thanks to the experience in providing these tests. For this reason, in this paper, we present and compare three algorithms that could be used for psychophysical measurements. We assume that the desired psychophysical capability can range from a max value to a minimal (lower) level. The test starts at level N and finishes when the user reaches his best capacity level[2].

The presented work is an extension of the paper [2]. We have extended the paper by introducing a new algorithm (the BESTN algorithm) and we have compared its performance with those of the already presented algorithms. Moreover, we have implemented a new scenario for the simulation in which we have considered that during a test (especially if it is long) the *attention* of the patient decreases.

The paper is organized as follows. In Sect. 2 we present the algorithms and the simulation protocol is introduced in Sect. 3. In Sect. 4 we answer a set of research questions about the features of the algorithms and we provide guidelines to choose the algorithm based on the test goal in Sect. 5. Related works are reported in Sect. 6.

2   Algorithms

In this section, we present the algorithms we have implemented to measure a psychophysical threshold: STRICTN, PEST, both well known in the literature and widely used, and two new ones, PESTN and BESTN, that try to improve the performances of the previous two.

All the proposed algorithms start from the assumptions that there are several *levels* of a given psychophysical capability, every person has a different *threshold* of such psychophysical capability, and the algorithm must evaluate this threshold. The basic idea behind all the proposed algorithms is the following. The

---

[2] The data and materials for all experiments are available at https://github.com/silviabonfanti/3d4ambAlgorithms.git.

test starts at *init* level, which corresponds to the easiest level (decided by the observer), and it is changed until the person is no longer able to answer correctly. The best reachable level that the person can achieve is called *target* and it corresponds to the most difficult level of the test. In this paper we assume that the *init* is greater than *target*, so for instance, the test starts from 10 and must reach 1 to measure the psychophysical capability. The level is therefore decremented until it reaches the minimum possible. However, not all the subjects can reach the *target* since some may have a limited psychophysical capability. The problem the algorithms try to address is to find the *threshold* of the single person, that we assume to between *init* and the *target*. To find such threshold, at every level the person is asked to guess the right answer at that given level, and after that the algorithm proceeds depending on the correctness of the answer. When the user finishes the test, the result can be: 1. PASSED at level X: the user has passed successfully the test and his psychophysical capability *threshold* is certified at level X. 2. FAILED: the user did not pass the test because the algorithm has found that he does not have the psychophysical capability.

The algorithms differ from one another in the following aspects: 1. when the user guesses right but the *target* i snot reached, what is the next tested level; 2. the number of right answers given at the *target* level to be certified; 3. the error management when the user does not guess the right answer; 4. the policy to interrupt the test and certify or not the level.

All the algorithms are explained in the next sections. All can be generalized in case the tests are performed using a different scale of levels, for instance by starting to 1 and going to a maximum value. Moreover, it is possible to start the test from a level which is not the easiest one.

2.1 STRICTN

The strict staircase algorithm, STRICTN, shown in Fig. 1, is well known in the literature and widely used (for instance [18]) since it can measure precisely the psychophysical threshold. However its main disadvantage is that it takes a lot of time, mostly when the difference between the starting threshold and target threshold is high. The test starts at the starting threshold `initThreshold`. If the user guesses the answer (`answer=RIGHT`) the `currentThreshold` (the threshold currently under test) is decremented. The algorithm stops in *PASSED* state when the `targetThreshold` is reached (`currentThreshold = targetThreshold`) and the user answers correctly N times, where N is equals to 3 or to a value chosen at the beginning of the test (`rightAnswersToCertify`). If the answer is `WRONG` the threshold is re-tested, if another error is performed the threshold is incremented and it becomes the new target (only higher levels can be certified at this point). A threshold is *PASSED* if the user responds correctly N times at that threshold. In the event that the person is not able to answer correctly N times the test result is *FAILED*.

The STRICTN algorithm generally requires long trials. To overcome the disadvantage of this, we have introduced the BESTN algorithm, explained in

---

Algorithm 1. STRICTN.

Input : initThreshold, targetThreshold, rightAnswersToCertify
Output: currentResult, currentThreshold

currentThreshold = initThreshold;
do
    | /* store the number of RIGHT/WRONG answers for each threshold   */
    | getAndStoreAnswer(currentThreshold, answer);
    | switch *answer* do
    | | case *RIGHT* do
    | | | if *currentThreshold* > *targetThreshold* then
    | | | | currentThreshold - -;
    | | | | currentResult = CONTINUE;
    | | | else
    | | | | /* compare the number of RIGHT answers at current threshold   */
    | | | | if *getNumAnswers(currentThreshold, RIGHT)* >=
    | | | | *rightAnswersToCertify* then
    | | | | | currentResult = PASSED;
    | | | | else
    | | | | | currentResult = CONTINUE;
    | | | | end
    | | | end
    | | case *WRONG* do
    | | | /* compare the number of WRONG answers at current threshold   */
    | | | if *getNumAnswers(currentThreshold, WRONG)* >= WRONG_TO_STOP
    | | | then
    | | | | if *currentThreshold* < *initThreshold* then
    | | | | | currentThreshold ++;
    | | | | | targetThreshold = currentThreshold;
    | | | | | currentResult = CONTINUE;
    | | | | else
    | | | | | currentResult = FAILED;
    | | | | end
    | | | else
    | | | | currentResult = CONTINUE;
    | | | end
    | end
while *currentResult* == *CONTINUE*;
return *[currentResult, currentThreshold]*

---

the next section, which reduces the number of right answers requested to certify a level.

2.2 BESTN

The key concept behind BESTN algorithm (see Algorithm 2) is that the user has to answer `rightAnswerToCertify` times correctly in the same threshold or in two consecutive thresholds. Moreover, this algorithm set the maximum answers (`RIGHT` or `WRONG`) possible for each threshold which is set to `answersToCertify` times. The test starts at `initThreshold`, if the person answer is `RIGHT` and the `currentThreshold` does not correspond to the `targetThreshold`, the threshold is decremented and the test `CONTINUE`s. In case the current threshold corresponds to the threshold to be certified (`currentThreshold=targetThreshold`) there are two different options:

– the user has answered correctly `rightAnswerToCertify` times in the current threshold (if current threshold is the lower certifiable) or the user has

---

Algorithm 2. BESTN.

Input   : initThreshold, targetThreshold, rightAnswersToCertify, answersToCertify
Output: currentResult, currentThreshold

currentThreshold = initThreshold;
do
   getAndStoreAnswer(currentThreshold, answer);
   switch *answer* **do**
      case *RIGHT* **do**
         if *currentThreshold* > *targetThreshold* **then**
            currentThreshold - -;
            currentResult = CONTINUE;
         else if *(getNumAnswers(currentThreshold, RIGHT) +*
         getNumAnswers(currentThreshold+1, RIGHT) >=
         rightAnswersToCertify) **then**
            currentResult = PASSED;
         else
            currentResult = CONTINUE;
         end
      case *WRONG* **do**
         if *getNumAnswers(currentThreshold, WRONG) == WRONG_TO_STOP*
         then
            if *currentThreshold* < *initThreshold* **then**
               currentResult = CONTINUE;
               currentThreshold ++;
               targetThreshold = currentThreshold;
            else
               currentResult = FAILED;
            end
         else if *getNumAnswers(currentThreshold) == answersToCertify* **then**
            if *currentThreshold* < *initThreshold* **then**
               if *(getNumAnswers(currentThreshold, RIGHT) +*
               getNumAnswers(currentThreshold+1, RIGHT) >=
               rightAnswersToCertify) **then**
                  currentResult = PASSED;
               else
                  currentResult = CONTINUE;
                  currentThreshold ++;
                  targetThreshold = currentThreshold;
               end
            else
               currentResult = FAILED;
            end
         else
            currentResult = CONTINUE;
         end
   end
while *(currentResult = CONTINUE)*;
return *[currentResult, currentThreshold]*

---

answered correctly `answersToCertify` times in two consecutive thresholds (current threshold and previous threshold): the test finishes in `PASSED` state.
– the user has not answer correctly enough times, so the test `CONTINUE`.

In case the user has answered `WRONG` enough times (`WRONG_TO_STOP`) at the same threshold and the current threshold is lower than the maximum certifiable threshold (`initThreshold`), the user can `CONTINUE` the test, the `targetThreshold` is set equals to the `currentThreshold`. Nevertheless, if the current threshold is equal to the `initThreshold`, the test stops and the test `FAILED`. When the second answer to current threshold

---

Algorithm 3. PEST.

---

    input : initThreshold, targetThreshold
    output: currentResult, currentThreshold

    currentThreshold = initThreshold;
    limitL = currentThreshold; limitR = targetThreshold;
    chance = 2;
    do
        getAndStoreAnswer(currentThreshold, answer);
        switch *answer* **do**
            case *RIGHT* **do**
                limitL = currentThreshold;
                currentThreshold = floor((limitL + limitR) / 2);
                if *limitL == limitR* **then**
                    currentResult = PASSED; currentThreshold = limitL;
                else
                    currentResult = CONTINUE;
                end
            case *WRONG* **do**
                if *currentThreshold == initThreshold OR limitL == limitR* **then**
                    if *chance > 0* **then**
                      chance−; currentResult = CONTINUE;
                    else
                      currentResult = FAILED;
                    end
                else
                  limitR = currentThreshold;
                  currentThreshold = ceil((limitL + limitR) / 2);
                  currentResult = CONTINUE;
                end
        end
    while *(currentResult = CONTINUE)*;
    return *[currentResult, currentThreshold]*

---

is wrong but the user has previously answered correctly `rightAnswerTo-Certify` the test finishes `PASSED`. If the second answer to current threshold is wrong and the previous conditions are not satisfied, the test `CONTINUE`s, the threshold is incremented and the new target threshold is equal to the `currentThreshold`. Finally, if the user answers `answersToCertify` times at current threshold (one correctly and one not) and the current threshold is equals to `maxThreshold`, the test finishes `FAILED`.

Although the required steps are decreased due to the improvement made compared to STRICTN algorithm, it still high. For this reason, the PEST algorithm, explained in the next section, has been introduced in the past, with the aim of reducing the number of required steps.

2.3 PEST

PEST (Parameter Estimation by Sequential Testing) algorithm (see Algorithm 3) has been proposed in [13]. This algorithm belongs to the adaptive methods family which are modified according to the moment-by-moment responses. The goal of PEST is to identify the psychophysical threshold with a minimum number of possible steps. The test starts at `initThreshold` and the goal is to reach the `targetThreshold`, the most difficult. Threshold of the test are into a window bounded by a left limit `limitL` and a right limit `limitR`. Initially, the variables `limitL` and `limitR` are set respectively to the starting level `initThreshold` and the `targetThreshold`. If the user answer is RIGHT the left limit is set to the current threshold and in the next step the tested threshold is equals to the round downward the mean between `limitL` and `limitR` to its nearest integer. The test continues until `limitL` and `limitR` correspond, the test finishes in PASSED state at current threshold. If the user answer is WRONG, the right limit is set to the current threshold and in the next step the tested threshold is equals to the round upward the mean between `limitL` and `limitR` to its nearest integer. Also in this case, the test continues until *limitL* and *lim-*

Algorithm 4. PESTN.

input : initThreshold, maxThreshold, targetThreshold, rightAnswersToCertify
output: currentResult, currentThreshold

do
    if *firstPhase* **then**
        if *answer* == *WRONG* **then**
            if *answers[limitL - 1] == 0 && currentThreshold == maxThreshold* **then**
                answers[limitL - 1]–;
            else if *answers[limitL - 1] == -1 && currentThreshold==maxThreshold*
            then
                currentResult=FAILED;
            else
                limitR = currentThreshold; limitsOneStep();
                currentThreshold = ceil((limitL+limitR)/2);
                answers[limitR - 1] - -;
            end
        else if *answer* == *RIGHT* **then**
            limitL = currentThreshold; limitsOneStep();
            currentThreshold = floor((limitL+limitR)/2);
            answers[limitL - 1] ++;
        end
    else
        if *answer* == *RIGHT* **then**
            answers[currentThreshold - 1] ++;
        else if *answer* == *WRONG* **then**
            answers[currentThreshold - 1] -= weight; weight = weight * 3;
        end
        if *answers[currentThreshold - 1] >= rightAnswersToCertify* **then**
            currentResult = PASSED;
        else if *(answers[currentThreshold - 1] <= -2) & (currentThreshold ¡*
        maxThreshold) **then**
            weight = 1; currentThreshold ++;
        else if *(answers[currentThreshold - 1] <= -2) & (currentThreshold ==*
        maxThreshold) **then**
            currentResult=FAILED;
        end
    end
while *(currentResult = CONTINUE)*;
return *[currentResult, currentThreshold]*

Function limitsOneStep:
    if *(limitL - limitR) == 1* **then**
        firstPhase = false; currentThreshold = limitR;
        if *limitR != 1* **then**
            weight = weight * 3;
        end
    end
end Function

itR correspond or `currentThreshold` reaches `initThreshold`, but if the user answers wrongly twice at `currentThreshold` the test finishes in *FAILED* state.

Compared to BESTN and STRICTN the number of steps required for PEST is significantly decreased, but at the end of the test, we are not sure that the certified threshold is the real threshold owned by the user. This is because the PEST algorithm requires only one correct answer to certify the target threshold, and it can be right just for randomness. For this reason, we have improved the PEST algorithm as explained in the next section.

2.4   PESTN

PESTN (presented in Algorithm 4) is based on PEST algorithm presented in Sect. 2.3. The main difference compared to the PEST algorithm is that a threshold is `PASSED` if the user answers correctly `rightAnswersToCertify` times at the threshold to be certified. The number of answers given at threshold N is saved into a vector `answers[]` at position N-1. Initially, the algorithm follows the PEST flow, until the set of certifiable thresholds is reduced to two consecutive levels. A `RIGHT` answer increments the number of right answers to the current threshold, a `WRONG` answer decrements the corresponding value. The test is `PASSED` if the user gives `rightAnswersToCertify` right answers at threshold i. In the case of two wrong answers at threshold i, the threshold is incremented until a higher threshold is certified or the threshold reaches the maximum certifiable. If the user does not answer correctly `rightAnswersToCertify` times at the same threshold, the test finishes in `FAILED` state.

3   Simulation Protocol

In this paper, we do not apply the algorithms to a specific case study, but we run simulation assuming that we have a test and we want to certify a psychophysical threshold. The test starts at level N, it is decremented if the user guesses the answer, otherwise the level is incremented. If the user is not able to guess any answer the test fails. The choice of the next level at each step follows one of the algorithms described in Sect. 2. To test the operation of the algorithms, we have executed the tests on virtual patients, automatically generated with software. We have simulated 48000 patients and using the proposed algorithms we tried to certify different level of the psychophysical threshold under certification. For each user, we randomly select the answer (`RIGHT` or `WRONG`). We have preferred `RIGHT` answers when the patient is at level i and his psychophysical threshold is greater or equal to i, `WRONG` answers when the level i of the test is more difficult compared to his psychophysical threshold. To decide the distribution of `RIGHT` and `WRONG` answer, we have simulated four scenarios by assigning a probability to the `RIGHT` and `WRONG` answers as shown in Table 1.

The first scenario, *Scenario 0*, we have assumed that the user gives the `RIGHT` answer if he has the current psychophysical threshold, otherwise, the answer is `WRONG`. This is the ideal scenario, but it does not happen in practice because the user may choose a different answer e.g. because it tries to guess. We have considered these cases by adding two scenarios: *Scenario 1* and *Scenario 2*. The difference is in the probability of giving the WRONG answer. The WRONG answer is selected with a probability of 0.9 in *Scenario 1* and 0.75 in *Scenario 2* when the user does not have the current psychophysical threshold. The RIGHT answer is selected with a probability of 0.9 if the user has the current psychophysical threshold. *Scenario 2* is likely to happen when the user has a limited set of answers, for instance four, and a randomly chosen answer has a not negligible possibility to be the right one even if the current psychophysical threshold is below his psychophysical level. The last scenario starts from *Scenario 1* and it considers the decreasing of the level of attention. During the screening performed to measure the stereoacuity presented in [3], we have noticed that after around 8 steps of the test, the users were annoying and their level of attention decreased. To simulate this situation, after 8 steps, we have increased the probability of giving a WRONG answer.

We have simulated all the algorithms with the same level of probabilities twice, in order to perform a *test-retest* assessment too. The goal is to evaluate test repeatability: the proposed algorithms guarantee the same level of certification in both simulations.

We have performed null hypothesis significance testing (NHST) for the evaluation and comparison of algorithms. NHST is a method of statistical inference by which an experimental factor is tested against a hypothesis of no effect or no relationship based on a given observation. In our case, we will formulate the null hypothesis following the schema that the algorithm X is no better than the others by considering the feature Y. Then, we will use the observations in order to estimate the probability or *p-value* that the null hypothesis is true, i.e. that the effect of X over the value Y is not statistically significant. If the probability is very small (below a given threshold), then the null hypothesis can be rejected.

Table 1. Probabilities of RIGHT and WRONG answers.

	S0	S1	S2	S3
Prob. RIGHT answer: currentLevel $\geq$ user psychophysical threshold	1	0.9	0.9	0.9
Prob. WRONG answer: currentLevel $<$ user psychophysical threshold or no psychophysical stimulus detection	1	0.9	0.75	0.9 (for the first 8 steps)
				0.75 (after 8 steps)

4   Analysis of the Results

After we have gathered all the data form the simulation, we have performed a statistical analysis by answering a sequence of research questions (RQs) in order to extract useful information. For each RQ, we have formulated a null hypothesis (H_0) which posits the opposite compared to what we expect.

RQ1: Which is the Algorithm that Minimizes the Number of False Positive/False Negative?

Besides measuring the psychophysical threshold of each person, the algorithm checks if that person has that psychophysical capability or not. The user may guess the right answer by chance, even if he or she is not actually capable of passing the test. On the other hand, we do not exclude that the patient gives the wrong answer even he or she has the desired capability. For these reasons, a test result could be *PASSED* when the patient does not have the capability, or *FAILED* even if the patient has the capability. These cases are called *false positive* and *false negative*. False positive is an error in the final result in which the test indicates the presence of the desired capability when in reality it is not present. Contrariwise, false negative is an error in which the test indicates the absence of the capability when the patient has it. We expect that one of the proposed algorithms minimize the number of false positive and false negative compared to the others.

To measure if an algorithm is better than the others in terms of false positive/false negative, we have introduced a statistical test called *Proportion Hypothesis Tests for Binary Data* [5]. The result of this test is the p-value, based on this value we have decided to reject/accept the null hypothesis. The p-value threshold chose to determine if the null hypothesis is accepted or not is 0.005, this value guarantees that the obtained results are statistically significant. We started from two null hypothesis, one for the false positive and the other for the false negative:

H0_FP: No algorithm is better than other in false positive minimization.
H0_FN: No algorithm is better than other in false negative minimization.

The p-values obtained are shown in Table 2, the p-value of Scenario 0 is not reported because this is ideal scenario in which no false positive/false negative are detected. Given the results we can reject both the H0_FN and H0_FP. This means that there is an algorithm which guarantees a lower rate of false negative and false positive compared to the others.

Table 2. Proportion Hypothesis Tests for Binary Data: p-value.

	S1	S2	S3
p-value FN	2.2e−16	2.2e−16	2.2e−16
p-value FP	1.58e−5	0.0001	0.0099

Furthermore, this is confirmed by the number of false positives and false negatives detected as reported in Table 3. The data proves that STRICTN guarantees a lower rate of false negatives, followed by the PESTN. Regarding the false positive, PEST and PESTN perform similarly well, while STRICTN suffers in the scenarios S2 and S3. BESTN instead while produces an acceptable number of false negatives, it suffers from an excess of false positives.

Table 3. Number of false positive and false negative.

Algorithm	False negatives			False positives		
	S1	S2	S3	S1	S2	S3
STRICTN	2	35	1	56	74	77
BESTN	16	77	15	101	103	91
PEST	70	178	73	55	57	57
PESTN	9	79	8	52	54	58

Furthermore, to compare the algorithms we measure the *sensitivity* and the *specificity*. The sensitivity of a test is also called the true positive rate (TPR) and is computed as TP/P where TP is the number of true positive and P is the number of positive results. The sensitivity is the probability that a person without the capability (positive) reaches *FAILED* result. The specificity of a test, also referred to as the true negative rate (TNR), is computed as TN/N where TN is the number of true negative and N is the number of negative results. The specificity is the probability that a person with the capability reaches *PASSED* result. The values are reported in Table 4. In our test we assume that the sensitivity is more important than the specificity, since we want to be minimized the cases where the capability is not present but the test is PASSED nonetheless.

Scenario S0 has the highest value of sensitivity and specificity (as expected) because it simulates the ideal situation in which all the patients have been certified with the target level and the patients without the capability have not been certified by the test. Since in terms of false negative there is an algorithm better than the other, we can notice that the sensitivity has different values based on the algorithm used and the scenario tested. The lowest value of sensitivity belongs to PEST algorithm in all scenarios, particularly in *Scenario 2*, while the algorithm with the highest value of sensitivity is STRICTN. The PESTN, although cannot perform well as the STRICTN, is very close to it. Regarding the specificity, PEST over performs the others, while BESTN is the worst.

RQ2: Which is the Algorithm that Minimizes the Number of Steps?

We have formulated the following null hypothesis to answer to RQ2:

H0: All the algorithms perform test with the same number of steps.

First of all, we have computed the average of steps for each algorithm and for each scenario (see Table 5). From the table, we can observe that STRICTN and BESTN algorithms are those with the higher average number of steps, PEST is

Table 4. Sensitivity and Specificity.

Algorithm	Specificity				Sensitivity			
	S0	S1	S2	S3	S0	S1	S2	S3
STRICTN	1	.8231	.8206	.8086	1	.9998	.9948	.9993
BESTN	1	.7707	.7375	.7827	1	.9982	.9864	.9984
PEST	1	.8098	.7786	.9072	1	.9875	.9738	.9894
PESTN	1	.8216	.8384	.8245	1	.9984	.9884	.9978

the algorithm with the lowest number of steps, while PESTN is in the middle. This can be confirmed by the Wilcoxon test [11]. We compare all the algorithms (in twos) to prove if one algorithm performs the test with fewer steps than the others. The p-value of Wilcoxon test are in Table 6, they have been computed under the hypothesis that the algorithm in the row takes fewer steps than the algorithm in the column. If p-value is less than threshold $t = 0.005$, the null hypothesis is disproved otherwise it is approved. In some cases, e.g. the PEST columns, the p-values are higher than the threshold t, and we can disprove the null hypothesis $H0$.

Table 5. The average of steps number.

Algorithm	S0	S1	S2	S3
STRICTN	11.1	12.2	12.4	12.3
BESTN	10.2	10.8	11.0	10.9
PEST	4.61	4.73	4.80	4.76
PESTN	6.54	7.93	8.15	7.90

Table 6. Wilcoxon test for number of steps comparison: p-value.

Algorithm	STRICTN	BESTN	PEST	PESTN
STRICTN	–	1	1	1
BESTN	<2.2e−16 (BESTN < STRICTN)	–	1	1
PEST	<2.2e−16 (PEST < STRICTN)	<2.2e−16 (PEST < BESTN)	–	<2.2e−16 (PEST < PESTN)
PESTN	<2.2e−16 (PESTN < STRICTN)	<2.2e−16 (PESTN < BESTN)	1	–

RQ3: Which is the Algorithm that Guarantees a Greater Number of Times in which the Measured Threshold is Equal to Target Threshold?

We start from the following null hypothesis.

H0: All the algorithms guarantee that the measured threshold is always not equal to the target threshold.

Given the target threshold (the one to be verified) and the measured threshold, we have computed the difference between them. Then, we have counted how many times they are different, the results are in Table 7.

All the algorithms in *S0* correctly certify the target value. In the other scenarios, since wrong answers are possible, sometimes the measured level is not equal to the target, especially for PEST algorithm. The more performing algorithm is the STRICTN because it runs sequentially all levels until the target is reached and it is required to guess three times the correct answer at the target level. The BESTN algorithm is slightly less performing than STRICTN.

Table 7. Times when measured threshold is equal to target threshold over 5,604 *PASSED* simulations - the *FAILED* tests are excluded.

	S0	S1	S2	S3
STRICTN	5,604	4,956	4,929	4,943
BESTN	5,604	4,466	4,608	4,582
PEST	5,604	2,155	2,223	2,123
PESTN	5,604	4,632	4,624	4,582

RQ4: Which is the Algorithm with the Minimum Difference between Target Level and Measured Level?

When the difference between the target level and measured level is not equal to zero, we are interested to know this value. To answers at this RQ, we start from the following null hypothesis:

H0: The difference between the target level and measured level is the same regardless of the algorithm.

The difference between target level and measured level is shown in Fig. 1, Fig. 2 and Fig. 3. In *Scenario 1*, the percentage of cases in which target and measured level are different for each algorithm simulation is the following: 27,00% PEST, 13,31% PESTN, 8,30% STRICTN (the percentage is computed over the 20.000 simulations for each algorithm). We have further investigated for each algorithm the difference between target and measured level. PEST algorithm

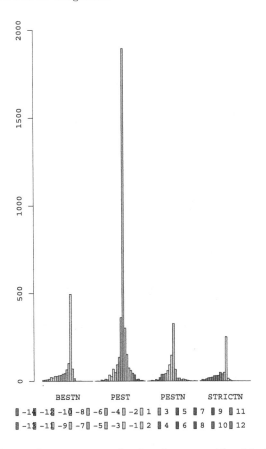

Fig. 1. Difference between target level and measured level in Scenario 1.

certifies user with one level plus or minus in 48,01% of cases and two levels plus or minus in 23,93% of cases. The difference between target and measured level is more than two levels in 28,06% of cases. While these two algorithms have a distribution centered on ±1 and ±2, PESTN and STRICTN distributions are centered on [−4, −1]. STRICTN certifies most of the tests (54,22%) with one level minus and 11,45% of them are certified with two levels minus. Furthermore, we have noticed that all the algorithms, except PEST, are "pessimists" because when the target and measured level are different, in many cases, they certify a higher level compared to the target. With the introduction of higher error probability, *Scenario 2*, the percentage of cases in which target and measured level are different for each algorithm simulation is the following: 42,25% PEST, 22,72% PESTN, 13,33% STRICTN (the percentage is computed over the 20.000 simulations for each algorithm). As expected, the percentages are higher compared to *Scenario 1* because the probability of the wrong answer has been incremented. The difference between target and measured level is centered on [−1, 3] for PEST algorithms and [−2, 2] for PESTN and STRICTN algorithms.

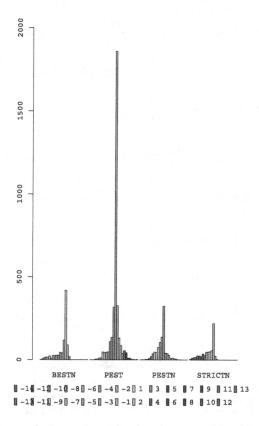

Fig. 2. Difference between target level and measured level in Scenario 2.

In details, PEST has 68,30% of cases in the [−1, 3] interval, while the percentage in interval [−2, 2] is 70,47% and 72,47%for PESTN and STRICTN respectively. S3 has values similar to S1, in some cases the difference is a little bit higher.

RQ5: Which is the Best Algorithm with the Best Performance in Test-retest?

Test-retest evaluates the repeatability of a test administered at two different times, T1 and T2. A test is repeatable if the measure does not change between the two measurements, under the hypothesis that in T1 and T2 the symptomatology is not changed.

We have started the analysis from the following null hypothesis:

H0: All the algorithms have the same performance in test-retest.

We have applied the Pearson Correlation Coefficient to measure the reliability of test-retest. The results are shown in Table 8. As expected, in *Scenario 0* the correlation is equal to 1 for all the algorithms because this scenario guarantees

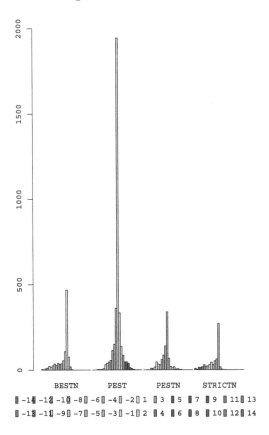

Fig. 3. Difference between target level and measured level in Scenario 3.

that for every simulation the certified level is always the target. In the other scenarios, the algorithm with the highest correlation is PESTN, which has good reliability coefficients (from 0.87 to 0.9). At the opposite, the algorithm with the lower correlation is PEST which has poor repeatability. Similarly to PESTN, BESTN and STRICTN have good reliability in all the scenarios.

5   Discussion

In the previous section, we have answered to a set of RQs to measure sensitivity and sensibility, number of steps, number of times that the measured level is equal to the target level, the difference between target level and measured level (when they are different), and the test-retest reliability. In this section, we want to discuss the results and provide some guidelines to choose the algorithm based on the test goal. For each RQ we have assigned a score from one to three (see Table 9), one is assigned to the algorithm which better satisfies the research question, three is assigned to the worst algorithm under analysis.

Table 8. Pearson correlation test-retest.

	S0	S1	S2	S3
STRICTN	1	0.88	0.85	0.85
BESTN	1	0.84	0.86	0.86
PEST	1	0.81	0.77	0.81
PESTN	1	0.90	0.87	0.88

Table 9. Comparison between RQs: which algorithm guarantee the best performance?

Algorithm	RQ1	RQ2	RQ3	RQ4	RQ5
STRICTN	1	4	1	1	2
BESTN	3	3	4	3	3
PEST	4	1	3	4	4
PESTN	2	2	2	2	1

STRICTN is the algorithm with best performance in guaranteeing the lowest number of false positive and false negative, target level, and measured level are the same most of the time and when they are different the difference is mostly ±1 level. The algorithm with worst performance is PEST. Nevertheless, the number of steps required for the test is very low, in most cases the target level is not equal to the measured level, and the test-retest reliability is the lowest. BESTN algorithm has similar performance to PEST, moreover it requires lot of steps to perform tests. When it is required an algorithm with good performance, but with a limited number of steps to complete the test, PESTN is a good compromise because it can be applied in around half of the steps compared to STRICTN. It has high sensitivity and sensibility, and the measured level is equal to the target in a large number of cases and when they are not equal the difference is minimal. Furthermore, it guarantees the best test-retest reliability.

Generally, we did not notice a big difference between *S1* and S3, in which we have included the decreasing of attention. This can be because we have considered tests with limited number of steps. We think that this scenario requires a more in-depth analysis, because, from our experience, when tests become long the attention (and also the patience) of patients decrease.

6   Related Work

In this section, we present the algorithms used in literature for the stereoacuity measurement. In papers [1,8] the authors apply the PEST algorithm to measure stereoacuity using the Freiburg Test and, as demonstrated also by our case study, the proposed algorithm allowed to save time during the stereoacuity measurement. We found that Staircase algorithm is often used in the literature, with some minimal differences. In papers [10,15–17], stereoacuity is measured using staircase, the disparity is increased/decreased of one level. The disparity is increased of one level and decreased of two levels in paper [6]. In paper [14], staircase is compared to book based clinical testing and the result is that the threshold measured with digital test is more reliable also due to the possibility to increase the number of levels of disparity.

A comparison among algorithms is presented in [9]. Also in that paper, the results show that faster converging maximum-likelihood procedures like PEST and BESTN offer some benefit over longer staircase procedures. especially when testing must be accomplished very quickly, as in testing animals or infants.

The necessity to devise new algorithm for testing infants and children is advocated in [7], where the authors consider how best to maximize speed, accuracy, and reliability.

7   Conclusion

In this paper we have presented four algorithms for the evaluation of psychophysical thresholds. The tests are performed on virtual patients, because it was very difficult to find a lot of patients available to perform a test many times. In the future we plan to define a protocol to test the algorithms on real patients, for example to measure the stereoacuity using our mobile application [4]. Our simulations show that the choice of the best algorithm to follow, depend on many factors. Algorithm like STRICTN performs generally well, except in cases in which the test cannot last so many steps. In those cases, other algorithms like our PESTN are more efficient.

References

1. Bach, M., Schmitt, C., Kromeier, M., Kommerell, G.: The Freiburg Stereoacuity test: automatic measurement of stereo threshold. Graefe's Arch. Clin. Exp. Ophthalmol. **239**(8), 562–566 (2001). https://doi.org/10.1007/s004170100317
2. Bonfanti, S., Gargantini, A.: Comparison of algorithms to measure a psychophysical threshold using digital applications: the stereoacuity case study. In: Pesquita, C., Fred, A.L.N., Gamboa, H. (eds.) Proceedings of the 14th International Joint Conference on Biomedical Engineering Systems and Technologies, BIOSTEC 2021, HEALTHINF, Online Streaming, 11–13 February 2021, vol. 5, pp. 78–86. SCITEPRESS (2021). https://doi.org/10.5220/0010204000780086
3. Bonfanti, S., Gargantini, A., Esposito, G., Facchin, A., Maffioletti, M., Maffioletti, S.: Evaluation of stereoacuity with a digital mobile application. Graefes Arch. Clin. Exp. Ophthalmol. **259**(9), 2843–2848 (2021). https://doi.org/10.1007/s00417-021-05195-z
4. Bonfanti, S., Gargantini, A., Vitali, A.: A mobile application for the stereoacuity test. In: Duffy, V.G. (ed.) DHM 2015. LNCS, vol. 9185, pp. 315–326. Springer, Cham (2015). https://doi.org/10.1007/978-3-319-21070-4_32
5. Fleiss, J.L., Levin, B., Paik, M.C.: Statistical Methods for Rates and Proportions. Wiley Series in Probability and Statistics, 3rd edn. Wiley, Hoboken (2003)

6. Hess, R.F., et al.: A robust and reliable test to measure stereopsis in the clinic. Invest. Opthalmol. Vis. Sci. **57**(3), 798 (2016). https://doi.org/10.1167/iovs.15-18690
7. Jones, P.R., Kalwarowsky, S., Braddick, O.J., Atkinson, J., Nardini, M.: Optimizing the rapid measurement of detection thresholds in infants. J. Vis. **15**(11), 2 (2015). https://doi.org/10.1167/15.11.2
8. Kromeier, M., Schmitt, C., Bach, M., Kommerell, G.: Stereoacuity versus fixation disparity as indicators for vergence accuracy under prismatic stress. Ophthalmic Physiol. Opt. **23**(1), 43–49 (2003). https://doi.org/10.1046/j.1475-1313.2003.00089.x
9. Leek, M.R.: Adaptive procedures in psychophysical research. Percept. Psychophys. **63**(8), 1279–1292 (2001). https://doi.org/10.3758/BF03194543
10. Li, R.W., et al.: Monocular blur alters the tuning characteristics of stereopsis for spatial frequency and size. R. Soc. Open Sci. **3**(9), 160273 (2016). https://doi.org/10.1098/rsos.160273
11. Noether, G.E.: Introduction to Wilcoxon (1945) individual comparisons by ranking methods. In: Kotz, S., Johnson, N.L. (eds.) Breakthroughs in Statistics. Springer Series in Statistics, pp. 191–195. Springer, New York (1992). https://doi.org/10.1007/978-1-4612-4380-9_15
12. Stevens, S.S.: Problems and methods of psychophysics. Psychol. Bull. **55**(4), 177–196 (1958)
13. Taylor, M.M., Creelman, C.D.: Pest: efficient estimates on probability functions. J. Acoust. Soc. Am. **41**(4A), 782–787 (1967)
14. Tidbury, L.P., O'Connor, A.R., Wuerger, S.M.: The effect of induced fusional demand on static and dynamic stereoacuity thresholds: the digital synoptophore. BMC Ophthalmol. **19**(1) (2019). https://doi.org/10.1186/s12886-018-1000-2
15. Ushaw, G., et al.: Analysis of soft data for mass provision of stereoacuity testing through a serious game for health. In: Proceedings of the 2017 International Conference on Digital Health, DH 2017. ACM Press (2017). https://doi.org/10.1145/3079452.3079496
16. Vancleef, K., Read, J.C.A., Herbert, W., Goodship, N., Woodhouse, M., Serrano-Pedraza, I.: Two choices good, four choices better: for measuring stereoacuity in children, a four-alternative forced-choice paradigm is more efficient than two. PLOS ONE **13**(7), e0201366 (2018). https://doi.org/10.1371/journal.pone.0201366
17. Wong, B.P.H., Woods, R.L., Peli, E.: Stereoacuity at distance and near. Optom. Vis. Sci. **79**(12), 771–778 (2002). https://doi.org/10.1097/00006324-200212000-00009
18. Zhang, P., Zhao, Y., Dosher, B.A., Lu, Z.L.: Evaluating the performance of the staircase and quick change detection methods in measuring perceptual learning. J. Vis. **19**(7), 14 (2019). https://doi.org/10.1167/19.7.14

Improving Teledermatology Referral with Edge-AI: Mobile App to Foster Skin Lesion Imaging Standardization

Maria João M. Vasconcelos[1(✉)] [iD], Dinis Moreira[1] [iD], Pedro Alves[1] [iD],
Ricardo Graça[1] [iD], Rafael Franco[2], and Luís Rosado[1] [iD]

[1] Fraunhofer Portugal AICOS, 4200-135 Porto, Portugal
maria.vasconcelos@fraunhofer.pt
[2] Shared Services of the Ministry of Health, Lisbon, Portugal
cnts@spms.min-saude.pt

Abstract. Every year, the number of skin cancer cases has been increasing which, consequently, increases the strain on the health care systems around the globe. With the growth of processing power and camera quality on smartphones, the investment in telemedicine and the development of mobile teledermatology applications can, not only contribute to the standardization of image acquisitions but also, facilitate early diagnosis. This paper presents a new process for real-time automated image acquisition of macroscopic skin images with the merging of an automated focus assessment feature-based machine learning algorithm with conventional computer vision techniques to segment dermatological images. Three datasets were used to develop and evaluate the proposed methodology. One comprised of 3428 images acquired with a mobile phone for this purpose and 1380 from the other two datasets which are publicly available. The best focus assessment model achieved an accuracy of 88.3% and an F1-Score of 86.8%. The segmentation algorithm obtained a Jaccard index of 85.81% for the SMARTSKINS dataset and 68.59% for the Dermofit dataset. The algorithms were deployed to a mobile application, available in Android and iOS, without causing any performance hindrances. The application was tested in a real environment, being used in a 10-month pilot study with six General and Family Medicine doctors and one Dermatologist. The easiness to acquire dermatological images, image quality, and standardization were referred to as the main advantages of the application.

Keywords: Mobile dermatology · Image acquisition · Image quality assessment · Feature extraction · Machine learning · Image segmentation

1 Introduction

Skin cancer is one of the most common malignancy in caucasian population with increasing incidence [3]. Awareness and screening campaigns and regular check-ups are crucial for the early detection and consequent improvement of treatment success rates, patient condition and diminish health costs [14].

The advances in mobile health (m-health) technologies allowed the development of several teledermatology solutions [8,27], essential for monitoring the evolution of skin

C. Gehin et al. (Eds.): BIOSTEC 2021, CCIS 1710, pp. 158–179, 2022.
https://doi.org/10.1007/978-3-031-20664-1_9

lesions or early detection of malignant lesions. Although dermoscopy is the standard procedure for the analysis of pigmented lesions [12], it requires specific equipment and it is only used by specialists, while general practitioners or patients frequently acquire macroscopic (close-up) images or clinical images with their smartphones. Nevertheless, specialists need to receive standardized information with guaranteed quality in order to provide reliable feedback or diagnosis, especially when dealing with clinical images [18].

Dermatological telereferral program has been in place in Portugal since 2014, with the goal to contribute to the early diagnosis of dermatological lesions and skin cancer, as well as to improve efficiency on dermatology consultations in the National Health Service (NHS). Order no. 005/2014 of Portuguese Health Director-General for teledermatological screening describes, as the name suggests, the procedures to be taken into consideration in the Portuguese NHS in the approach of patients with dermatological pathologies. It contains details about the type of information (metadata and images) that should be collected by the general practitioner from the Primary Care Units (PCU) in order for the dermatologist in the Hospital to be able to properly select (triage) the type of consultation and priority needed (teleconsultation or presential). Since 2018, Order No. 6280/2018, of 28 June, determined that every first access to a dermatology specialist consultation should follow the dermatological telereferral program rules. In order to take pictures of the lesions, doctors primarily used digital cameras and more recently have been using smartphones to later manually attach the images to the patient's clinical process. According to the doctors feedback, it is very common the dermatologists receive images that do not have enough quality for clinical purposes and general practitioners say that this manual process of attaching the images is time consuming and prone to errors.

The present work integrates a larger project, DermAI, that aims to improve the existing Teledermatology processes between PCUs and Dermatology Services in the NHS for skin lesion referral. We envision two major goals: (a) to support doctors in PCUs through the development of a computer vision-based mobile application that fosters image acquisition standardization and (b) to assist dermatologists in the referral process for booking specialist consultations in the hospital through the adequate prioritization of cases [7].

This research addresses DermAI first goal towards the implementation and test of a mobile application that standardizes the image acquisition to be later integrated with the national health registry system, specifically for dermatological telereferral. We focus on the description of the automated image acquisition of macroscopic skin images through mobile devices, that was primarily presented in [23]. In this paper, details are provided concerning the complete mobile application developed as well as the results of the usage of the mobile application in a real environment.

2   Related Work

With the evolution of mobile technologies the development of applications that use the device's camera for image acquisition of skin lesions has increased [8]. Even though smartphones cameras have embedded auto-focus systems, which frees the users from having to manually focus, external factors such as small camera movements during the image acquisition, poor or inconsistent illumination may originate low quality images such as blurred images. Additionally, and due to the fact that the lens' aperture on mobile devices is usually small, a longer exposure time is required which consequently increases the chances of occurring the mentioned small camera movements. Therefore, this simple factor may lead to the inability of the dermatologist to provide a clinical decision due to the poor quality of the image. In [9], a set of quality standards for tele-dermatology in the UK were presented regarding image quality, resolution and more specifically focus. This image quality standards mention that images for teledermatology assessment should be a minimum size of 2000×1500 pixels or 3 megapixels, acquired using electronic flash and with a focusing distance no closer than 20cm to the lesion.

Several papers and applications resort to the smartphone auto-focus function to obtain a focused image of a skin lesion [6]. The mobile applications, Spotmole and DermPic [22, 24], also appear to use the smartphone's auto-focus function for addressing this issue, however neither application does a verification of the image sharpness or quality. The former asks the user to manually confirm if the photo has an adequate quality while the latter just assumes its focus, thus depending on the user's subjectivity and proficiency with the application. In overall, using auto-focus function is sufficient to get a focused image, but when it comes to medical devices and procedures, a higher fidelity degree is thus required. This requisite is not only important to improve the monitoring and diagnosis ability of skin lesions, but also to highlight the need to assess the quality of the images acquired by these applications [10, 17].

In [1] a methodology for the automatic focus assessment on dermoscopic images acquired with smartphones was presented. A combination of 90 different focus metrics and their relative values between the original and an artificially generated blurred image served as basis for the training of a decision tree model. A global accuracy of 86.2% was attained regarding the focus status of the acquired images in dermoscopic images. More recently, in [11], the authors compared the use of several different smartphone cameras, as well as two Digital Single-Lens Reflex cameras and a professional medical camera (Medicam 1000 s) for dermoscopy image acquisition. Image sharpness, resolution and color reproduction were measured and the attained results showed that some smartphones' render overly saturated colors and may apply some over-sharpening methods to the picture which can alter the characteristics of the object being photographed.

Regarding studies focused in close-up or clinical images, in [31], the authors develop a methodology for the real-time acquisition of quality verified skin lesions from a video taken with a mobile device camera. They concluded that acquiring focused images with smartphones' camera is feasible, being the best results obtained when using the Brenner Gradient focus metric. In the proposed method the skin lesion is segmented using the grey image, followed by the application of a median filter and Otsu method for automatic threshold detection. For the study, 60 images from melanoma and benign lesions were used to build and test the system and implemented in an iOS app. Similarly, [8] developed a popular application, Skin Vision App, that uses a special camera module for the acquisition of quality skin lesion images. The authors claimed that this camera module reduced the number of blurry photos, on average, by about 52%.

Regarding skin lesions segmentation, most methods in the literature were proposed for dermoscopic images, while for macroscopic images still lacks further research [2, 15, 19, 25, 29]. One of the main reasons for that is closely related with the small amount of available datasets that include annotated images of macroscopic images. Also, most studies focus on pigmented lesions [19, 25, 29] and do not consider non-pigmented lesions that are also very common [2, 15]. Examples of methodologies vary from threshold-based techniques [29], usage of unsupervised dictionary learning methods [19], active contour model without edges and a support vector machine method [25]. In terms of segmentation performance, [25] obtained an XOR error of 16.89% and [25] evaluated the correctness of the segmentation based on the visual assessment of a specialist which reached a 94.36% of correctly segmented images. More recently, the usage of deep learning methods was reported [2, 15]. The highest reported performance obtained, in the deep learning methods, was in [2] with 82.64% Jaccard index in a pigmented lesions database and 81.03% in a non-pigmented lesions database. However, most of the works mentioned previously do not apply the methods in real-time apart from [1, 8, 29, 31].

3   Macroscopic Image Acquisition Pipeline

The presented pipeline enables the automated acquisition process of macroscopic skin lesions using smartphones, being proposed in [23]. It is comprised by an image processing methodology that is divided into three main modules: the preview focus assessment module, the segmentation module and the acquired picture focus assessment module, as depicted in Fig. 1.

The automated image acquisition process starts by checking if each upcoming camera preview frame image has enough quality and focus for the purpose, followed by the segmentation of the skin lesion. This segmentation step is automatic, not requiring any user interaction, and it is only performed after guaranteeing the quality and adequacy on a certain number of consecutive camera preview frames images. Finally, the acquired picture is again evaluated in terms of its focus and quality by the focus assessment module, before being presented to the user.

3.1   Datasets

Macroscopic Image Quality Assessment Dataset. A dataset of focused and non-focused images, named the Macroscopic Image Quality Assessment (MacroIQA) dataset, was collected. This dataset served as basis to create and assess the image quality and focus ability of the model in macroscopic skin lesions images.

The MacroIQA dataset is composed of a total of 3428 macroscopic images of skin moles from 19 different caucasian subjects. 10 different smartphones, ranging from low to high-end models, were used to acquire these images. This variability was extremely important for ensuring the overall robustness of the proposed solution since we aimed to create a model which can be independent of quality of a given smartphone camera and/or model. Thus, this dataset contains at least one blurred and one focused image for each skin mole and smartphone. For each acquisition, both camera preview and captured

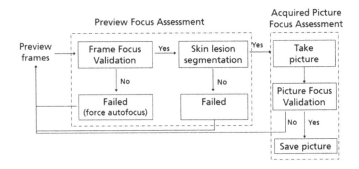

Fig. 1. System architecture diagram for the automated mobile image acquisition of macroscopic skin lesions [23].

images were stored and used for different purposes: (i) in the preview stage, the goal is to assess the image in terms of image stabilization, standardization and overall quality, before starting the skin mole automated segmentation; (ii) in the acquired stage, the goal is to assess the image in terms of focus and quality, assuring that the final image that is stored in the system is suitable for further diagnosis purposes. Additionally, it is worth noticing that the preview images (1280 × 720 px) have a smaller resolution compared to the acquired images (1920 × 1080 px), The latter fact should be taken into account when developing the overall system since the analysis of the smaller resolution preview images analysis may constitute an additional challenge. A summary of the amount of collected images per type and class is provided in Table 1.

Along the data collection process, different aspects were taken into account in order to assure proper variability of the skin moles images among the recruited voluntary participants. Thus, skin moles images were acquired from subjects with different genders and skin tones (phototypes varying from I to V) and with different sizes, shapes and colors, as well as with the presence or absence of hair. This variability in the dataset guarantees that all the selected features and trained models will be able to cope with all of these differences, therefore improving the robustness and suitability of the proposed solution to be used in any case and deployed in a real life scenario. Some illustrative examples of skin lesions are presented in Fig. 2.

In respect to the image annotations, each collected image was labelled as being focused and not focused by non-specialists in this area and therefore, can be subjective and prone to human error. With this in mind, three independent annotators performed the labelling of the entire dataset, being the final label of each image defined by majority voting.

Table 1. Image type distribution in the MacroIQA dataset.

Images	Focused	Non-Focused	Total
Preview	734	977	1711
Acquired	705	1012	1717
Total	1439	1989	3428

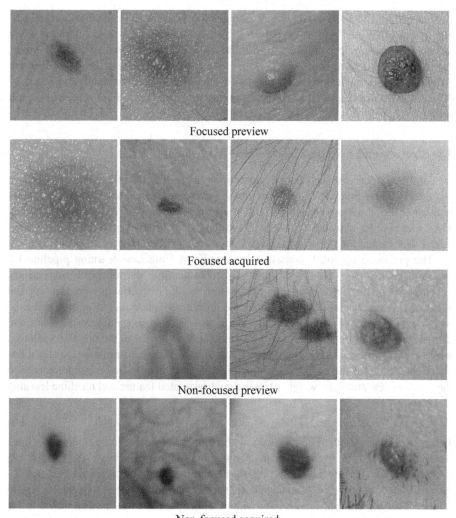

Focused preview

Focused acquired

Non-focused preview

Non-focused acquired

Fig. 2. Illustrative focused and non-focused images of skin moles present in the MacroIQA dataset.

Macroscopic Segmentation Datasets. Two datasets, Dermofit image Library [21] and SMARTSKINS dataset [33], were used to develop and test the proposed segmentation pipeline.

The Dermofit dataset has 1300 high-quality color skin lesions, acquired with traditional cameras, and their corresponding binary segmentation masks highlighting the lesion area. Of this 1300 images, 819 are benign and 481 are carcinogenic images which span across 10 different classes based on gold standard diagnosis provided by dermatology experts.

The SMARTSKINS dataset was acquired at the Skin Clinic of the Portuguese Institute of Oncology of Porto involving 36 subjects. This dataset was acquired with two different mobile devices and it comprises several subsets captured in different years. For this work we selected a subset of 80 melanocytic lesions that have two different ground truths for the lesion area (i.e. segmentation masks were manually generated by different annotators), as well as medical annotations regarding ABCD score and overall risk.

3.2 Preview and Acquired Image Focus Assessment

One of the most critical aspects of this pipeline is to evaluate an image in terms of focus and quality, independently of being an image with a smaller resolution from the camera preview or the actual acquired image with higher resolution acquired by the smartphone. Thus, and in order to achieve this goal, an independent feature-based machine learning model was trained for assessing preview frame and acquired images, respectively.

The proposed approach consisted in a traditional machine learning pipeline for assessing each image. This pipeline, described in detail in the following subsections, is composed by the steps: image pre-processing, feature extraction, model training and validation. Moreover, it is intended that the proposed system must run in a real-time and in a wide range of different smartphones, with varying processing capabilities and cameras, highlighting the need of overall robustness and speed of the proposed solution while dealing with limited computational resources. The latter limitation greatly influenced the design of the machine learning pipeline, specifically by giving preference to the usage of few and light-weighted image quality-related feature and machine learning models.

Image Pre-processing. The first step of the pipeline was a resizing operation. Since different devices were used during the acquisition, the original image was resized to a fixed resolution. The preview frame and the acquired images were resized to 1280×720 px and 1920×1080 px, respectively. Then, each image was cropped to a central square with 35% of the original image size (width). This operation was used to decrease the processing time of each image and also to discard non-interest regions (as the background) from the original. This cropped image is the one later used in the feature extraction step and for decision making. Afterwards, this square region image is converted to the grayscale colorspace, followed by the generation of a blurred version of it. The generation of this artificially blurred image from the original one is quite important when extracting the image-related features, since a blurred image generally has soft edges, less color variation and brightness, meaning that pixels belonging to the same area will have, in their correspondent grayscale image, identical color values and features if the original image is non-focused and more variable ones if the original is a perfectly focused image. Thus, the impact of this operation, in an already non-focused image is significantly smaller compared to a focused one, which may help its differentiation [1,13]. The generation of the artificially blurred image is obtained by applying a mean filter to the grayscale image, as described in [13].

Feature Extraction. For each image in the dataset, a set of several state-of-the-art image quality related features were extracted. Most of the focus-related metrics used in this study were already reported in [1,32]. In addition to that, some extra features were computed, such as gradient based functions (Thresholded absolute gradient; Tenengrad variance), DCT-based functions (DCT Reduced Energy Ratio; Modified DCT) and other relevant functions (Image contrast; Vollath's standard deviation; Helmli and Scheres Mean Method), which are detailed in [26,30]. The complete set of features extracted were described in [23].

For each grayscale and artificially blurred image pair, these focus assessment-related features were computed independently. Additionally, and following [1] study, a new subset of features was derived based on their relative estimated values. This new set of features consisted in computing the difference and the quotient between the values obtained for each feature between the grayscale and artificially blurred image. Ultimately, a feature vector of a total of 504 metrics was obtained for each input image, by merging all the extracted absolute and relative aforementioned focus features.

Model Training and Optimization. In order to automatically capture focused macroscopic skin lesions and to cope with the difference in terms of image quality between preview and acquired images, two independent and robust models were trained: the preview images and the acquired images focus assessment. Therefore, the MacroIQA dataset was divided into two different sub-datasets, one consisted of only preview frame images and the other consisted of only acquired images, which were then used for solving each task.

The optimization and selection of the best machine learning pipeline was accomplished using a Feature-based Machine Learning (FbML) tool [20]. This tool is based on the open-source project *auto-sklearn* [16], and allows a search space initialization and pipeline optimization via meta-learning (search for similar datasets and initialize hyperparameter optimization algorithm with the found configurations). Moreover, an extensive list of options are available when using this tool for data pre-processing (balancing, imputation of missing values, re-scaling), feature transformation, and feature and classifier selection. Thus, and for each sub-dataset, several machine learning pipelines, with different steps, were explored using the following options/parameters:

1. **Scalers:** Standardization (zero mean and unit variance); Min-Max Scaling; Normalization to unit length; Robust Scaler; Quantile Transformer; None.
2. **Feature transformation/selection:** Principal component analysis (PCA); Univariate Feature Selection; Classification Based Selection (Extremely Randomized Trees and L1-regularized Linear SVM); None.
3. **Classifiers:** K-Nearest Neighbors; Linear and Non-linear Support Vector Machines; Decision Trees; Random Forest; Adaboost.
4. **Validation Strategy:** 10-Fold Cross Validation.
5. **Optimization metric:** ROC-AUC.

Given the limited computational capabilities of some smartphone models, the need of real-time feature computation and also providing real-time feedback to the user regarding the focus level, specially for the camera preview frames images, an additional feature reduction step was employed. Thus, the authors defined a constraint of using a maximum of three different features for each classification task. For each trained and optimized machine learning pipeline, all combinations of three features were evaluated, using an iterative leave-one-session-out validation approach. This choice ensured that only a maximum of three features are selected per model, reducing the processing time associated with the computation of the features values, without compromising the overall classification results. The leave-one-session-out for validation will ensure an adequate overall robustness of the algorithm to variability presented in the data.

3.3   Lesion Segmentation

The current work is based on the developments made in [29], given their requirement of developing an automated acquisition process of macroscopic skin images method for real-time usage on mobile devices. The methodology presented on the referred work was, to the extent of our knowledge, only tested on the SMARTSKINS dataset, whose composition is primarily of pigmented skin lesion images (e.g. melanocytic nevus), where the inside area of the pigmented skin lesions usually has a darker coloration than the surrounding skin. Given that the Dermofit dataset is majorly composed of non-pigmented skin lesions (e.g. basal and squamous cell carcinomas), optimizations were possible in order to improve the performance of the previously mentioned approach for non-pigmented skin lesions.

Regarding the pre-processing, the previously proposed algorithm transforms the image to grayscale followed by a median blur filter that smooths the image's structures. Here, three different pre-processing techniques were tested: i) Brightness and Contrast Adjustment; ii) Mean Shift Color Enhancement; and iii) Grayscale Sharpening. These steps are explained in the following subsections, as well as the optimizations implemented regarding segmentation and filtering procedures.

Brightness and Contrast Adjustment. The adjustment of both brightness and contrast was done by applying a constant gain, α, and bias, β, to the original image. These variables work as a histogram range amplifier and range shift, respectively. This procedure had previously been successfully used in [28]. The parameters are automatically calculated with the following assumptions: the desired histogram range is 255; the minimum and maximum intensity values used to stretch the histogram are calculated using only the intensities with more than 1% frequency. Figure 3.B shows the effect of this process which might result in a significant increase in pixel intensity and, therefore, lead to unrealistic colors that render the image unsuitable for clinical decision purposes. However, the increased contrast accentuates the lesion's edges which can facilitate the detection of the lesion area.

Mean Shift Color Enhancement. The second pre-processing method step consists on a smoothing procedure using Mean Shift Filter (MSF). Given the previous results presented in [28], the edge preserving qualities of the filter and the ability to homogenize color intensities, this method was of particular interest. The downside of the MSF is the fact that it can be a computationally heavy method. Therefore, the trade-off between the improvements in the segmentation and the added processing time will be evaluated. This step can be observed in Fig. 3.C.

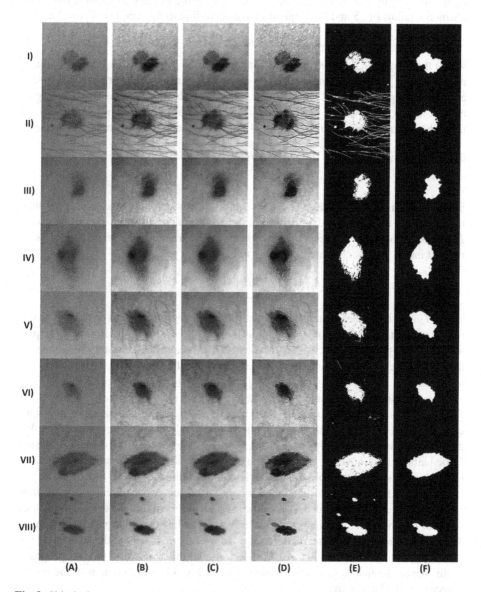

Fig. 3. Skin lesion segmentation and filtering: (**A**) Original image; (**B**) Brightness and contrast adjustment; (**C**) Mean shift color enhancement; (**D**) Grayscale sharpening; (**E**) Adaptive thresholding; (**F**) Morphological operations, hole filling and area filtering.

Grayscale Sharpening. A grayscale sharpening step was chosen to increase the sharpness and contrast of the skin mole. This was achieved with the usage of an unsharped mask, obtained by combining the target image after going through a Gaussian filter with a window radius of 15 and the original image according to the weights of Eq. (1):

$$I_{Shar} = 1.5 \times I_{Gray} - 0.5 \times I_{Gau} - (0.75 \times I_{Gray} \odot 0.2 \times I_{Lap}), \qquad (1)$$

where the image I_{Gray} is the grayscale image after the brightness and contrast adjustment and I_{Shar} is the sharpened image (see Fig. 3.D). Since the unsharp mask can cause artifacts on edge borders, a Laplacian component was also added to the sharpening procedure. This component is responsible for avoiding double edges and was obtained through an element-wise multiplication ($\odot$) of the original image with the Laplacian of the original image using the following kernel: $\begin{bmatrix} 0 & 1 & 0 \\ 1 & -4 & 1 \\ 0 & 1 & 0 \end{bmatrix}$.

Segmentation and Filtering. The segmentation method follows the work presented in [29] which is based on adaptive thresholding. Considering the pre-processed image I_{Shar}, obtained after the previous step of grayscale sharpening, the corresponding segmented image I_{Seg} is obtained according to Eq. (2):

$$I_{Seg}(x, y) = \begin{cases} 0 & \text{if } I_{Shar}(x, y) > T_{Shar}(x, y) \\ 255 & \text{otherwise} \end{cases}, \qquad (2)$$

where T_{Sharp} is the mean intensity value of the square region centered on the pixel location (x, y) with a side value of W_{Side} minus the constant C. In comparison with the previously work, given the effectiveness of the new three pre-processing steps in increasing the contrast between the skin lesion and its surrounds, the thresholding parameters had to be adapted, namely $C = 45$ and $W_{Side} = \max\{I_{width}, I_{height}\}$, (Fig. 3.E).

It is possible to see some small irregularities in the segmented skin lesions in Fig. 3.E. To clean the contours, an opening morphological operation with an elliptical structuring element of size 7 was applied, followed by a hole-filling procedure. We can see the advantages of this step in Fig. 3, changes from (E) to (F), where in lesion II the hairs were removed, in lesion III the contour of the lesion was smoothed and, for example, in lesion IV the holes inside the lesion were filled.

Finally, a filter threshold is applied where any object whose area is smaller than 10% of the image are discarded. An additional perk of this filtering is the assurance that the skin lesion has an adequate size, since if the user has the smartphone far from it, the segmentation will be discarded, forcing the user to approximate the smartphone to the target lesion. Due to the nature of the lesions and the acquisition process proposed in this paper, the final result, which can be seen in Fig. 3.F, is the contour of the binary object with the largest area.

4   Mobile Application

To foster the standardization of image acquisition in dermatology in the Portuguese NHS a mobile application that follows order no. 005/2014 for teledermatological screening was built, and its prototype put into use.

This application allows the proper acquisition of different dermatological images - macroscopic, anatomical, full body and dermoscopic - depending on the type of lesion (extensive, small or pigmented) to be referenced for dermatology consultation in the Portuguese NHS Hospitals (see Fig. 4). It allows the automatic acquisition of macroscopic images of skin lesions in an easy and intuitive manner, while providing real-time feedback to the user about the level of focus during and after the acquisition process (see Fig. 4c). Moreover, in the event of the developed automated image acquisition not being able to detect the skin mole, the user is always able to acquire an image by changing the image acquisition to a manual mode. In the manual acquisition mode, all previously described methods (Sect. 3.2) are still applied, apart from the automatic segmentation of the skin lesion. In the manual mode, as the name suggests, the user is always responsible for the pressing of the camera button which triggers the image capturing process. Regarding the acquisition of anatomic, full body, and dermoscopic images, focus assessment is also performed, which has been previously described in other works, namely for anatomic and full body. The used focus metric is the same as the one described in [13] and the dermoscopic image acquisition algorithm was previously detailed in [1].

The mobile application runs offline in Android and iOS smartphones and was developed to minimize errors and facilitate image acquisition. The photos are stored locally in the application storage environment and made available for the healthcare practitioners to export them to their computers to annex them to the referral process. To guarantee the quality of the images the application can only be used in smartphones with Android 5.0 (API level 21) or above or with iOS 8.0 or above. We also recommend the usage of smartphones with a camera with more than 8MP. To properly evaluate the usability and suitability of this mobile application in a real environment, a pilot was run on different PCUs and one Dermatology Service, whose results will be detailed in the following section.

5 Results and Discussion

5.1 Macroscopic Image Acquisition Pipeline Results

Preview Focus Assessment Results. One of the major challenges of the proposed macroscopic image acquisition pipeline is the focus assessment of preview frame images. These images are of reduced resolution and yet, still provide the most valuable information to the user. The real-time analysis can provide prompt feedback and guidance to the user throughout the process of acquiring the skin mole image. Thus, making this type of visual feedback quite important to the user throughout the process, as depicted in Fig. 4c. The preview focus assessment model was trained using a subset of the MacroIQA dataset, composed only by focused and non-focused preview frame images. The optimized machine learning pipeline was found via the optimization approach detailed on Sect. 3.2, consisted in applying a scaling operation (*Standard Scaler*) on the three selected features to have zero mean and unit variance, and a *Random Forest* (number of trees: 100) classifier. Furthermore, the three selected features for the preview images focus assessment were: *Standard Deviation of the Normalized Variance*,

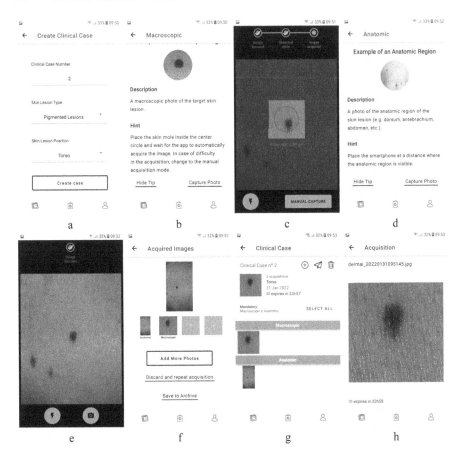

Fig. 4. Application screenshots of DermAI mobile application: clinical case creation (a); acquisition tips for macroscopic and anatomic images (b, d); image acquisition for macroscopic and anatomic images (c, d); complete case (g) and macroscopic image detail (h).

Maximum of the Laplace Diagonal and *Maximum of Laplacian Filter*, all extracted from the grayscale image.

The focus assessment results of the preview frame images are presented in Table 2. As it can be seen, an overall accuracy of 88.3%, sensitivity of 89.9% and a specificity of 87.1% were attained for correctly classifying if a certain preview frame image is actually focused or not. Only three different features were used, all extracted from the preview frames grayscale images, demonstrating the model's capability of effectively provide accurate and reliable predictions for assessing the image focus and quality. The chosen features demonstrated to be enough for having a fast characterization of pixel values intensity changes and discontinuities in the camera preview frames images. Moreover, it is also worth mentioning that given the high number of camera preview frames images per second, it's smaller resolution and the need of providing real-time feedback to the user, the proposed model is quite accurate and suitable for use, given its purpose.

Table 2. Preview image focus assessment classification results of the best performing model [23].

Metric	Accuracy	Sensitivity	Specificity	F1-Score
Results (%)	88.3	89.9	87.1	86.8

Lesion Segmentation Results. The influence of the new pre-processing steps on the segmentation approach is here presented. As previously mentioned, in Sect. 3.3, the MSF can be computationally heavy which would render this technique unusable in real-time. However, its potential improvements in the segmentation performance could be crucial. Thus, a comparative study was conducted where the segmentation performance and processing time were evaluated. Table 3 shows the results of the optimization pipeline with and without the MSF step.

It is possible to observe in Table 3 that the proposed optimizations had a great improvement in the segmentation performance on the Dermofit dataset (45.20% for the method proposed in [29] against 67.87% or 68.59%, depending on the usage of MSF). This improvement is mostly due to the fact that the new methodology has a higher performance on non-pigmented skin lesions, whereas for pigmented skin lesions, the SMARTSKINS dataset, there were slight improvements. Regarding the use of MSF, only few classes had a small improvement (3), while others did not. Provided that the processing time is almost 70 times slower using MSF, there is no justification for its use in real-time. Considering this trade-off, this step was not integrated in the pipeline in the mobile application.

Table 3. Jaccard index (%) of the segmentation results for both datasets, using: i) the Ros15 method [29]; and ii): the proposed method, with and without MSF [23].

Dataset	Ros15 method	Proposed with MSF	Proposed without MSF
Dermofit Dataset			
Actinic Keratosis	11.91	33.27	36.50
Basal Cell Carcinoma	26.86	51.65	53.08
Dermatofibroma	57.76	76.84	75.056
Haemangioma	74.33	73.44	74.22
Malignant Melanoma	68.24	74.85	72.75
Melanocytic Nevus	51.25	79.29	79.81
Pyogenic Granuloma	73.99	74.18	73.41
Seborrhoeic Keratosis	39.93	73.71	74.08
Squam. Cell Carcinoma	35.52	49.13	52.54
Full dataset	45.20	67.87	68.59
SMARTSKINS Dataset			
Ground Truth #1	84.59	86.11	86.44
Ground Truth #2	82.73	85.30	85.18

Acquired Images Focus Assessment Results. The ultimate goal of the proposed pipeline is to evaluate the image focus and quality of the acquired macroscopic skin mole picture. These images are of utmost interest for the dermatologists, since it carries the fundamental information and it's the basis for deriving a potential diagnosis. Thus, ensuring that a given image is focused and has enough quality is crucial to the process, not only for medical reasoning but also to avoid storing pictures with insufficient quality, that latter on will be discarded.

The acquired images focus assessment model was trained using a subset of the MacroIQA dataset, only composed by focused and non-focused skin moles acquired macroscopic images. The optimized machine learning pipeline was found via the optimization approach detailed on Sect. 3.2, and for this case, consisted in applying the same type of scaling operation as obtained for the preview images *Standard Scaler*, together with the use of the *Adaboost* (n_estimators = 77) classifier. Furthermore, the three selected features for the acquired picture focus assessment were: *Difference between Standard Deviation of the Thresholded Absolute Gradient of gray and blur image, Division between the Standard Deviation of the Sum Modified Laplacian of blur and gray image, Quotient between the mean DCT Enery of blur and gray image.*

The focus assessment results of the acquired pictures are presented in Table 4. As it can be seen, an overall accuracy of 86.8%, sensitivity of 88.7% and a specificity of 85.6% were attained for correctly identifying if a certain acquired skin mole picture is focused or not. Moreover, only three different features, that combined information both from the gray and artificially generated blurred images, were used. These features proved to be able to correctly evaluate the focus and quality of the acquired skin mole pictures. These relative features are based on differences and ratios between features values extracted from the gray and blur images, providing a way for having a robust characterization and comparison of pixel values intensities within focused and non-focused images, as previously reported in the literature [1]. Given the existing variability in the dataset in terms of skin mole's shape, color, texture, size or subject's gender, age and skin phototype, the obtained results for the focus assessment of the acquired skin mole pictures demonstrated to be quite accurate and robust, confirming the suitability of using the proposed solution in a real life scenario.

Table 4. Acquired images focus assessment classification results of the best performing model [23].

Metric	Accuracy	Sensitivity	Specificity	F1-Score
Results (%)	86.8	88.7	85.6	84.7

5.2 Trial Results

In order to evaluate the quality of the images acquired with the mobile application, validate the focus and acquisition algorithms as well as the usability of the mobile application, a trial was run in four PCUs and one Dermatology Department of the Portuguese NHS. The trial protocol was submitted and approved by the Health Ethical Committee from Unidade Local de Saúde (ULS) Guarda and informed consents were obtained both from doctors and patients.

PCU Doctors Feedback. The previously described mobile application was used between November 2020 and August 2021 by six General and Family Medicine doctors from four PCUs and the images evaluated by one dermatology specialist. Before the trial started, the authors provided an online workshop to present the project and explain the mobile application functionalities in a two hour session. The clinicians could choose to use their personal smartphone or a smartphone provided by the project. At the end of the trial, the participants were asked to answer a questionnaire and later the results were presented and discussed with the participating doctors. The results obtained will be detailed here.

A total of six General and Family Medicine doctors used the mobile application during the trial. Two doctors used the smartphone provided by the project and four used their own smartphone. The doctors' age ranged between 33 and 62 years (mean age 42 years) and 13.8 years of experience in the field. All doctors had a smartphone and experience with its usage. 83% of the doctors participated in the training session and at the end of the trial, when asked about the importance of the session, 67% considered the training essential while 33% considered optional.

Before using the mobile application, half of the participants used their personal smartphones to take the pictures, while the other half used a digital camera, both smartphone or camera or none. In 2021, the majority of the participants (80%) indicated to reference patients once or twice per month, while in 2019, the most common was to refer patients three or four times per month. This drop in the referrals is mainly due to Covid-19 pandemic, since patients mostly approach PCU for urgent situations.

When asked about the percentage of referrals being returned from the dermatology service in 2019 or while using the application, a drop was mentioned. In 2019, 50% of the doctors indicated that 1% to 25% of the referrals were returned. After using the application, only 17% referred that 1% to 25% of the referrals were returned. Previously, the return motives were frequently due to bad image quality, no image attached or technical problems.

67% of the participants considered the process of exporting the images simple and that it was easy to find the images on the smartphone. One participant mentioned that the process could be improved, namely by automatically exporting the images to the referral system.

67% of the participants considered recommending the mobile application to their colleagues and agree that it improves the quality of the acquired images. The mentioned application advantages are: "efficiency and speed", "image acquisition in the correct format and size", "easiness of focus", "image quality improvement and standardization" and "grouping by clinical case". Regarding disadvantages, the doctors mentioned the lack of complete integration with the referral system and asked to diminish the number of steps on the mobile application.

During the pilot, only one doctor stopped using the mobile application, mentioning having troubles acquiring the images. The System Usability Scale (SUS) [5] was used to measure the perceived ease of use of the system, since it is widely used, reliable, and easy to administer. At the end of the trials, each participant filled in the SUS questionnaire, answering each question on a 5-point Likert scale. We analysed the results according to the adjective rating scale proposed by Bangor, Kortum, and Miller [4].

The mean value of the SUS questionnaire was 72.1, which according to the authors classifies the system as Good. Among the six participants who filled in the SUS, only one participant rated the system as Poor. All the others gave the system a positive rating.

After presenting the results to the participating PCU doctors, they corroborated the results. As main advantages of the mobile application it was mentioned the easiness of acquisition and image quality, while as disadvantage, the mobile application not being fully integrated with the referral system.

Dermatology Feedback. During the 10 month trial, a total of 31 cases were referred to the Dermatology Services. This short number of cases is justified by the Covid-19 pandemic, as patients refrained from consulting the health services unless it was urgent. The cases were mostly from female patients (68%) and older adults, as it can be observed in Fig. 5.

A dermatologist specialist annotated all cases by indicating the consultation type to follow up the case, being either through teleconsultation or in-person and the priority level of the consultation (see Fig. 5) as well as the differential diagnosis of the referred cases. Around 60% of the referenced cases were further booked with in-person consultation. Different benign and malign differential diagnosis were mentioned, including Actinic and Seborrheic Keratosis, Non-neoplastic Nevus, Dermatofibroma, Solar Lentigo, Basal Cell Carcinoma and Other Malignant Neoplasm.

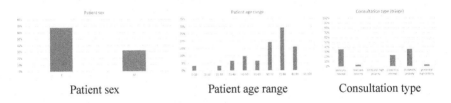

Patient sex   Patient age range   Consultation type

Fig. 5. Distribution of referred cases regarding patient sex, age range and specialist consultation type.

Regarding the images, the doctor annotated the focus and overall image quality considering four levels (bad, acceptable, good and very good). The reported results can be seen in Fig. 6 and illustrative examples of macro images with different focus levels are depicted in Fig. 7. Within the 31 cases a total of 37 and 33 macroscopic and anatomic images were sent, respectively. It is worth mentioning that the mobile application forces the acquisition of at least one macro and one anatomic image. In terms of focus, 73% of the macro images were considered very good, 11% good, 14% acceptable and 3% bad (3% corresponding to one image). Regarding the image quality in general, 65% of the macro images were very good, 16% good, 14% acceptable and 5% bad (5% corresponding to two images). In terms of focus, 73% of the anatomic images were considered very good, 21% good, and 6% bad (6% corresponding to two images). Concerning the image quality in general, 55% of the anatomic images were very good, 30% good, 9% acceptable and 6% bad (6% corresponding to two images).

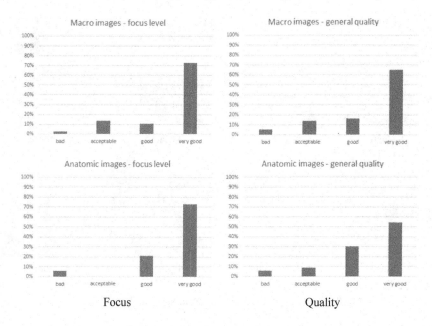

Fig. 6. Distribution macro and anatomic images of referred cases regarding focus and general quality.

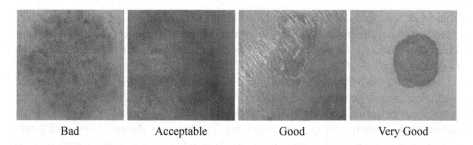

Fig. 7. Examples of macro images with different focus levels.

For the anatomic images the reason for the slightly worse results regarding the overall quality is the presence of clothes which hinders the doctor's analysis or the image being taken too far away from the lesion.

After presenting the results in the focus group, the dermatologist indicated that the usage of the mobile application by the PCU doctors benefited the triage work in the hospital, as an improvement of the lesion definition and focus was verified, and more standardization of the information shared (see Fig. 8). It was also mentioned that receiving both macro and anatomic images from the lesion is advantageous for their work, as it is possible to have clear information about the lesion and surrounding skin. By looking at the age and sex distribution of the patients the doctor confirmed that it translated the reality in dermatology consultations, as well as the lesions type variability.

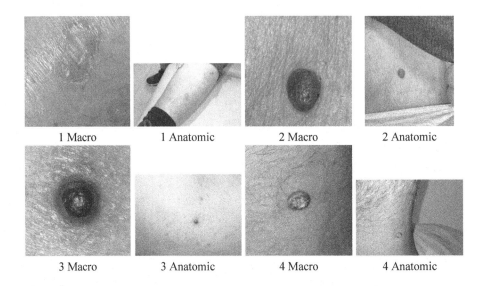

| 1 Macro | 1 Anatomic | 2 Macro | 2 Anatomic |

| 3 Macro | 3 Anatomic | 4 Macro | 4 Anatomic |

Fig. 8. Examples of image standardization for different cases.

6   Conclusion and Future Work

This work was motivated by the perks of Mobile Teledermatology such as an easier referral or monitorization in health care processes and facilitation of early diagnosis. The methodologies presented aim to help develop a standardization of image acquisition in dermatology.

Regarding the presented approach that analyses the preview images, the proposed methodology was proven to be suitable for real-time use without hindrances to the smartphone performance and obtained an accuracy and F1-score of 88.3% and 86.8%, respectively. These results are very promising demonstrating the capability of differentiating focused from non-focused images while maintaining the proper function of the application.

Following the preview focus analysis, a segmentation algorithm was developed to be able to run in real-time to not only find the skin lesion but also to segment it. A pre-process pipeline consisting of brightness and contrast adjustment, mean shift color enhancement, and grayscale sharpening, was implemented and tested to increase the easiness and ability to segment the lesion. An adaptative thresholding algorithm was used to segment the lesion followed by morphological operations to help clean and increase the segmentation performance. This entire pipeline was tested on two different datasets, Dermofit and SMARTSKINS, covering both pigmented and non-pigmented skin lesions. The pipeline obtained a Jaccard index of 68.59% and 86.44%, respectively, with the latter result surpassing the literature.

Similarly to the analysis of the preview focus, a similar approach was taken to evaluate the focus of the acquired images. An accuracy of 86.8% and an F1-score of 84.7% was obtained. This second verification increases the robustness of the entire process and helps ensuring the quality of the acquired images resulting in an increased number of suitable images for clinical purposes.

An embedded Android and iOS application with the proposed methodology were developed, in order to test the viability of the proposed approach in a real life scenario. Empirically, the obtained results through the real-time usage of the developed applications seem to be in line with the results here described, being more than sufficient for its overall use in practice.

To confirm the initial tests, a pilot study was run. The study lasted 10 months with six General and Family Medicine doctors and one dermatology specialist using the application, whether in their personal smartphone or in one provided to them. As main advantages of using the mobile application, doctors mention the easiness to acquire dermatological images as well as image quality improvement and standardization. Regarding the usability of the mobile application, a mean value of 72.1 was obtained in the SUS questionnaire, indicating good usability.

With the presented solution we aim to contribute to PCU service improvement, by ensuring that the gold-standard guidelines are being followed, enabling a quick and intuitive acquisition of dermatological data and automatically assessing image quality. The proposed solution also improves Hospital Dermatology Services by providing quality information to specialists. Finally this work contributes to the society with healthcare processes optimization through Artificial Intelligence and m-Health technologies' integration and impact assessment in a real operational environment.

As future work, the number of steps required to complete an image acquisition will be reduced and improved, as suggested by the doctors as well as the full integration with the NHS referral system.

Acknowledgements. This work was done under the scope of project "DERM.AI: Usage of Artificial Intelligence to Power Teledermatological Screening", and supported by national funds through 'FCT—Foundation for Science and Technology, I.P.', with reference DSAIPA/AI/0031/2018. The authors thank doctors from Unidade Local de Saúde da Guarda that participated in the trial.

References

1. Alves, J., Moreira, D., Alves, P., Rosado, L., Vasconcelos, M.: Automatic focus assessment on dermoscopic images acquired with smartphones. Sensors (Switzerland) **19**(22), 4957 (2019). https://doi.org/10.3390/s19224957
2. Andrade, C., Teixeira, L.F., Vasconcelos, M.J.M., Rosado, L.: Deep learning models for segmentation of mobile-acquired dermatological images. In: Campilho, A., Karray, F., Wang, Z. (eds.) ICIAR 2020. LNCS, vol. 12132, pp. 228–237. Springer, Cham (2020). https://doi.org/10.1007/978-3-030-50516-5_20
3. Apalla, Z., Nashan, D., Weller, R.B., Castellsagué, X.: Skin cancer: epidemiology, disease burden, pathophysiology, diagnosis, and therapeutic approaches. Dermatol. Ther. **7**(1), 5–19 (2017)
4. Bangor, A., Kortum, P., Miller, J.: Determining what individual SUS scores mean: adding an adjective rating scale. J. Usability Stud. **4**(3), 114–123 (2009)
5. Brooke, J.: SUS: a retrospective. J. Usability Stud. **8**(2), 29–40 (2013)

6. Börve, A., et al.: Smartphone teledermoscopy referrals: a novel process for improved triage of skin cancer patients. Acta Dermato-Venereologica **95** (2014). https://doi.org/10.2340/00015555-1906

7. Carvalho, R., Morgado, A.C., Andrade, C., Nedelcu, T., Carreiro, A., Vasconcelos, M.J.M.: Integrating domain knowledge into deep learning for skin lesion risk prioritization to assist teledermatology referral. Diagnostics **12**(1) (2022). https://doi.org/10.3390/diagnostics12010036

8. de Carvalho, T.M., Noels, E., Wakkee, M., Udrea, A., Nijsten, T.: Development of smartphone apps for skin cancer risk assessment: progress and promise. JMIR Dermatol. **2**(1), e13376 (2019)

9. Commissioning PC: Quality standards for teledermatology using 'store and forward' images (2011). https://sad.org.ar/wp-content/uploads/2020/12/Teledermatology-Quality-Standards.pdf. Accessed 15 Nov 2022

10. Dahlén Gyllencreutz, J., Johansson Backman, E., Terstappen, K., Paoli, J.: Teledermoscopy images acquired in primary health care and hospital settings - a comparative study of image quality. J. Eur. Acad. Dermatol. Venereol. **32**(6), 1038–1043 (2018). https://doi.org/10.1111/jdv.14565

11. Dugonik, B., Dugonik, A., Marovt, M., Golob, M.: Image quality assessment of digital image capturing devices for melanoma detection. Appl. Sci. (Switzerland) **10**(8), 2876 (2020). https://doi.org/10.3390/APP10082876

12. Errichetti, E., Stinco, G.: Dermoscopy in general dermatology: a practical overview. Dermatol. Ther. **6**(4), 471–507 (2016)

13. Faria, J., Almeida, J., Vasconcelos, M.J.M., Rosado, L.: Automated mobile image acquisition of skin wounds using real-time deep neural networks. In: Zheng, Y., Williams, B.M., Chen, K. (eds.) MIUA 2019. CCIS, vol. 1065, pp. 61–73. Springer, Cham (2020). https://doi.org/10.1007/978-3-030-39343-4_6

14. Ferlay, J., et al.: Estimating the global cancer incidence and mortality in 2018: GLOBOCAN sources and methods. Int. J. Cancer **144**(8), 1941–1953 (2019)

15. Fernandes, K., Cruz, R., Cardoso, J.S.: Deep image segmentation by quality inference. In: 2018 International Joint Conference on Neural Networks (IJCNN), pp. 1–8. IEEE (2018)

16. Feurer, M., Klein, A., Eggensperger, K., Springenberg, J., Blum, M., Hutter, F.: Efficient and robust automated machine learning. In: Advances in Neural Information Processing Systems, pp. 2962–2970 (2015)

17. Finnane, A., et al.: Proposed technical guidelines for the acquisition of clinical images of skin-related conditions. JAMA Dermatol. **153**(5), 453–457 (2017). https://doi.org/10.1001/jamadermatol.2016.6214

18. Finnane, A., Dallest, K., Janda, M., Soyer, H.P.: Teledermatology for the diagnosis and management of skin cancer: a systematic review. JAMA Dermatol. **153**(3), 319–327 (2017)

19. Flores, E., Scharcanski, J.: Segmentation of melanocytic skin lesions using feature learning and dictionaries. Expert Syst. Appl. **56**, 300–309 (2016)

20. Gonçalves, J., Conceiçao, T., Soares, F.: Inter-observer reliability in computer-aided diagnosis of diabetic retinopathy. In: HEALTHINF, pp. 481–491 (2019)

21. EI Ltd: Dermofit image library - Edinburgh innovations (2019). https://licensing.eri.ed.ac.uk/i/software/dermofit-image-library.html. Accessed 11 June 2019

22. Lubax, I.: Dermpic (2019). https://apps.apple.com/app/dermpic-dermoscopy/id1413455878?src=AppAgg.com (mobile software)

23. Moreira, D., Alves, P., Veiga, F., Rosado, L., Vasconcelos, M.: Automated mobile image acquisition of macroscopic dermatological lesions. In: Proceedings of the 14th International Joint Conference on Biomedical Engineering Systems and Technologies - HEALTHINF, pp. 122–132. SCITEPRESS-Science and Technology Publications, Lda (2021)

24. Munteanu, C.: Spotmole (2016). https://play.google.com/store/apps/details?id=com. spotmole&hl=en (mobile software)
25. Oliveira, R.B., Marranghello, N., Pereira, A.S., Tavares, J.M.R.: A computational approach for detecting pigmented skin lesions in macroscopic images. Expert Syst. Appl. **61**, 53–63 (2016)
26. Pertuz, S., Puig, D., Garcia, M.A.: Analysis of focus measure operators for shape-from-focus. Pattern Recogn. **46**(5), 1415–1432 (2013). https://doi.org/10.1016/j.patcog.2012.11. 011
27. Rat, C., et al.: Use of smartphones for early detection of melanoma: systematic review. J. Med. Internet Res. **20**(4), e135 (2018)
28. Rosado, L., Da Costa, J.M.C., Elias, D., Cardoso, J.S.: Mobile-based analysis of malaria-infected thin blood smears: automated species and life cycle stage determination. Sensors **17**(10), 2167 (2017)
29. Rosado, L., Vasconcelos, M.: Automatic segmentation methodology for dermatological images acquired via mobile devices. In: Proceedings of the International Joint Conference on Biomedical Engineering Systems and Technologies, vol. 5, pp. 246–251. SCITEPRESS-Science and Technology Publications, Lda (2015)
30. Santos, A., Ortiz de Solórzano, C., Vaquero, J.J., Pena, J.M., Malpica, N., del Pozo, F.: Evaluation of autofocus functions in molecular cytogenetic analysis. J. Microscopy **188**(3), 264–272 (1997)
31. Udrea, A., Lupu, C.: Real-time acquisition of quality verified nonstandardized color images for skin lesions risk assessment - a preliminary study. In: 2014 18th International Conference on System Theory, Control and Computing, ICSTCC 2014, pp. 199–204. Institute of Electrical and Electronics Engineers Inc. (2014). https://doi.org/10.1109/ICSTCC.2014.6982415
32. Vasconcelos, M.J.M., Rosado, L.: No-reference blur assessment of dermatological images acquired via mobile devices. In: Elmoataz, A., Lezoray, O., Nouboud, F., Mammass, D. (eds.) ICISP 2014. LNCS, vol. 8509, pp. 350–357. Springer, Cham (2014). https://doi.org/ 10.1007/978-3-319-07998-1_40
33. Vasconcelos, M.J.M., Rosado, L., Ferreira, M.: Principal axes-based asymmetry assessment methodology for skin lesion image analysis. In: Bebis, G., et al. (eds.) ISVC 2014. LNCS, vol. 8888, pp. 21–31. Springer, Cham (2014). https://doi.org/10.1007/978-3-319-14364-4_3

Towards Interpretable Machine Learning Models to Aid the Academic Performance of Children and Adolescents with Attention-Deficit/Hyperactivity Disorder

Caroline Jandre[1]($\boxtimes$) [ID], Marcelo Balbino[1] [ID], Débora de Miranda[2] [ID], Luis Zárate[1] [ID], and Cristiane Nobre[1] [ID]

[1] Department of Computer Science, Pontifical Catholic University of Minas Gerais, Minas Gerais, Brazil
caroline.jandre@sga.pucminas.br, marcelobalbino@gmail.com, {zarate,nobre}@pucminas.br
[2] Department of Pediatrics, Federal University of Minas Gerais, Minas Gerais, Brazil
debora.m.miranda@gmail.com

Abstract. Educational Data Mining (EDM) integrates numerous auxiliary techniques in capturing, processing, and analyzing school data, with the aim of monitoring and evaluating the process of acquiring knowledge. This assessment and closer monitoring of the student can positively help the learning of students with Attention Deficit Hyperactivity Disorder (ADHD), as they are more likely to have school difficulties, especially in the basic subjects: arithmetic, writing, and reading. Therefore, this work, which is an extension of the article by Jandre et al., seeks to complement the prediction of the results found with the VTJ48 and JRip algorithms that lead to high or low performance of de students whit ADHD in the three basic disciplines, adding the analysis of Random Forest, SVM, and ANN models, in addition to the application of the SHAP method to explain the output of the best model obtained, in case it is not explicitly interpretable. With the results obtained, it can be seen that the best prediction for the arithmetic discipline was performed by Random Forest and SVM (tied); in writing it was the ANN; and in reading it was the VTJ48. In addition, among the features that lead students with ADHD to have a high or low school performance are factors related to parental behavior, student gender, mother's education level, and family financial situation, among others.

Keywords: Interpretability · Machine learning · SHAP · Academic performance · School performance · ADHD · Children · Adolescents

1 Introduction

The search for models for the efficiency and quality of improved teaching and learning stimulated the creation of an area known as Educational Data Mining (EDM), which integrates numerous auxiliary techniques in capturing, processing, and analyzing school data, with the objective of monitoring and evaluating the knowledge acquisition process. All this analysis enables solutions that support the decision-making process in educational environments [39], may lead to the construction of a more inclusive environment. This change can positively impact the learning of students with Attention-Deficit/Hyperactivity Disorder (ADHD), as they are more likely to experience school difficulties, disruptive behaviors, and negative interactions with their colleagues, teachers, and parents [33], circumstances that can be softened with directed interventions.

Present in the Diagnostic and Statistical Manual of Mental Disorders (DSM), o ADHD is defined by harmful levels of inattention, disorganization, and/or hyperactivity and impulsivity, which can impact the social, emotional, and academic functioning of the individual, as well as their family [5,33]. Population surveys suggest that ADHD occurs in most cultures in about 5% of children, being more frequent in males. When it occurs in girls, they usually show more characteristics of inattention [5,25].

Since ADHD is not a definitive factor for poor school performance [12], it is essential to identify which other characteristics can enhance or minimize losses in the academic environment. This work is an extension of the article by Jandre et al. [19] that aimed to find classification rules that best describe school performance in arithmetic, writing, and reading (subjects that are part of the first phase of elementary school, provided for in the International Standardized Classification of Education [43]) of students with ADHD, using two classification algorithms: JRip, which generates rules directly from the dataset, and C4.5, a decision tree algorithm.

The objective of this work is to complement the prediction of the results found, adding the analysis of Machine Learning (ML) models: Random Forest (RF), Support Vector Machine (SVM), and Artificial Neural Network (ANN), as these tend to present better performance when compared to other algorithms. In addition, the SHapley Additive exPlanations (SHAP) method will be applied to explain the output of the best model obtained.

As it is an extension, the methodology of the initial stage of data mining, used in this work, followed the one applied in the work of Jandre et al. [19]: we used the same initial database with 266 children and adolescents and 255 features; same pre-processing as the base; and the same three approaches for feature selection: 1) *Genetic Algorithm (GA)*, which works to select the smallest subset of features, representative and relevant, seeking a higher quality model [31]; 2) *RF*, an ensemble algorithm, combining decision trees, which lists the features in order of importance; and 3) feature selection performed by a *specialist in ADHD and literature information* [4].

The article follows the following structure: in Sect. 2, the theoretical foundation is presented, which brings the main concepts related to work. The works related to the theme are covered in Sect. 3. Section 4 presents the methodology used, with a detailed description of the database and the pre-processing steps. Section 5 presents the discussions regarding the results found. Finally, in Sect. 6, the final considerations in this article are exposed.

2 Background

2.1 Attention-Deficit/Hyperactivity Disorder

The term ADHD appeared for the first time in the DSM, in its version III-R, but it was in the DSM-IV that it became known with its three subtypes: *predominantly inattentive,* when symptoms related to inattention are more accentuated; *predominantly hyperactive/impulsive*, in which the traits linked to hyperactivity and impulsivity are more significant; or *combined*, an association of inattentive, hyperactive and impulsive behaviors, this subtype being what is present in about 62% of people with ADHD [7,25,32].

Is discussed that the cause of ADHD is multifactorial, ranging from biological to environmental aspects, and that the disorder is related to the dysregulation of the neurotransmitters dopamine and noradrenaline. If these neurotransmitters act unsatisfactorily in the frontal lobe and its connections, attention, planning, organization, impulse control, focusing/filtering stimuli, among other functions, are affected, which would explain the symptoms of ADHD [26].

The diagnosis of ADHD is often complex, as there is not a specific test sufficient to define the existence of the disorder, making its identification happen through clinical-behavioral criteria. Furthermore, in 30 to 50% of cases, people with ADHD also have other types of disorders, called comorbidities, which makes the accuracy of symptoms even more ambiguous [23,29].

The treatment for ADHD, it usually requires a comprehensive and multimodal approach, including pharmacotherapy, behavioral measures, and environmental modifications, to reduce behavioral symptoms, as well as providing an improvement in the quality of life of the individual and his/hers relatives [33].

It is noteworthy that the school environment is considered of great help in the cognitive and socio-emotional development of the human being [36]. Thus, the educational institution can help students with ADHD to overcome their academic difficulties, creating strategies that contribute to the inclusion process and ensuring that these students are not at a disadvantage about other people who do not have the disorder [10,26].

2.2   Features Selection with Genetic Algorithm

Two methods stand out for dimensionality reduction in terms of the number of features: 1) *compression of features*, which encodes or transforms the data to obtain a compact representation of the originals, as is the case with Principal Component Analysis; 2) *features selection*, which identifies and discards irrelevant, not very relevant or redundant features. Among the strategies for selecting features, the following stand out: 1) *exponential* (represented by exhaustive search); 2) *sequential* (represented by direct sequential selection); 3) *random* (represented by GA) [31].

Genetic algorithm is a heuristic optimization and search technique based on the principles of genetics and the mechanisms of natural selection [15]. The technique was introduced by Holland [18] and popularized by Goldberg [14] and is based on the Darwinian maxim that *"The better an individual adapts to his environment, the greater his chance of surviving and generating descendants"* [24].

Algorithm 1 is a simplified representation of the GA evolution process. The proposal is to work with a population composed of many individuals to evolve according to a criterion defined by the *fitness* function. The individual is represented by the chromosome, a data structure representing the possible solutions to the problem. The process begins by randomly generating a set of chromosomes, constituting the initial population. This population is evaluated through the fitness function, which determines how well the individual has adapted to the problem. Next, individuals are submitted to the evolution-ary process that involves selecting parents and genetic operators. The selection consists of finding the most suitable individuals (parents) and letting them pass their genes on to the next generation. Once the parents are selected, they are submitted to genetic opera-tors (mutation and crossover) to generate new individuals (children). The new individu-als are evaluated by the function *fitness* and passed on to the next generations following the principle of natural selection until the stopping criterion is met.

Algorithm 1. GA Pseudocode.

$t \leftarrow 0$;
$InitializePopulation(P(t))$;
$fitness(P(t))$;
while *not* *Stopping Criteria* **do**
    $parents \leftarrow Selection(P(t))$;
    $children \leftarrow CrossoverMutation(parents)$;
    $P(t) \leftarrow P(t) + children$;
    $fitness(P(t))$;
    $P(t+1) \leftarrow NewPopulation(P(t))$;
    $t \leftarrow t + 1$;
end

2.3 Interpretability

ML systems have become increasingly common in high-risk problems that profoundly impact human life and society. Models have supported issues where a correct decision is essential [38]. Given this, there was a movement in the scientific community searching for increasingly better models from the point of view of predictive performance. Much research has been directed in this direction, and relevant results have been obtained, mainly through the so-called "black-box" methods [1].

However, having a model with high predictive performance is only a partial solution to the problem in many domains. In high-risk scenarios, such as the health area, for example, the decision-maker feels insecure without an explanation of the results of the model [42]. Therefore, it is necessary to present elements that allow developers and users to understand the system's decisions better, increasing confidence in the results and, when necessary, allowing the perception of incorrect decisions.

Faced with the need to explain the results generated by ML models, the scientific community has begun to turn its attention to the design of methods that aim at inter-pretability. To this end, one can make use of intrinsically interpretable models (e.g., decision tree) or methods that provide *post hoc* explanations for the predictions made by complex models [20].

As illustrated in Fig. 1, interpretability methods present a new perspective for ML solutions by adding an explanation model(g) to the original prediction model(f). The idea is to generate an interpretable approximation of the original model [28].

For this purpose, Lundberg and Lee [27] present SHAP, a tool based on cooperative game theory to interpret ML models. The approach uses *SHAP values* as a way to measure the importance of each feature in a prediction. Thus, each feature impacts a

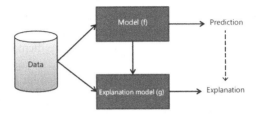

Fig. 1. How an explanation model is used in predicting interpretation [28].

given instance by a value that can be positive, negative, or zero. The authors created a version applicable to any model called *Kernel SHAP* and some specific versions for certain types of models such as *Linear SHAP*, *Low-Order SHAP*, *Max SHAP*, *Deep SHAP* and the *SHAP Tree Explainer*.

3   Related Works

The literature has been progressing about research focused on EDM, with works aimed at acquiring knowledge on educational topics, such as student performance prediction [2], learning through remote teaching [16], among other issues related to the school environment.

The work of Wandera et al. [44] revealed characteristics associated with good academic performance in high schools in South Africa, using Logistic Regression, Light Gradient Boosting (LightGBM), and tree-based algorithms. The database used combined sources related to community research, students' school performance, among other information. The SHAP and odds ratios were used to explain the model results and provide information on the relationships between the variables. The Logistic Regression and LightGBM models outperformed the decision tree model, and the significant characteristics presented by SHAP indicate that the availability of potable water in the community, the situation of the schools' bathrooms, the possibility of using cellular internet by students, among other variables, impact the school performance of students.

Souza and dos Santos [39] used a database that addresses the performance in Mathematics and Portuguese of students in secondary education in two Portuguese schools. The objective was to compare consolidated techniques within the scope of the EMD, with the Deep Learning technique. The ML algorithms chosen were: Naïve Bayes, Decision Tree, RF, and SVM. For Deep Learning, the MultilayerPerceptron (MLP) architecture was used. The authors point out that the Decision Tree was the second most accurate model, reaching 87% accuracy, and that, due to its simplicity of application and processing speed, it can be a promising alternative. Regarding the prediction of school performance, the authors found the grades and the number of student absences as the main features. However, they emphasize that the influence of other elements cannot be ruled out, such as the experience of adversities by the students, but that, due to the lack of information in the questionnaires that evidence what motivated the students' grades and attendance, it is only possible to say that the influential features are those related to their school performance.

The literature also reveals that ML methods have been widely used in research related to ADHD and have generated important advances in the search for knowledge associated with this disorder.

Anuradha et al. [3] conducted a study for diagnosing ADHD in 100 children aged 6 to 11 years using the SVM algorithm. The database was collected through the students' responses to a questionnaire and medical diagnoses indicating whether the children had ADHD. The work used GA to features selection in order to identify the essential features and increase the accuracy of the model. The study achieved an 88.7% success in diagnosing ADHD, which was considered a satisfactory result from the authors.

Rahadian et al. [35] used GA to improve a Learning Vector Quantization 2 Neural Network (LVQ2NN) method to classify data about the type of ADHD in patients. The GA was used to optimize the weight vector in the training process. The tests performed without the GA reached 80% of correctness, while the model with the GA improved the performance to 89.5%.

Therefore, this work is in line with the literature, as it uses algorithms frequently used in other articles, and techniques for interpretability and selection of known features. However, there is still not a wide range of studies relating data on the lives of people with ADHD and EDM. Thus, this extension of the article by Jandre et al. [19] may contribute to more findings focused on this area of interest.

4 Materials and Methods

4.1 Description of the Database

The database was made available by the Department of Pediatrics of the Federal University of Minas Gerais - Brazil. The sample consists of 266 students (instances), aged between 6 and 18 years. Among them, 196 are diagnosed with ADHD and 70 have a negative diagnosis.

The database, based on 225 characteristics (features), it was built from the individual and family responses present in the questionnaires. Also, interviews were conducted with those responsible and patients who are followed up at the hospital linked to the college. The base contains information on health, financial conditions, parental care, education, among others, in addition to the notes for the arithmetic, writing, and reading tests of each present in the database.

4.2 Pre-processing

With the aim to improve the quality of the data, the pre-processing of the database was performed through the steps described below.

1. Exclusion of instances that did not present the grade of the Test of School Performance (TSP) [40] in arithmetic, writing, or reading.
2. Transformation of the grades obtained in the TSP, comparing them with the average grade of a Brazilian state, in High and Low performance. For this, the Standards Tables present in the TSP manual were used. The tables in the manual for the classification of notes range from the 1st to the 6th grade, which corresponds from the

2nd to the 7th year in the current academic category. Therefore, the years before the 2nd year were classified according to the classification criteria of the 2nd year, and those after the 7th year followed the classification parameters of the 7th year.

3. Exclusion of irrelevant features (e.g., name and telephone number), and those who presented the same information or were complementary (e.g., age in months and age in years), concatenating them and maintaining only one feature.

4. Transformation of features belonging to the same category into a single feature (e.g., Conduct Disorder and Opposition Disorder are part of Behavior Disorders, so a single feature called "Behavior Disorders" has been created, which indicates whether the individual has "Conduct Disorder" or "Opposition Disorder").

5. Filling in the missing data by the average, in numerical data, or by mode, in categorical features.

6. Binarization of non-ordinal nominal features, that is, they were coded as the presence or absence of the characteristic.

7. Random manual separation of 15% of each class's instances to carry out the tests.

8. Balancing of 85% of the remaining data using the SpreadSubsample algorithm present in the Waikato Environment for Knowledge Analysis - WEKA[1] The SpreadSubsample algorithm follows the undersampling approach, randomly reducing instances of the majority class. Uniform distribution was applied. After balancing, the Randomize filter was executed in order to shuffle the instances.

Thus, Table 1 shows the total number of instances, of each class, for testing and creating models, after the pre-processing steps. It should be noted that the separation of the instances for testing was carried out before the database was balanced.

Table 1. Number of balanced instances for creating the model and unbalanced for the tests [19].

Discipline	Training/Validation		Test	
	High	Low	High	Low
Arithmetic	59	59	11	29
Writing	50	50	09	31
Reading	39	39	08	27

As for the features, at the end of the pre-processing, 130 remained to represent the base. Figure 2 presents an overview of the database, with the categories of data and the number of features in each category, in the form "Number of initial features/Number of features after pre-processing".

4.3 Dimensionality Reduction with Genetic Algorithm, Random Forest, and Specialist

A combination of three methods - GA, RF, and specialist - was used to select the essential features in learning among the 130 features present in the database.

---

[1] WEKA is open source software issued under the GNU General Public License that contains a collection of ML algorithms [13]. Available at http://www.cs.waikato.ac.nz/ml/weka.

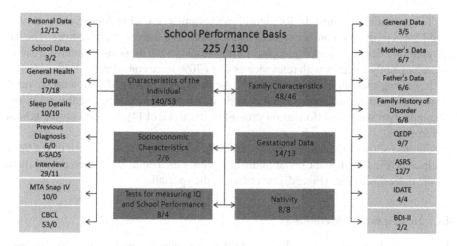

Fig. 2. Overview of the database, grouped by categories [19].

The Non-dominated Sorting Genetic Algorithm II (NSGA-II) algorithm was chosen to find the best subset of features maximizing your fitness, in this case, the F-Measure. To evaluate the F-Measure, the K-Nearest Neighbors (KNN) classifier was used. His choice was motivated by the low computational cost for adjusting his parameters. In this work, the parameter k (number of closest neighbors) was adjusted, varying its value range [1–10]. GA was implemented in the Python language, using the DEAP library, available from Université Laval [11].

Aiming at the adequate definition of the necessary parameters for the experiments' execution, intervals of values were analyzed, having as a stopping criterion the number of GA generations. For each set of parameters, 10 different random seeds were used. Table 2 shows the ranges of values used.

Table 2. Range of parameter values [19].

Population initialization	Random
Representation	Binary
Crossover operator	Two Points
Crossover probability	70%, 75%, 80% and 85%
Mutation operator	One Point
Mutation probability	1%, 5% and 10%
Population size	100, 300 and 500
Number of generations	100, 300 and 500
Crossover selection method	Tournament ($size = 2$)
Composition of the new generation	Non-dominated individuals
Stopping criteria	Number of generations

To automatically adjust the RF algorithm's parameters, CVParameterSelection[2] was used [21], varying the number of trees and features, and the depth of the trees. The RF calculates the feature's importance, indicating which are the most important for creating the model. Only features with relevance as from 70% were considered.

Regarding specialist, the knowledge of the medical expert in ADHD, who provided the database and is a collaborator in this work, was used to finalize the features selection, in conjunction with the information present in the work of [4], focused on the school performance.

Figure 3 shows the features selected by GA and RF, separated for each of the three disciplines (Figs. 3a, b and c). The figure also shows the features considered important, for the three disciplines (Fig. 3d), according to the specialist.

4.4   Description of Methods

To assist in discovering the rules that lead the student to obtain a high or low performance, the VTJ48 algorithm (tree algorithm) and the JRip (rule algorithm) were used. VTJ48 [41] has the same functioning as J48, developed by Quinlan [34], which is a Java adaptation of C4.5. That is, the VTJ48 also builds a decision tree from the instances, but its difference is that it automatically adjusts the confidence for pruning and the minimum number of instances per leaf. JRip is a Java implementation of the Ripper algorithm, proposed by [9] as an optimized version of the IREP algorithm. JRip constructs the rules seeking to represent the model as compactly as possible with as much information of the data; that is, it seeks to consistently explain which features are relevant to the pattern(s) found in the database, with the minimum of rules.

Regarding the "black-box" algorithms, RF, MLP, and Sequential Minimal Optimization (SMO) were used. WEKA's RF is an extension and improvement of bagging for decision trees, and can be used for classification or regression [6]. RF uses the voting system, combining the response of several trees, to determine the class of an instance. MLP is an implementation of ANN. This algorithm follows a flow that starts at the input layer and goes through n layers, until reaching the output layer (which represents a given problem), using backpropagation to classify the instances [30]. The SMO is an implementation to train an SVM classifier, which aims to find the hyperplane that presents the greatest distance between the existing classes in the database, maximizing its separation [17].

Two strategies were used to deepen the understanding of the model and consequently the comprehension of the features that impact the performance in arithmetic, reading, and writing: 1) if the best predictive model of performance is the decision tree, which is intrinsically interpretable, we use the rules obtained through the tree; 2) if the best model is based on one of the "black-box" algorithms, we propose to perform the interpretability using the SHAP approach.

About SHAP, as shown in Sect. 2.3, the tool generates an explanation model from the classification model. The explanation model takes as input a sample of data and performs interpretability for the predictions of this sample. We chose to apply the explanation model to the same set of instances in which the classification model tests were

---

[2] Available in the WEKA tool.

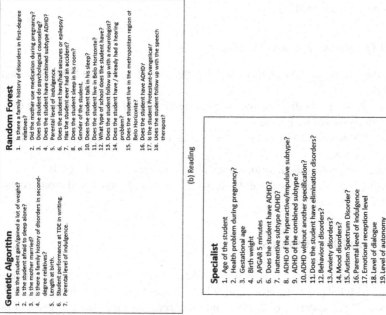

Fig. 3. Description of the features of the three databases, considering the three selection methods [19].

applied. The graphs generated by SHAP allow us to identify and understand the most relevant features for the predictions.

4.5 Model Quality Assessment Metrics

To evaluate the quality of the obtained models, Precision, Recall, and F-Measure metrics were used.

Precision[3] is the percentage of instances correctly classified in a class, out of all those that were classified in the class.

Recall[4] is the percentage of instances of a class that have been correctly predicted to belong to the class.

F-Measure[5] represents the harmonic mean between Precision and Recall.

All classifiers were built and validated using the k-fold cross-validation process, with $k = 10$ [22].

5 Results and Discussions

Figures 4, 5, 6, 7, and 8 present the results of the model creation and testing phase of the RF, MLP, SMO algorithms, JRip, and VTJ48, respectively. The values refer to the experiments with the selection of the GA and the insertion of the characteristics of the RF and specialist. The results are presented by discipline and by the algorithm. We chose to make a graph for each algorithm to highlight their behavior in each experiment separately. It is noteworthy that in the experiments in which the features were selected only by the GA, the number of features used in the prediction of arithmetic, writing, and reading performance was only 16, 29, and 7, respectively. In the experiments in which the features are a combination of the non-identical ones present in the selection of the GA, RF, and Specialist, 51 features remained for arithmetic representation, 54 for writing, and 43 for reading.

Analyzing the basis used for the test and observing the F-Measure metric, it can be seen that the RF algorithm, Fig. 4, obtained better results: with the features selected by GA, RF, and Arithmetic Specialist; and that in writing and reading, the two versions of the base achieved the same result.

The MLP, observing Fig. 5 and following the same analysis parameter, also stood out, in arithmetic, with the GA, RF, and Specialist versions, especially when compared to the high class, which is the original minority class, and, consequently, the one with the greatest difficulty for prediction. In the writing discipline, the best results were also obtained by the combination of GA, RF, and Specialist. However, in reading, the version with features only selected by the GA obtained the best results.

Analyzing the SMO algorithm (Fig. 6), again the version of GA, RF, and Specialist had the best result in arithmetic. In writing, there was no difference between the versions. In reading, the best result was obtained with the features selected by the GA.

---

[3] $Precision = \frac{VP}{VP+FP}$.

[4] $Recall = \frac{VP}{VP+FN}$.

[5] $F-Measure = \frac{2 \times Recall \times Precision}{Recall+Precision}$.

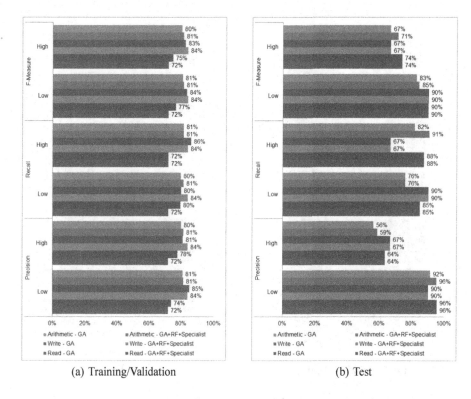

(a) Training/Validation   (b) Test

Fig. 4. RF algorithm result.

There was a tie between the two versions of the base in arithmetic, when analyzing the JRip algorithm (Fig. 7). Writing excelled with the version of features selected by GA, and reading with those selected by GA, RF, and Specialist.

Finally, in the VTJ48 algorithm, observing Fig. 8, it can be seen that in arithmetic the version with the features selected by AG, RF, and Specialist was the one with the best result. In writing and reading, it was the GA-only version that stood out.

After this investigation, it is noted that: in arithmetic, the version of the base with the features selected by the GA, RF, and Specialist was the one with the best use, as it presented the best result in 4 of 5 evaluated algorithms, and tied for 1, that is, it was not the worst result at any time; in writing, the best version depends on the algorithm applied, as there was a tie in results in 2 algorithms, a superior result with GA, RF, and Specialist in 1, and only with the features selected by the GA in 2 algorithms. In reading, it can be said that the best version is the one with the features selected only with GA, as it presented a superior result in 3 algorithms, tied in 1, and was inferior in 1 algorithm.

To identify which algorithm had the best prediction in each of the disciplines, another comparison was performed, analyzing only the F-Measure metric, in the test phase, with the bases of the best version previously reported in the description of the

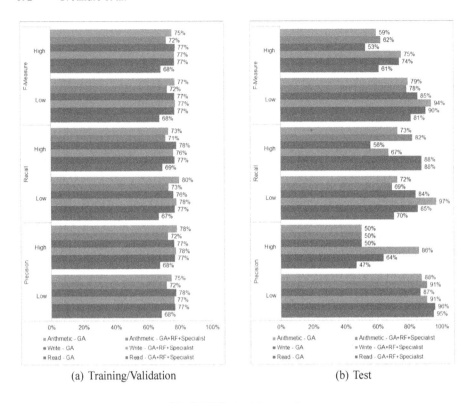

(a) Training/Validation   (b) Test

Fig. 5. MLP algorithm result.

results of each of the algorithms (during the analysis of Figs. 4, 5, 6, 7, and 8). Figure 9 presents the new comparison.

After analyzing Fig. 9, it is noted that, in reading, the algorithm with the highest performance was VTJ48, which is a Decision Tree algorithm; in writing it was the MLP, which is an ANN implementation; and in arithmetic there was a tie between the RF (ensemble algorithm) and the SMO (implementation to train an SVM classifier).

Note that to find the best results described, the following settings were used:

– **VTJ48, in the reading base, with features selected only by the GA:** minimum number of instances per sheet = 2; confidence limit for pruning = 0.5.
– **MLP, in the base of writing, with features selected by GA, RF, and Specialist:** learning rate = 0.4; momentum = 0.3; number of epochs = 600; number of hidden layers = 39.
– **RF, in the arithmetic base, with features selected by GA, RF, and Specialist:** number of trees = 100; number of features = 8; maximum depth of trees = 4.
– **SMO, in the arithmetic base, with features selected by GA, RF, and Specialist:** complexity constant = 2; kernel = puk.

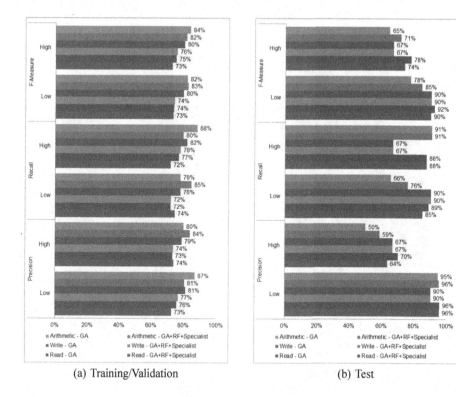

(a) Training/Validation   (b) Test

Fig. 6. SMO algorithm result.

5.1 VTJ48 Rules and Interpretability Using SHAP

In the experiments, with the reading base, the algorithm that had the best performance was the VTJ48, which already allows exploring its rules explicitly. Therefore, the Table 3 Table presents the rules found that explain the reasons for a student to have a high or low performance in the reading discipline, with coverage from 10%. Coverage is the percentage of instances that the rule classifies correctly, out of all instances of the class.

Table 3. Generated rules and coverage [19].

Read		
Number	Rule	Coverage
1	If writing performance = low and indulgence $\leq$ 15 then **Low**	80%
2	If writing performance = high then **High**	44%
3	If writing performance = average and fear of sleeping alone = no then **High**	26%

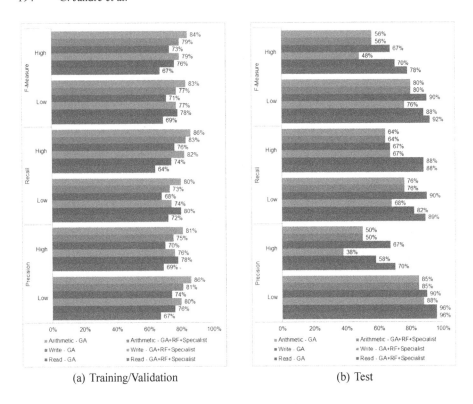

(a) Training/Validation   (b) Test

Fig. 7. JRip algorithm result.

Analyzing the rules found in reading, it is noted that the performance in writing has a strong influence on the student's performance in this discipline, especially in rule 2, where if the student does well in writing, he also does well in reading. However, the influence of some other features on reading performance is also observed. Rule 1, for example, with coverage of 80%, points to the importance of the parental behavior, because if the student has a low writing performance and his parents are less indulgent (the highest present value in the base is 24), that is, generally do not forgive mistakes or praise successes, their reading performance will also below. This observation indicates that family support is essential, especially in times of difficulty. Rule 3 suggests that when writing performance is average, and the student is not afraid to sleep alone, he has a high reading performance. One of the justifications for fear of sleeping alone may be linked to phobic anxiety, which causes a lack of confidence, security, and support, leading to feelings of helplessness, fragility, and dependence [37]. Therefore, not being afraid to sleep alone can represent certain self-confidence, which results in a positive performance.

On the other hand, in arithmetic and writing, the best performance was obtained through "black-box" algorithms, which implies restrictions on the interpretability of model decisions. In several problems, as is the case in the present research, limitations in the interpretability of decisions undermine the confidence in the model and its consequent use in practice. Furthermore, the opportunity for knowledge discovery is also reduced.

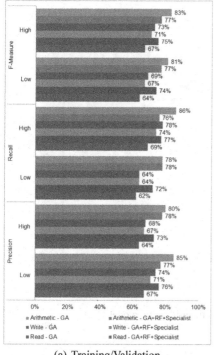
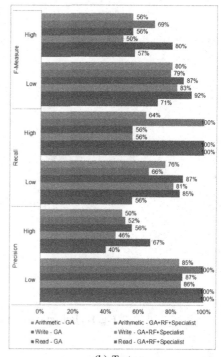

(a) Training/Validation   (b) Test

Fig. 8. VTJ48 algorithm result.

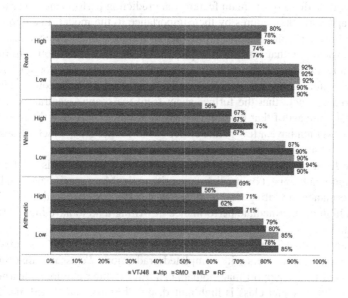

Fig. 9. Comparison between algorithms.

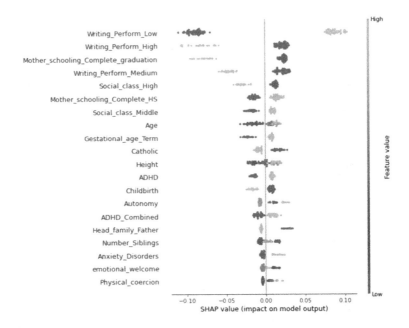

Fig. 10. Impact of features on the arithmetic model.

Thus, we chose to use SHAP to deepen our understanding of model decisions and identify the features with the most significant impact on predicting performance in arithmetic and writing. Figure 10 exemplifies one of the graphs from the tool. It presents an overview of the effects of the main features on predicting performance in arithmetic.

The graph sorts the features by their importance to the model. Each point present on the line of a particular features represents an instance and, consequently, a student that was impacted by that features. If a point is on the right side relative to the central axis, such a feature moves the student closer to the low class. The dot color represents the feature's value in the instance (red for higher values, blue for lower values). It is also important to note that the further away from the graph's central axis, the more significant the impact of that feature for a given instance. Note that the features at the bottom of the graph have a few points closer to the central axis, which means that this feature has a little significant effect on the model.

We see from the graph in Fig. 10 that performance in writing is the feature with the most significant impact on prediction in arithmetic. More specifically, students with lower performance in writing tend to have lower performance in arithmetic. Also, students with high or intermediate performance in writing tend to have high performance in arithmetic.

The graph shows the importance of the mother's schooling, with a positive and significant influence on mothers with completed graduation. We assume that this feature may be related to the support that mothers can offer to their children's learning. Similarly, the family's social class is highlighted, possibly associated with the resources provided to students that require financial support, especially in the case of students with ADHD.

Furthermore, the graph indicates the importance of "Age" on the features with the most significant impact. To delve deeper into the behavior of a particular feature, SHAP has the graph present in Fig. 11. In this case, we can observe the effect of age on predicting performance in arithmetic. It is possible to observe a trend of more outstanding academic difficulty of the student in this subject with the advancement of school years, especially from the age of nine (positive SHAP *values* for the Lower class). We believe that this influence of age is related to the fact that younger children are beginning school life and thus are little impacted by academic activities. As years go by, the difficulty level of the activities increases, which can cause learning problems and, consequently, lead to a worsening in academic performance.

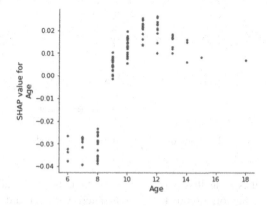

Fig. 11. Impact of age on arithmetic.

Other features are listed but with less importance. Among these, the features "ADHD" and "combined ADHD" stand out, indicating that although ADHD impacts academic performance in arithmetic, other features have a more significant influence. It is noteworthy that over the years, the characteristics of ADHD may have become more evident, which is probably why this feature is not as prominent in this analysis since there are children of early school age.

About the writing model, Fig. 12 shows the list of the most important prediction features in this discipline. There is a relationship between performance in writing and the other disciplines present in the database, so students with lower performance in arithmetic and reading also tend to have low performance in writing and vice-versa.

Next, the graph shows the importance of the feature ADHD, in which having ADHD is a complicating factor for performance in writing. The gender feature also stands out, indicating that being male makes the prediction of lower performance closer while being female contributes to higher performance. The fact that the male gender tends to low performance may indicate a reproduction of social stereotypes in which girls are said to be quieter, and boys are rowdy and undisciplined, which leads to a negative evaluation of the child's behavior and influences the final grade [8]. Other features complete the list but with less importance.

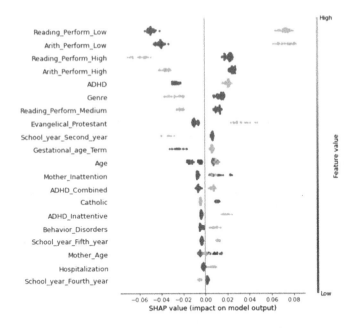

Fig. 12. Impact of features on the writing model.

After analysis, it is clear that performance in students can be affected by factors related to parental behavior, circumstances associated with fear and insecurity (sleeping alone), mother's education, family's financial conditions, gender, age, and student's height, in addition to their performance in other disciplines. ADHD also impacts performance, but generally less so than other aspects of an individual's life. Therefore, a multifactorial approach must be taken so that students with ADHD can improve their academic performance.

6   Final Considerations

As much as society is paying more attention to issues related to ADHD, there is still little knowledge disseminated to the population about the characteristics and implications of the disorder. The judgments that children and adolescents with ADHD are normally affected by can lead to the exclusion of these people, resulting in low self-esteem and anti-sociability. In addition, if the student with ADHD receives due attention from parents and school members, it is possible to change the prognosis considered unfavorable. Therefore, it becomes significant to identify which characteristics influence the individual's academic experience to alleviate their difficulties.

In this work, three algorithms considered "black-box" (RF, MLP, and SMO) and two considered "white-box" (VTJ48, and JRip) were used. With the results, it is noticed that explicitly interpretable algorithms do not always lose in performance, because, in the reading base, it was the VTJ48 that obtained the best prediction result. Therefore, the use of the "white-box" method proved to be positive in this context. In arithmetic and writing, the association of the "black-box" and SHAP algorithms was efficient, as it was possible to achieve good predictions and, later, identify the most significant features for academic performance, deepening the understanding of the model decisions and contributing to increasing knowledge about the problem in question. According to the observations made, some factors are more relevant than whether or not the student has ADHD. This is an indication that the disorder itself does not indicate how the student's academic performance will be, as the environmental and emotional factors in which he is involved directly affect his attainment of academic knowledge.

Regarding dimensionality reduction, the two versions of the database (one only with features selected by GA, and another with features selected by GA, RF, and Specialist), contributed to a good predictive result, with each version having its own contribution more directed to one or another discipline.

In future work, to identify other factors that may affect the performance of students with ADHD, we intend to evaluate new approaches for balancing, since the use of different instances can contribute to new discoveries. In addition, it is considered to investigate what the results would be like if the problem were treated as multi-label. In other words, it is intended to evaluate the quality of the models in the prediction of student performance in all subjects, jointly.

Acknowledgements. This study was financed in part by the Coordination for the Improvement of Higher Education Personnel - Brasil (CAPES) - Finance Code 001. The authors thank the National Council for Scientific and Technological Development of Brazil (CNPq - Conselho Nacional de Desenvolvimento Científico e Tecnológico) and the Foundation for Research Support of the Minas Gerais State (FAPEMIG). The work was developed at the Pontifical Catholic University of Minas Gerais, PUC Minas in the Applied Computational Intelligence laboratory - LICAP.

References

1. Abdul, A., Vermeulen, J., Wang, D., Lim, B.Y., Kankanhalli, M.: Trends and trajectories for explainable, accountable and intelligible systems: an HCI research agenda. In: Proceedings of the 2018 CHI Conference on Human Factors in Computing Systems, pp. 1–18. Association for Computing Machinery, New York (2018). https://doi.org/10.1145/3173574.3174156
2. Ahmed, A., Elaraby, I.S.: Data mining: a prediction for student's performance using classification method. World J. Comput. Appl. Technol. **2**(2), 43–47 (2014)
3. Anuradha, J., Tisha, Ramachandran, V., Arulalan, K.V., Tripathy, B.K.: Diagnosis of ADHD using SVM algorithm. In: Proceedings of the Third Annual ACM Bangalore Conference, COMPUTE 2010, Association for Computing Machinery, New York (2010)
4. Araújo, A.P.d.Q.C.: Avaliação e manejo de criança com dificuldade escolar e distúrbio de atenção. Jornal de Pediatria **78**, S104–S110 (2002)
5. American Psychological Association et al.: DSM-5: Manual diagnóstico e estatístico de transtornos mentais. Artmed Editora (2014)
6. Brownlee, J.: How to use ensemble machine learning algorithms in Weka (2016). https://machinelearningmastery.com/use-ensemble-machine-learning-algorithms-weka/. Accessed 08 Apr 2022
7. Cardoso, L., Mollica, A.M.V., Sales, A.M., Araújo, L.C.: O lúdico e a aprendizagem de crianças com transtorno de déficit de atenção/hiperatividade. Revista Científica FAGOC-Multidisciplinar **3**(2) (2019)

8. Carvalho, M.P.d.: Por que tantos meninos vão mal na escola? critérios de avaliação escolar segundo o sexo. Cadernos de Pesquisa (2007)
9. Cohen, W.W.: Fast effective rule induction. In: Twelfth International Conference on Machine Learning, pp. 115–123. Morgan Kaufmann (1995)
10. Cortez, M.T., Pinheiro, Â.M.V.: TDAH e escola: incompatibilidade? Paidéia **13**(19) (2018)
11. Fortin, F.A., De Rainville, F.M., Gardner, M.A.G., Parizeau, M., Gagné, C.: Deap: evolutionary algorithms made easy. J. Mach. Learn. Res. **13**(1), 2171–2175 (2012)
12. Frazier, T.W., Youngstrom, E.A., Glutting, J.J., Watkins, M.W.: ADHD and achievement: meta-analysis of the child, adolescent, and adult literatures and a concomitant study with college students. J. Learn. Disabil. **40**(1), 49–65 (2007)
13. Garner, S.: Weka: the Waikato environment for knowledge analysis. In: Proceedings of the New Zealand Computer Science Research Students Conference (1995)
14. Goldberg, D.E.: Genetic algorithms in search. In: Optimization, and Machine Learning (1989)
15. Haupt, R.L., Haupt, S.E.: Practical Genetic Algorithms. Wiley, Hoboken (2004)
16. He, W.: Examining students' online interaction in a live video streaming environment using data mining and text mining. Comput. Hum. Behav. **29**(1), 90–102 (2013). https://doi.org/10.1016/j.chb.2012.07.020. Including Special Section Youth, Internet, and Wellbeing
17. Hearst, M.A., Dumais, S.T., Osuna, E., Platt, J., Scholkopf, B.: Support vector machines. IEEE Intell. Syst. Appl. **13**(4), 18–28 (1998)
18. Holland, J.: Adaptation in natural and artificial systems: an introductory analysis with application to biology. Control Artif. Intell. (1975)
19. Jandre, C., Santos, B.C., Balbino, M., de Miranda, D., Zárate, L.E., Nobre, C.: Analysis of school performance of children and adolescents with attention-deficit/hyperactivity disorder: a dimensionality reduction approach. In: HEALTHINF, pp. 155–165 (2021)
20. Kaur, H., Nori, H., Jenkins, S., Caruana, R., Wallach, H., Wortman Vaughan, J.: Interpreting interpretability: understanding data scientists' use of interpretability tools for machine learning. In: Proceedings of the 2020 CHI Conference on Human Factors in Computing Systems, pp. 1–14 (2020)
21. Kohavi, R.: Wrappers for performance enhancement and oblivious decision graphs. Ph.D. thesis, Stanford University, Department of Computer Science, Stanford University (1995)
22. Kohavi, R.: A study of cross-validation and bootstrap for accuracy estimation and model selection. In: Proceedings of the 14th International Joint Conference on Artificial Intelligence, IJCAI 1995, vol. 2, pp. 1137–1143. Morgan Kaufmann Publishers Inc., San Francisco (1995)
23. Koltermann, G.: Sintomas de TDAH, desempenho neurocognitivo e nível socioeconômico em crianças de 3° e 4° anos do ensino fundamental. Mestrado em psicologia, Universidade Federal do Rio Grande do Sul, Porto Alegre (2018)
24. de Lacerda, E.G., de Carvalho, A.: Introdução aos algoritmos genéticos. Sistemas inteligentes: aplicaçoes a recursos hídricos e ciências ambientais **1**, 99–148 (1999)
25. Larroca, L.M., Domingos, N.M.: TDAH-investigação dos critérios para diagnóstico do subtipo predominantemente desatento. Psicologia Escolar e Educacional **16**(1), 113–123 (2012)
26. de Lima, C.B., Coelho, C.L.M.: Transtorno de déficit de atenção/hiperatividade-um olhar sob a perspectiva da educação especial inclusiva. Cadernos de Pesquisa em Educação **20**(47), 172–192 (2018)
27. Lundberg, S.M., Lee, S.I.: A unified approach to interpreting model predictions. In: Guyon, I., et al. (eds.) Advances in Neural Information Processing Systems, vol. 30, pp. 4765–4774. Curran Associates, Inc. (2017)
28. Mokhtari, K.E., Higdon, B.P., Başar, A.: Interpreting financial time series with SHAP values. In: Proceedings of the 29th Annual International Conference on Computer Science and Software Engineering, CASCON 2019, pp. 166–172. IBM Corporation (2019)

29. Moreira, S.C., Barreto, M.A.M.: Transtorno de déficit de atenção e hiperatividade: conhecendo para intervir. Revista Práxis 1(2) (2017)
30. de Pádua Braga, A., de Leon Ferreira, A.C.P., Ludermir, T.B.: Redes neurais artificiais: teoria e aplicações. LTC Editora, Rio de Janeiro (2007)
31. Pappa, G.L., Freitas, A.A., Kaestner, C.A.: A multiobjective genetic algorithm for attribute selection. In: Proceedings of the 4th International Conference on Recent Advances in Soft Computing (RASC 2002), pp. 116–121. Nottingham Trent University, Nottingham (2002)
32. Phelan, T.: TDA/TDAH - Transtorno de Déficit de Atenção e Hiperatividade - Sintomas, Diagnósticos e Tratamentos: Criancas e Adultos. M. Books, São Paulo (2004)
33. Pongwilairat, K., Louthrenoo, O., Charnsil, C., Witoonchart, C., et al.: Quality of life of children with attention-deficit/hyper activity disorder. J. Med. Assoc. Thai. 88(8), 1062–1066 (2005)
34. Quinlan, R.: C4.5: Programs for Machine Learning. Morgan Kaufmann Publishers, San Mateo (1993)
35. Rahadian, B.A., Dewi, C., Rahayudi, B.: The performance of genetic algorithm learning vector quantization 2 neural network on identification of the types of attention deficit hyperactivity disorder. In: 2017 International Conference on Sustainable Information Engineering and Technology (SIET), pp. 337–341 (2017)
36. Rangel Júnior, É.d.B., Loos, H.: Escola e desenvolvimento psicossocial segundo percepções de jovens com tdah. Paidéia 21(50), 373–382 (2011)
37. da Rocha Antony, S.M.: Os ajustamentos criativos da criança em sofrimento: uma compreensão da gestalt-terapia sobre as principais psicopatologias da infância. Estudos e pesquisas em Psicologia 9(2), 356–375 (2009)
38. Rudin, C.: Stop explaining black box machine learning models for high stakes decisions and use interpretable models instead. Nat. Mach. Intell. 1(5), 206–215 (2019)
39. Souza, V.F., dos Santos, T.C.B.: Processo de mineração de dados educacionais aplicado na previsão do desempenho de alunos: Uma comparação entre as técnicas de aprendizagem de máquina e aprendizagem profunda. Revista Brasileira de Informática na Educação 29, 519–546 (2021)
40. Stein, L.M.: TDE: teste de desempenho escolar: manual para aplicação e interpretação, pp. 1–17. Casa do Psicólogo, São Paulo (1994)
41. Stiglic, G., Kocbek, S., Pernek, I., Kokol, P.: Comprehensive decision tree models in bioinformatics. PLoS ONE 7(3), e33812 (2012). https://doi.org/10.1371/journal.pone.0033812
42. Tjoa, E., Guan, C.: A survey on explainable artificial intelligence (XAI): toward medical XAI. IEEE Trans. Neural Netw. Learn. Syst. 1–21 (2020). https://doi.org/10.1109/TNNLS.2020.3027314
43. UNESCO Institute for Statistics: International standard classification of education: ISCED 2011. UNESCO Institute for Statistics Montreal, Quebec (2012)
44. Wandera, H., Marivate, V., Sengeh, M.D.: Predicting national school performance for policy making in South Africa. In: 2019 6th International Conference on Soft Computing Machine Intelligence (ISCMI), pp. 23–28 (2019). https://doi.org/10.1109/ISCMI47871.2019.9004323

Requirements for Implementing Digital Health Terminology Standards in Uganda's Electronic Medical Records-Based Health Information Systems

Achilles Kiwanuka[1,2] and Josephine Nabukenya[1(✉)]

[1] Makerere University, Kampala, Uganda
josephine@cit.ac.ug
[2] Medical Research Council/Uganda Virus Research Institute and London School of Hygiene and Tropical Medicine Uganda Research Unit, P.O. Box 49, Entebbe, Uganda

Abstract. Uganda's Ministry of Health has implemented numerous electronic-based Health Information Systems. Huge financial investments towards implementing the system are supported by the Uganda government and Health Development Partners. Despite the investments, health information systems in the country are still fragmented and non-interoperable. Non-interoperability is caused by scanty practices and/or implementation of the digital health standards (data and interoperability) and limited to non-compliance of monitoring these standards in the implementation of the healthcare interventions. Addressing the digital health standards challenges will support the effective implementation of the healthcare interventions. Accordingly, this paper focuses on requirements for data and interoperability standards, specifically terminology standards, for Uganda's Health Information Systems using HIV information systems as a case study. Using expert opinion of stakeholders responsible for standardization in Uganda's digital health eco-system, the digital health terminology standards requirements were validated. Requirements for implementing digital health terminology standards constitute; mapping of healthcare business processes, developing terminology services, having functional governance structures, and terminology standards capacity building.

Keywords: Digital health · Terminology standards · Electronic health information systems

1 Introduction

Uganda's Ministry of Health (MoH) has implemented numerous electronic-based Health Information Systems (EHIS) including OpenMRS, mTrac, Integrated Clinic Enterprise (ICEA), and District Health Information Software 2 (DHIS2) among others, that are used for reporting, documenting and managing HIV and TB patients [1]. The information systems are expected to improve health data management; however, many information systems are yet to realize their full potential due to non-interoperable data sitting in siloed health information systems. This has resulted into challenges of ineffective use for decision making and policy development [2]. Despite the heavy investments in Information Communication Technologies (ICT) [3, 4], EHIS are still not adequately used; this is partly caused by disparate, un-interoperable fragmented EHIS in varying health system levels and lack of common data interoperability and terminology standards to facilitate unambiguous sharing of data consistently across the health system [1, 5, 6]. According to the *Institute of Electrical and Electronics Engineers*, a *standard* is a document specifying features of a product or process [7].

Interoperability can be defined as information standardised sharing among two or more health information systems through the business processes using ICT systems [8]. Interoperability is classified into technical, syntactic and semantic [9]. This study focused on the semantic interoperability classification. *Semantic interoperability* is the unambiguous interpretation of exchanged data between humans to humans, humans to computers and computers to computers while ensuring that the meaning is maintained [10]. Nilsson and Sandin also define semantic interoperability as entailing information exchange with uniform interpretation across stakeholders. [11]. Amongst the levels of interoperability, semantic is a challenge because of its domain-specific nature [12] and the absence of data and interoperability standards [13, 14]. Health systems must adopt consistent clinical messaging and data standards that provide a framework and language for communicating shared meaning [15]. While utilizing standards, there is a decrease in health workers' concerns over patient data safety and professional liability [16, 17]. The uniform interpretation of medical words, that is semantic codes, should cut across all health workers that interface with data [18].

Opportunities to improve healthcare by reusing data are often missed due to lack of standards implementation [19] and the limited interoperability of digital health applications [20]; worse still, the requirements and/or processes for implementing the data and interoperability standards are not well-documented. Whereas requirements are conditions over environmental situations, requirements specifications are provide enough information to build an artifact without additional environment knowledge [21]. Challenges of implementing the terminology and classification standards include inadequate compliance monitoring, insufficient participation of key stakeholders, inadequate technical expertise, financial constraints and weak leadership or governance [19]. Interoperability issues can be addressed through having uniform medical coding and digital health data standards [22]. Specifically, adoption of a standard terminology is essential for the achievement of complete interoperability in healthcare [23].

The commonly used terminology and classification standards are International Classification of Diseases - ICD [24], Systematized Nomenclature of Medicine - SNOMED [25] and Logic Observation Identifiers, Names and Codes – LOINC [26]. The ICD is the global health information standard for mortality and morbidity statistics, and it has been translated into 43 languages [27]. SNOMED is an international clinical reference terminology used in over 50 countries [28] and can potentially improve patient safety, data quality, and enhance semantic interoperability [22]. LOINC provides a universal coding system for reporting laboratory and other clinical observations [29]. Implementation of such standards is a prerequisite for the smart healthcare [30].

Existing research shows that utilization of data standards in health information systems, supports better health delivery and outcomes [15]. Despite the presence of internationally available terminology standards, many developing countries, including Uganda, are yet to establish what it takes to effectively implement terminology standards to achieve semantic interoperability. This research draws on challenges affecting data and interoperability standards [19, 31] in using HIV-based electronic medical records systems in Uganda; from which a set of requirements for implementing digital health terminology standards to achieve semantic interoperability is derived.

2 Methodology

2.1 Study Design

A cross-sectional study design was adopted to generate the requirements [19, 32], which were validated using expert opinion [1, 33]. The process followed the four stages of user requirements analysis which include information gathering, user needs identification, envisioning and evaluation and lastly requirements specifications [34]. Importantly, the HIV electronic-based information systems were chosen as a case study due to their numerous funding sources to support reporting donor-driven data and routine health information management system indicators [35]. The requirements validation exercise involved stakeholders at both national and sub-national levels of Uganda's health system. The study covered the Central, Western and West Nile administrative regions of Uganda.

2.2 Study Respondents

Expert opinion was obtained from the respondents. The selection criteria for inclusion of the respondents necessitated that they had been actively involved in the digital health sphere of Uganda for at least 5 years and/or had participated in the stakeholder validation workshop to understand the challenges of digital health in Uganda. The stakeholder validation meeting enabled respondents to have a background of the derived requirements and validate them from an informed perspective. 47 purposively selected information rich respondents participated in the validation exercise (see Table 1). The respondents represented the full spectrum of digital health stakeholders in the country and increased heterogeneity of the study findings.

2.3 Data Collection and Analysis

A stakeholder meeting was gathered that included various digital health stakeholders to present the requirements and allow them to seek clarification, if any, about the requirements. The stakeholders were sent an online google form with yes/no options and an alternative to give additional information for the requirements. The data was then exported to Microsoft Excel and analyzed using descriptive statistics and then presented using bar graphs. The cut-off for accepting the requirements was pre-set at 90%.

Table 1. Categorization of the respondents who validated the Requirements.

Categorization	Number of respondents
Academicians	3
Biostatisticians	5
Clinicians	5
Digital Health NGOs	4
Health Development Partners	2
Health Facility Administrators	5
ICT Personnel	1
Laboratory Personnel	3
Monitoring and Evaluation Personnel	3
Medical Recorders	3
Nurses	6
Pharmacy Personnel	2
Policy Makers	4
Research Institutions	1

2.4 Ethical Clearance

Ethical clearance to interact with the study participants was obtained from the Makerere University School of Public Health Research Ethics Committee (REC) and/or Institutional Review Board (IRB). Informed consent was also obtained from the participants before completing the online form.

3 Findings

The validated terminology services requirements are classified as as functional and non-functional requirements [36]. This classification helps to differentiate between functionalities of the system and system attributes [37].

3.1 Functional Requirements for Implementing Digital Health Terminology Services

The functional requirements describing what the digital health standards implementation framework should do are presented in Fig. 1. All the functional requirements validated scores were above 90%.

The digital health terminology services implementation framework shall specify which terminology standards to adopt across all business domains. This requirement addresses the lack of nationally adopted standards across all business domains of healthcare.

The digital health terminology services implementation framework mapping of existing national codes to international terminology standards addresses the need to contextualise the international standards to suit the local context. International standards cannot be used *as is* because of design actuality differences. During the mapping process, not all national codes will match the international standards and thus a need for a mechanism to handle such mismatches. These processes would then lead to an accessible repository of all terminology standards implemented in the country.

The digital health terminology services implementation framework shall have an evaluation process for evaluating terminology standards adoption. The process shall be essential to ascertain digital health applications compliance with the international terminology standards to aid semantic interoperability. The evaluation process shall base on the guidance provided to digital health application developers.

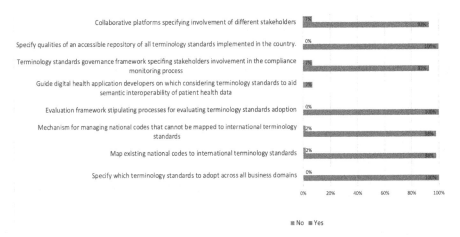

Fig. 1. Functional requirements for terminology services implementation.

Stakeholder involvement is important in not only implementing terminology services but also monitoring their compliance. The digital health terminology services implementation framework shall have a terminology standards governance framework specifying stakeholders' involvement in the compliance monitoring process. Additionally, there should be collaborative platforms for involving different stakeholders in the digital health terminology processes.

3.2 Non-functional Requirements for Implementing Digital Health Terminology Services

A non-functional requirement is a description of the artifact's attributes or behaviours and constraints on the system's behavior system [37, 38]. The derived non-functional requirements are summarised in Table 2. All the functional requirements scored over 90% in the validation (Table 3).

Table 2. Non-functional requirements for implementing digital health terminology services.

Non-functional requirements	Challenge addressed
Digital health applications shall be designed using approved terminology standards	Implementation of different standards that might deter semantic interoperability
Adopted standards shall have open licenses to enable use by multiple stakeholders without license restrictions	Proprietary standards are costly to be implemented in Uganda, just like many low- and middle-income countries
A health data reference model describing healthcare processes shall be part of the terminology services	Lack of clear business processes in the health sector
The Ministry of Health shall have guidelines for accessing the terminology services and terminology standards	Inaccessibility of standards by health workers and stakeholders leading to non-implementation of standards
The terminology services shall have hard copy and online user guide that explain all functionalities and implementation guides	Inaccessibility of guidance on using terminology services

Table 3. Non-functional requirements for implementing digital health terminology services (cont.).

Non-functional requirements	Challenge addressed
The terminology services shall have stable electricity and internet connections and with reliable backup connections to avoid disruption of services	Unstable power supply and internet
The terminology services shall be implemented as service modules	Business continuity in case one or more services fail
The terminology services shall maintain unique user identification and password for everyone who uses the services	User and access control
The terminology services shall be able to accommodate new disease or health codes as they are approved by statutory bodies	Dynamic indicators definitions
The Ministry of Health shall build capacity of health workers in digital health terminology services	Lack of awareness, knowledge and skills of terminology services amongst health care workers

4   Discussion

The study focused on generating and validating requirements for digital health terminology services. To understand the requirements better and their relationships, the requirements have been condensed into four (see Fig. 2). The themes are mapping healthcare business processes, developing terminology services, governance structures and capacity building.

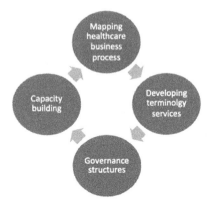

Fig. 2. Requirements for implementing digital health terminology standards.

4.1 Mapping Healthcare Business Processes

Mapping in health improves understanding of complex systems and contextualization of digital health interventions to suit the local context [39]. However, before mapping takes place, understanding of both the local and international context should be considered [5]. Much as some respondents mentioned that there is no requirement of having health data reference models, mapping of healthcare processes to understand the information flows in health services is paramount [40, 41].

Semantic interoperability requires implementation of terminologies and clinical-content models [42] for the uniform interpretation of clinical data [43]. There are a number of digital health applications in Uganda [44] that could benefit from process mapping while aligning their applications with terminology standards. Over 93% of the respondents concurred the need of having guidelines for application developers to implement terminologies in their digital health solutions. The drive to digital solutions, unlike paper-based information systems, also supports mapping of different terminology standards [45–47].

4.2 Developing Terminology Services

Developing terminology services for any national health information system should build on what is already existing internationally and locally through conducting a landscape analysis. The lack of guidelines on which terminology standards to adopt deters implementation of standards. Guidelines should be explicit about the terminology standards, and semantic interconnection modes, across the data and business domains of healthcare. Adebesin and Kotzé developed a process of a process for digital health standards selection [48] that stakeholders could use to select which standards are appropriate for their interventions.

Clinical terminology services can solve challenges of adoption of terminology standards [49]. The MoH should have a terminology standards framework to guide selection and regulation of terminology standards and services in the country because multiple standards pose a challenge to standardization [50].

4.3 Governance Structures

The MoH should have comprehensive guidelines for terminology services, implementing terminology standards and capacity building of digital health coding. The structures should include collaborative platforms where all stakeholders can participate in the development, review and monitoring compliance of digital health terminology standards. Such platforms maybe physical or virtual through seminars, workshops or web interfaces. To support continuous interaction, there should be centralized (online) resources for all stakeholders.

Having guidelines in place doesn't necessarily mean that stakeholders will comply. There should be structures, with resources, to monitor implementation and compliance to the terminologies while implementing digital health solutions. One of the resources that is lacking in terms of numbers and quality is the human resources. The government should not only have structures but also train staff who are going to manage the same structures. Regulation of digital health developers is crucial to know which applications are being implemented. There should be criteria to assess whether any given application meets the minimum terminology standards to be implemented in health services. Implementation of the standards should be monitored through continuous review to ensure that guidelines are being followed [5].

4.4 Capacity Building

Many health workers do not receive adequate information technology training. On being employed, they face computers at their workplaces. A study conducted in the Western part of the Uganda indicated that 59% of the health staff were unskilled in computer applications [51]. Besides, there is limited terminology expertise among health workers. This shows the need to need organize on-job training of health workers not only in terminology standards but also general ICT skills. Efforts in build terminology standards knowledge and skills should be guided by a roadmap for nationwide sensitization amongst stakeholders followed by official launching of the approved strategies.

Capacity building should involve sensitizing all relevant stakeholders on digital health terminology standards to improve meaningful data exchange and sharing. This should also extend to incorporating the terminology training to in health workers' training curricula and workshops organized for health workers in service. Online fora for specific terminologies could be used by health workers coupled by efforts by the MoH to strengthen digital health implementation in the country.

5 Conclusion

This study identified four requirements' categories for implementing digital health terminology standards in Uganda's Electronic Medical Records-based health information systems which are mapping of healthcare business processes, developing terminology services, having functional governance structures, and terminology standards capacity building. The requirements can be used to design and implement a process model for implementing the terminology services and thus improving on the semantic interoperability of health information systems. The researchers recommend using the requirements to design a process framework for contextualizing and implementing digital health terminology standards using available international terminology standards. Future work should also focus on other approaches of semantic interoperability approaches such as ontology to better understand semantics of disease data [52].

References

1. Ministry of Health. Uganda National eHealth Strategy 2017–2021. Uganda: Ministry of Health (2017)
2. Henriksson, D.K., Peterson, S.S., Waiswa, P., Fredriksson, M.: Decision-making in district health planning in Uganda: does use of district-specific evidence matter? Health Res. Policy Syst. **17**(1), 1–11 (2019)
3. Nagwovuma, M., Ndagire, L., Eilu, E.: Performance Evaluation for electronic health information systems in Uganda. In: 2021 IST-Africa Conference (IST-Africa). IEEE, pp. 1–8 (2021)
4. Kruk, M.E., Rabkin, M., Grépin, K.A., Austin-Evelyn, K., Greeson, D., Masvawure, T.B., et al.: 'Big push'to reduce maternal mortality in Uganda and Zambia enhanced health systems but lacked a sustainability plan. Health Aff. **33**(6), 1058–1066 (2014)
5. Alunyu, A.E., Nabukenya, J.: A conceptual model for adaptation of ehealth standards by low and middle-income countries. J. Health Inform. Afr. **5**(2) (2018)
6. Egwar, A.A., Ssekibuule, R., Nabukenya, J.: Status of resources for information technology to support health information exchange in resource-constrained settings. In: HEALTHINF2020, pp. 463–471 (2020)
7. Institute of Electrical and Electronics Engineers. IEEE Standard Computer Dictionary: A Compilation of IEEE Standard Computer Glossaries. New York: The Institute of Electrical and Electronics Engineers (2010)
8. European Commission. New European Interoperability Framework: Promoting seamless services and data flows for European public administrations. Luxembourg: Publications Office of the European Union Luxembourg (2017)
9. Kubicek, H., Cimander, R., Scholl, H.J.: Layers of Interoperability. Organizational Interoperability in E-Government: Lessons from 77 European Good-Practice Cases, pp. 85–96. Springer Berlin Heidelberg (2011). https://doi.org/10.1007/978-3-642-22502-4
10. Xiao, G., Guo, J., Da Xu, L., Gong, Z.: User interoperability with heterogeneous IoT devices through transformation. IEEE Trans. Industr. Inf. **10**(2), 1486–1496 (2014)
11. Nilsson, J., Sandin, F.: Semantic interoperability in industry 4.0: survey of recent developments and outlook. In: 2018 IEEE 16th International Conference on Industrial Informatics (INDIN). IEEE, pp. 127–132 (2018)
12. Liyanage, H., Krause, P., De Lusignan, S.: Using ontologies to improve semantic interoperability in health data. BMJ Health Care Inform. **22**(2) (2015)
13. Mukasa, E., Kimaro, H., Kiwanuka, A., Igira, F.: Challenges and strategies for standardizing information systems for integrated TB/HIV services in Tanzania: a case study of Kinondoni municipality. Electron. J. Inf. Syst. Dev. Countries. **79**(1), 1–11 (2017)
14. Marghoob, A.A.: Standards in dermatologic imaging. JAMA Dermatol. **151**(8), 819–821 (2015)

15. Dixon, B.E., Vreeman, D.J., Grannis, S.J.: The long road to semantic interoperability in support of public health: experiences from two states. J. Biomed. Inform. **49**, 3–8 (2014)
16. Benavides-Vaello, S., Strode, A., Sheeran, B.C.: Using technology in the delivery of mental health and substance abuse treatment in rural communities: a review. J. Behav. Health Serv. Res. **40**(1), 111–120 (2013)
17. Jennett, P.A., Scott, R., Affleck Hall, L., Hailey, D., Ohinmaa, A., Anderson, C., et al.: Policy implications associated with the socioeconomic and health system impact of telehealth: a case study from Canada. Telemed. J. E Health **10**(1), 77–83 (2004)
18. Braa, J., Sahay, S., Lewis, J., Senyoni, W.: Health information systems in indonesia: understanding and addressing complexity. In: Choudrie, J., Islam, M.S., Wahid, F., Bass, J.M., Priyatma, J.E. (eds.) ICT4D 2017. IAICT, vol. 504, pp. 59–70. Springer, Cham (2017). https://doi.org/10.1007/978-3-319-59111-7_6
19. Kiwanuka, A., Bagyendera, M., Wamema, J., Alunyu, A., Amiyo, M., Kambugu, A., et al.: Establishing the state of practice about data standards in monitoring healthcare interventions for HIV in Uganda's EMR-based health information systems. In: HEALTHINF, pp. 200–211 (2021)
20. Beerenwinkel, N., Fröhlich, H., Murphy, S.A.: Addressing the computational challenges of personalized medicine (Dagstuhl Seminar 17472). Dagstuhl Reports: Schloss Dagstuhl-Leibniz-Zentrum fuer Informatik (2018)
21. Jackson, M.: The meaning of requirements. Ann. Softw. Eng. **3**(1), 5–21 (1997)
22. Lee, D., de Keizer, N., Lau, F., Cornet, R.: Literature review of SNOMED CT use. J. Am. Med. Inform. Assoc. **21**(e1), e11–e19 (2014)
23. Iroju, O., Soriyan, A., Gambo, I., Olaleke, J.: Interoperability in healthcare: benefits, challenges and resolutions. Int. J. Innov. Appl. Stud. **3**(1), 262–270 (2013)
24. World Health Organization. International statistical classification of diseases and related health problems: Tabular list. World Health Organization (2004)
25. Bhattacharyya, S.B.: Introduction to SNOMED CT. Springer, Cham (2015). https://doi.org/10.1007/978-981-287-895-3
26. Huff, S.M., Rocha, R.A., McDonald, C.J., De Moor, G.J., Fiers, T., Bidgood, W.D., Jr., et al.: Development of the logical observation identifier names and codes (LOINC) vocabulary. J. Am. Med. Inform. Assoc. **5**(3), 276–292 (1998)
27. World Health Organization: FAQs for ICD-11 (2021). https://www.who.int/classifications/icd/revision/icd11faqs.pdf. Accessed 20 Dec 2021
28. Lee, D., Cornet, R., Lau, F., De Keizer, N.: A survey of SNOMED CT implementations. J. Biomed. Inform. **46**(1), 87–96 (2013)
29. McDonald, C.J., Huff, S.M., Suico, J.G., Hill, G., Leavelle, D., Aller, R., et al.: LOINC, a universal standard for identifying laboratory observations: a 5-year update. Clin. Chem. **49**(4), 624–633 (2003)
30. Chang, V., Cao, Y., Li, T., Shi, Y., Baudier, P.: Smart healthcare and ethical issues. In: 1st International Conference on Finance, Economics, Management and IT Business: SciTePress, pp. 53–59 (2019)
31. Adebesin, F., Kotzé, P., van Greunen, D., Foster, R.: Barriers & challenges to the adoption of E-Health standards in Africa (2013)
32. Kiwanuka, A., Mercy, A., Josephine, N.: Constraints to and enablers for contextualising digital health terminology standards in Uganda's health services: a qualitative case study. Submitted for publication (2022)
33. Remy, C., Bates, O., Dix, A., Thomas, V., Hazas, M., Friday, A., et al.: Evaluation beyond usability: Validating sustainable HCI research.In: Proceedings of the 2018 CHI Conference on Human Factors in Computing Systems, pp. 1–14 (2018)

34. Maguire, M., Bevan, N.: User requirements analysis. In: Hammond, J., Gross, T., Wesson, J. (eds.) Usability. ITIFIP, vol. 99, pp. 133–148. Springer, Boston, MA (2002). https://doi.org/10.1007/978-0-387-35610-5_9

35. Ministry of Health. The Second National Health Policy: Promoting People's Health to Enhance Socio-economic Development. Kampala: Ministry of Health - Uganda; 2010

36. Glinz, M.: A glossary of requirements engineering terminology. Version 1.6. International Requirements Engineering Board, IREB (2014)

37. Koelsch, G.: Requirements Writing for System Engineering. Springer, Cham (2016). https://doi.org/10.1007/978-1-4842-2099-3

38. Glinz, M.: On non-functional requirements. In: 15th IEEE International Requirements Engineering Conference (RE 2007). IEEE, p. 21–26 (2007)

39. Antonacci, G., Lennox, L., Barlow, J., Evans, L., Reed, J.: Process mapping in healthcare: a systematic review. BMC Health Serv. Res. 21(1), 1–15 (2021)

40. Aftab, S., Mehmood, Y., Ahmad, F., Javed, Y., Hussain, M., Afzal, M.: Mapping integrating the healthcare environment (IHE) to business process execution language for people (BPEL 4PPL). In: 2009 IEEE 13th International Multitopic Conference. IEEE, pp. 1–6 (2009)

41. Antonacci, G., Reed, J.E., Lennox, L., Barlow, J.: The use of process mapping in healthcare quality improvement projects. Health Serv. Manag. Res. 31(2), 74–84 (2018)

42. Goossen, W., Goossen-Baremans, A., Van Der Zel, M.: Detailed clinical models: a review. Healthcare Inform. Res. 16(4), 201–214 (2010)

43. Knaup, P., Bott, O., Kohl, C., Lovis, C., Garde, S.: Section 2: patient records: electronic patient records: moving from islands and bridges towards electronic health records for continuity of care. Yearb. Med. Inform. 16(01), 34–46 (2007)

44. Kabahuma, C., Nabukenya, J.: Managing patient identification in Uganda's health facilities: examining challenges and defining requirements for a national client registry. J. Health Inform. Afr. 6(2), 26–35 (2019)

45. Banda, J.M., Evans, L., Vanguri, R.S., Tatonetti, N.P., Ryan, P.B., Shah, N.H.: A curated and standardized adverse drug event resource to accelerate drug safety research. Sci. Data 3(1), 1–11 (2016)

46. Bousquet, C., Souvignet, J., Sadou, E., Jaulent, M-C., Declerck, G.: Ontological and non-ontological resources for associating medical dictionary for regulatory activities terms to SNOMED clinical terms with semantic properties. Front. Pharmacol. 975 (2019)

47. Yuksel, M., Gonul, S., Laleci Erturkmen, G.B., Sinaci, A.A., Invernizzi, P., Facchinetti, S., et al.: An interoperability platform enabling reuse of electronic health records for signal verification studies. BioMed. Res. Int. 2016 (2016)

48. Adebesin, F., Kotzé, P.: A process for developing an e-health standards selection method artefact using design science research. J. Des. Res. 15(3–4), 258–287 (2017)

49. Metke-Jimenez, A., Steel, J., Hansen, D., Lawley, M.: Ontoserver: a syndicated terminology server. J. Biomed. Semant. 9(1), 1–10 (2018)

50. Oderkirk, J.: Readiness of electronic health record systems to contribute to national health information and research (2017)

51. Muhaise, H., Kareeyo, M.: Electronic health information systems critical implementation issues (E-HMIS): district health information software version. 2 in the greater Bushenyi, Uganda. Am. Acad. Sci. Res. J. Eng. Technol. Sci. 34(1), 205–212 (2017)

52. Liaw, S.-T., Taggart, J., Yu, H., de Lusignan, S., Kuziemsky, C., Hayen, A.: Integrating electronic health record information to support integrated care: practical application of ontologies to improve the accuracy of diabetes disease registers. J. Biomed. Inform. 52, 364–372 (2014)

Multi-class Detection of Arrhythmia Conditions Through the Combination of Compressed Sensing and Machine Learning

Giovanni Rosa[1], Marco Russodivito[1], Gennaro Laudato[1(✉)],
Angela Rita Colavita[2], Luca De Vito[4], Francesco Picariello[4],
Simone Scalabrino[1,3], Ioan Tudosa[4], and Rocco Oliveto[1,3]

[1] STAKE Lab – University of Molise, Pesche, IS, Italy
{giovanni.rosa,marco.russodivito,gennaro.laudato,
simone.scalabrino,rocco.oliveto}@unimol.it
[2] ASREM, Campobasso, CB, Italy
angelarita.colavita@asrem.org
[3] Datasound srl, Pesche, IS, Italy
{rocco,simone}@datasound.it
[4] Department of Engineering, University of Sannio, Benevento, BN, Italy
{devito,fpicariello,ioan.tudosa}@unisannio.it

Abstract. Medical technologies in the form of wearable devices are an integral part of our daily lives. These devices are devoted to acquire physiological data to provide personal analytics and to assess the physical status of assisted individuals. Nowadays, thanks to the research effort and to the continuously evolving technologies, telemedecine plays a crucial role in healthcare. Electrocardiogram (ECG) is one of the source signal that has been widely involved in telemedicine and therefore the need for a quick and precise screening of ECG pathological conditions has become a priority for the scientific community. Based on the above motivation, we present a study aimed at evaluating the applicability of an highly accurate detector of arrhythmia conditions to be used in combination of a compressed version of the ECG signal. The advantage of using a technique of Compressed Sensing (CS) relies on a faster detection of the approach, due to the lower complexity of the method's workflow. We conducted an experimental study to determine if such a detector, working on compressed ECG signal, can achieve comparable results with the original approach applied to the uncompressed signal. The results demonstrated that with a Compression Ratio equal to 16 it is possible to achieve classification metrics around 99%, therefore showing a high suitability of the approach to be involved in contexts of Compressed ECG.

Keywords: Machine learning · Compressed sensing · Automatic detection · ECG · Arrhytmia

C. Gehin et al. (Eds.): BIOSTEC 2021, CCIS 1710, pp. 213–235, 2022.
https://doi.org/10.1007/978-3-031-20664-1_12

1   Introduction

Wearable technologies are becoming more and more present in our daily lives as devices used for tracking activities, customizing user's daily experiences, and monitoring people's health status [58]. The wearable devices fit into the Internet-of-Things (IoT) paradigm, as things equipped with microchips, sensors and wireless communication capabilities [6]. A particular application is directed to the ones called Wearable Health Devices (WHDs) which uses various sensing technologies to collect measurements for body temperature, motion/posture, heart rate, electrocardiogram (ECG), blood pressure, respiration wave, and many other parameters [15, 62]. WHDs populate a subclass of IoT called Internet-of-Medical-Things (IoMT) [36]. The adoption of WHDs allows medical practitioners to increase the efficiency of the diagnosis and reduce its costs [27]. This is possible due to the availability of heterogeneous computing on WHDs and cloud-based data storage for further assessment and long-term monitoring of the health status [1].

Many examples of IoMT systems have been recently proposed [13,36,39, 44,63], such as the *ATTICUS* system [7]. This is a system dedicated to the ambient-assisted living based on the analysis of vital and behavioral data thanks to an innovative remote monitoring system. The signals are acquired through a smart T-shirt [7,14] and then sent to an Ambient Intelligence device. All the devices of ATTICUS are capable of (i) predicting anomalous situations (*e.g.,* atrial fibrillation episodes) and (ii) communicating them to a central Decision Support System (DSS) for the final confirmation.

The high quantity of information generated and transmitted by WHDs (*e.g.,* the ones that acquire real-time multi-lead ECG) raised the necessity of adopting compression techniques to reduce the usage of both memory and bandwidth. Domain Transform Methods (DTM) can ensure the production of compressed ECG signals with low loss in terms of clinical information. Such methods, however, increase the local computational load, which results in increased the power consumption. Since WHDs are powered by relatively small batteries, they suffer from limited autonomy. Using lossy compression methods based on Compressed Sensing (CS) — in particular, digital CS methods — allows to alleviate power consumption problems. Such methods require low computational load on microprocessors during the ECG signal compression step. In this case, the aim of ECG signal compression is to reach maximum efficiency of data reduction without loss of diagnostic information [12]. Previous studies have demonstrated that the adoption of CS algorithms is a solution for WHDs only if the diagnostic information (*e.g.,*, ECG morphology) is neither distorted nor lost [53]. If the original ECG signals show sign of a medical conditions, it is possible to devise detection techniques able to directly detect them on the compressed signals [9]. Examples of conditions that can be detected on compressed signals include ventricular ectopic beat, supraventricular ectopic beat, fusion of a normal and a ventricular ectopic beat [38]. However, to the best of our knowledge, there is no approach able to automatically detect arrhythmia conditions on compressed ECG signals.

Among the many conditions for which WHDs could be beneficial, arrhythmia is probably one of the most spread and dangerous. Arrhythmia is a condition in which the heart beats are irregular, excessively rapid or slow. Atrial and ventricular arrhythmias are the two forms of arrhythmias [52]. Even if some arrhythmias are generally regarded to be innocuous, other arrhythmias, particularly ventricular arrhythmias, are extremely deadly. Indeed, ventricular arrhythmias can lead to abrupt cardiac arrest if they are not treated with extreme care and monitored continuously [16].

In this paper, we introduce NEAPOLIS, a NovEl APproach for the autOmatic reaL-time beat-to-beat detectIon of arrhythmia conditionS. NEAPOLIS aims at detecting Bundle Branch Block (BBB), Premature Ventricular Contractions (PVC) and Atrial Premature Beats (APB), and it was designed with the requirements to provide a real-time and accurate detection of such conditions. Thanks to the developments of this extended work, NEAPOLIS is now capable of working with both uncompressed and compressed ECG signals. The set of features is the same regardless the input signal; indeed, we use a combination of state-of-art features (derived from statistics computed on the RR information and from the morphological description of a heartbeat to describe both an uncompressed and a compressed ECG signal.). As for the former, we evaluated the features directly on the sample of the ECG signal. As for the latter, instead, we integrated in the approach a CS technique based on a Deterministic Binary Block Diagonal (DBBD) matrix as sensing matrix and we calculated the features from the signal in the compressed domain.

This paper is an extension of our HEALTHINF'21 work [56]. The novel contribution we provide in this extension is the following:

1. We introduce an extended version of NEAPOLIS which is able automatically classify not only uncompressed ECG signals (like in our previous work), but also compressed ones; we achieve this goal by re-designing the set of features used in our previous work and adopting a CS technique based on a Deterministic Binary Block Diagonal (DBBD) matrix;
2. We evaluate NEAPOLIS on the Physionet MIT-BIH arrhythmia database, by compressing the original signals with several Compression Ratio (CR) factors.

The rest of the paper is structured as follows: Sect. 2 first describes the arrhythmia conditions and their incidence on the population and then recall the main steps of the original version of NEAPOLIS; in the second part of the section, a brief description of the state-of-the-art methods for the detection in the compressed domain is offered together with a detailed description of the chosen method as CS algorithm for NEAPOLIS. Section 4.1 reports on the design of the study to experiment NEAPOLIS in the compressed domain and Sect. 4.2 contains the details on the results achieved by the approach. Finally Sect. 5 concludes the paper and highlights the future works.

2   Background and Related Work

2.1   The Arrhythmia Conditions

A bundle branch block can be defined as an abnormality of the electrical conduction system of the heart [18]. In case the defect is originated in the left or right ventricles the blocks are further classified into Right BBB (RBBB) and Left BBB (LBBB). Scientific research studies have reported that BBB has been observed in 8% to 18% of subjects with acute myocardial infarction. It has also been associated with an increased risk of complete heart block and sudden death [34,48]. Before the involvement of thrombolytic treatment—that limits infarct size, improves ventricular morphology and function, and decreases mortality—several studies had reported on the incidence of RBBB in patients with acute myocardial infarction [45]. The range of incidence rate was found to be between the 3% and 29% [11,32]. In a recent study, conducted on 1015 patient where 38%of them had ST elevation myocardial infarction (STEMI), RBBB was documented in 8% of patients while LBBB in 4% of patients [19]. Also, both left and right BBB have been associated with increased in-hospital and long-term mortality in patients with acute non-ST elevation myocardial infarction (NSTEMI) [33]. RBBB are present with a incidence rate of 7% for those with NSTEMI. It was also found that RBBB is usually the manifestation of infarctions. These latter are often accompanied by heart failure, complete AV block, arrhythmias, and a high mortality rate [4,47,55]. With regard to the LBBB, the incidence in the general population is low, approximately 0.6% of subjects developing it over 40 years [10,28]. The incidence rate changes if considering patients with chronic heart failure. Indeed, approximately one third of these patients have left bundle branch block (LBBB) on their 12-lead ECG [5,59].

Premature ventricular complex (PVC) is characterized by early depolarization originating from ventricles. PVC is an electrocardiogram (ECG) finding that is commonly found in the general population and is associated with structural heart disease and an increased risk of sudden death [2,43]. In the absence of structural heart disease, frequent PVCs have traditionally been considered a benign phenomenon, only requiring medical attention when symptomatic. This understanding has undergone a substantive evolution over the last decade. So-called benign PVCs are now known to have malignant potential in susceptible patients and can manifest as triggers for ventricular fibrillation (VF) and sudden cardiac death [29]. Scientific research studies have reported that PVCs are present in more than the 6% of middle-aged adults, based on a 2-minute ECG [61].

Ranging from 20% to 25% of ischemic strokes occur due to embolic complications caused by atrial fibrillation [17,25]. In addition, for patients that have experienced ischemic stroke or transient ischemic attacks, in presence of AF they can be exposed to recurrent strokes [65]. Therefore, it is vital to detect paroxysmal atrial fibrillation after stroke or transient ischemic attack and involve anticoagulation treatment in such patients [26,66]. This diagnose typically includes a 24 h continuously monitoring. One of the clues that can lead to a early diagnosis of paroxysmal atrial fibrillation are the occurrence of atrial premature beats (APB). APBs are observed frequently in normal subjects and patients with a variety of diseases. They are manifested as an interruption in the heart rhythm with a premature beat having a narrow QRS complex [60]. Indeed, in 24-hour ECG recordings frequent APB are correlated to an increased incidence of paroxysmal AF in patients with ischemic stroke [64].

2.2   Automatic Detection of Arrhythmia Conditions

In literature there are different set of features for capturing both temporal and morphological carachteristics of ECG signals. Zhao et al. [70] proposed an approach for the extraction of features that allows a reliable heart rhythm recognition. They basically used two techniques for the features generation: wavelet was used to extract the coefficients of the transform and autoregressive modelling (AR) to obtain the temporal structures of ECG waveforms. Then, wavelet and AR coefficients were concatenated together to form the feature vector for the classification. They evaluated a large set of outputs that include also our target conditions, but they chose to experiment the method on a subset of the available recordings from the MIT-BIH Arrhythmia[1], a freely accessible and common database of the scientific literature with annotation at heartbeat level. The results showed that the approach provided good performances of classification reaching an accuracy of 99.68%.

Li et al. [41] proposed a method for ECG classification using entropy on Wavelet packet decomposition (WPD) and Random Forest. The authors also experimented the devised method on the MIT-BIH Arrhythmia database but with a different output because they conducted another kind of experiment, focused on a medical standard, *i.e.,* the EC57:1998 standard [3]. The authors stated that although the coefficients by Discrete Wavelet Transform (DWT) or WPD can reveal the local characteristics of an ECG signal, the number of such coefficients is usually so huge that it is hard to use them as features for classification directly. Therefore, they extracted some high-level features from these coefficients for better classification. In the proposed method, they chose the entropy as high level features extractor from a DWT. The results reported on an obtained overall accuracy approximately equal to 94.61%.

Another very important set of features is the one proposed by Leonarduzzi et al. [40], *i.e.,* a set of features derived from the multifractal analysis. The authors stated that this analysis highly suits the analysis of the Heart Rate Variability (HRV) fluctuations, since it gives a description of the singular behavior of a signal. Therefore, the main features of this work are based on the multifractal wavelet leader estimates of the second cumulant of the scaling exponents and the range of Holder exponents, or singularity spectrum. The results demonstrated how these features can be involved in a tool for a precise detection of myocardial ischemia.

Many works from the scientific literature have involved the Fast Fourier Transform (FFT) in their methods for the classification of ECG segments. For instance, Haque et al. [24] proposed a combination of FFT-based and wavelet features. The main findings achieved by the authors was that the wavelet can provide better indicators—rather than the FFT—of small abnormalities in ECG signals.

There are various approach for automatic arrhythmia conditions based on machine learning techniques, as described by [20]. In Table 1 we report some of

---

[1] https://archive.physionet.org/physiobank/database/mitdb/.

the most recent and best performing approaches in literature based on different machine learning techniques, including also neural networks and transfer learning. For example, Yildirim et al. [68] presented a new deep learning model for ECG classification using network-based wavelet sequences, called DBLSTM-WS. Their approach was evaluated on the detection of five different heartbeat types, including Left Bundle Branch Block (LBBB) and Right Bundle Branch Block (RBBB), with an accuracy score of 99.39%. Yildirim et al. [69] proposed an approach where they combine a convolutional auto-encoder (CAE), to reduce the signal size of arrhythmic beats, with a LSTM classifier. As a result, ECG signals were compressed by an average 0.70% percentage root mean square difference (PRD) rate, with an accuracy score over 99.11% was observed. Moreover, Li et al. [42] proposed a deep learning-based method of cardiac arrhythmia episodes using deep residual networks (ResNet). Their approach was evaluated with both single and 2-lead ECG signals. The resulting classification accuracy is 99.06% for single lead ECG and 99.38% for 2-lead ECG. Zheng et al. [71] proposed an automatic approach that takes as input ECG signal images, from where using a combined deep learning model composed of CNN-LSTM, can classify 8 different heartbeat types from MIT-BIH database. Their approach achieved an overall accuracy score of 99.01%. Sahoo et al. [57] proposed an automatic approach using an QRS complex features combined with the multiresolution wavelet transform to calssify four types of heartbeats. The overall accuracy achieved is 98.39% using SVM. Osowski et al. [49] proposed a recognition system based on SVM for heartbeat classification. Using Higher Order Statistics (HOS) combined with Hermite, their approach achieves an overall accuracy of 98.18%.

There are also approaches that exploit the advantages of Transfer Learning, with an embedded feature extraction using ECG signal images. For example, Isin et al. [30] proposed AlexNet, a transferred deep convolutional network that can classify up to three different cardiac conditions with a recognition rate of 98.51%. Also, Pal et al. [50] proposed CardioNet that can classify 29 types of arrhythmia conditions from MIT-BIH database with a total accuracy score of 98.92%.

Pandey et al. [52] proposed a relevant work on automatic detection of Arrhythmia conditions. Their approach provides a complete automatic detection of five heartbeat types, including the LBBB, RBBB and PVC. The approach is based on a single Long Short-Term Memory (LSTM) Neural Network as model. The inputs to the model were based on higher-order statistics, wavelets, morphological descriptors, and R-R intervals. Thus, 45 features were in charge of describing the electrocardiogram signals. In details, to extract the features, the authors designed a temporal window of 180 samples sized (half of a second on the MIT-BIH Arrhythmia). The window was centered on each R peak, previously obtained thanks to the annotations of each R wave position available from this database. The features have been evaluated only inside this interval. A 2-fold cross validation was used to evaluate the accuracy of the classification: The entire MIT-BIH arrhythmia database was divided in two folds, i.e., two sub-dataset. Their LSTM model was trained on 40% (80% of 50%) sub-dataset, and

Table 1. Summary of the approaches for the automatic detection of arrhythmia conditions proposed in literature.

Study	Heartbeat classes	Features	Technique	Overall accuracy
Yildirim et al. [68]	5	End-to-end, DWT	DBLSTM-WS	99.39%
Yildirim et al. [69]	5	Encoded features	CAE-LSTM	99.11%
Li et al. [42]	5	End-to-end	ResNet	99.06%
Zheng et al. [71]	8	End-to-end	CNN-LSTM	99.01%
Sahoo et al. [57]	4	QRS, DWT	SVM	98.39%
Osowski et al. [49]	13	HOS, Hermite	SVM	98.18%
Li et al. [41]	5	WPE, RR	RF	94.61%
Isin et al. [30]	3	AlexNet	CNN	98.51%
Pal et al. [50]	29	DenseNet	CardioNet	98.92%
Pandey et al. [52]	5	Temporal, Morphological	LSTM	99.37%

10% (20% of 50%) sub-dataset was dedicated to a preliminary validation phase. The remaining 50% of the data set was used for testing. After the performance evaluation, the model obtained an overall accuracy equal to 99.37%.

The main difference between NEAPOLIS and the described approaches is that we allow a real-time classification, also achieving a fast and lightweight performing classification. This was mainly due to the features vector of NEAPOLIS that was basically composed of near real-time features and a low-complexity model for the classification. Indeed, Neural Networks are usually more expensive in terms of resources compared to classical machine learning algorithms, also some the described studies does not follow the AAMI standard for the validation of their approach (as the case of the work proposed by Li *et al.* [41]). In the context of this study, we also evaluate the effectiveness of those features in the context of compressed ECG signals.

2.3   Detection in the Compressed Domain

In this section, a brief description of the state of the art of works evaluating the accuracy of heart disease detectors in the compressed domain is presented.

The utilization of CS in WHD based monitoring may provide a solution for detection of atrial fibrillation from compressed ECG signals. This detection approach may reduce the time required for digital signal processing algorithms applied on raw (or reconstructed after compression) ECG signals. For example, the problem that persists in existing methods utilized for the detection of atrial fibrillation pathology from compressed ECGs is related to the unsatisfactory classification performance of the used algorithms, especially in where high CR is required [9]. In literature, investigations regarding the applied detection algorithms from compressed ECGs are reported and in the following, a brief review is presented.

The authors of the work proposed in [9] implemented a deep learning method which is able to detect the atrial fibrillation directly from compressed samples of ECG signals without performing the reconstruction step. This method makes use of the measurement matrix (i.e., the sensing matrix) utilized during ECG signal compression to initialize the first layer of a deep neural network in order to obtain a prior information which leads thereafter to obtain an improved classification performance of the desired pathological (e.g., the presence of atrial fibrillation) issue on the investigated ECG signal. Furthermore, the reported experimental results in [9] describe an accuracy of 97.52% and an F1 score of 98.02% for a CR = 10%, and on the other side, the method was assessed against of a CR = 90% reporting a reduction of the accuracy to 6.77% and F1 to 5.31%, respectively.

The work proposed in [37] dealt with an approach that retrieves vital information from a digital compressed single-lead electrocardiogram (ECG) signal by combining Machine Learning and Compressed Sensing. This study was focused on the identification of R-peak occurrences from compressed ECG. The results demonstrated that the use of CS in combination with a ML technique achieve results comparable to the ones applied to the uncompressed ECG signal.

In the work proposed in [38], a heartbeat morphology classifier was presented. This method worked on compressed ECG signals and signal compression was realized through 1-bit quantization. The authors then experimented several machine learning techniques to classify the heartbeats from compressed ECG signals. The obtained results showed that the tool exhibited comparable results with other similar methods that performed the same detection but on uncompressed ECG signals.

2.4 The Compressed Sensing Algorithm

The CS algorithm here adopted is based on a Deterministic Binary Block Diagonal (DBBD) matrix as sensing matrix. In particular, in case of ECG, the DBBD in combination with the Discrete Cosine Transform (DCT) dictionary matrix has been demonstrated to outperform the others CS techniques based on sensing matrix randomly built [54]. Another CS technique for ECG is proposed in [53]. In this case, the sensing matrix is chosen such that the vector of compressed samples is obtained from a sort of cross-correlation between the ECG signal and a vector consisting of ones where the ECG signal has a high contribution and zero elsewhere. Even if the approach of [53] outperforms the DBBD-based method in terms of reconstruction quality, it requires more steps for its implementation, i.e. the determination of the vector containing ones and zero according to a threshold defined from a percentile of the ECG amplitude distribution and also the transmission of this vector to the host. For this reason, in this paper, the DBBD technique has been adopted being more easy for its implementation on low-power device with low computational capabilities.

In general, the CS can be modelled as multiplication between the column vector $\mathbf{x}$ of N acquired samples at Nyquist rate and a $M \times N$ sensing matrix $\mathbf{\Phi}$:

$$\hat{\mathbf{y}} = \mathbf{\Phi} \cdot \mathbf{x} \tag{1}$$

The $\mathbf{y}$ vector will contain the M compressed samples.

In the case of DBBD, the sensing matrix $\mathbf{\Phi}$ is defined as:

$$\hat{\mathbf{\Phi}} = \begin{bmatrix} \mathbf{1}_{CR} & \mathbf{0}_{CR} & \cdots & \mathbf{0}_{CR} \\ \mathbf{0}_{CR} & \mathbf{1}_{CR} & \cdots & \mathbf{0}_{CR} \\ \vdots & \cdots & \ddots & \vdots \\ \mathbf{0}_{CR} & \cdots & \mathbf{0}_{CR} & \mathbf{1}_{CR} \end{bmatrix} \tag{2}$$

where, $CR = N/M$ is the compression ratio, $\mathbf{1}_{CR}$ and $\mathbf{0}_{CR}$ are row vectors of CR ones and zeros, respectively. According to (2), the CR must be an integer, otherwise, the sensing matrix *Phi* cannot be built.

Usually, in the literature, the reconstruction phase is performed with the aim of estimating $\mathbf{x}$ from the compressed vector $\mathbf{y}$, according to the sensing matrix $\mathbf{\Phi}$, and a dictionary matrix $\mathbf{\Psi}$. In particular, $\mathbf{\Psi}$ is selected according to a specific domain where the signal can be represented by few K non zero coefficients. The first reconstruction step consists in estimating these coefficients (i.e. $\hat{\boldsymbol{\theta}}$) by solving:

$$\hat{\boldsymbol{\theta}} = \arg \min_{\boldsymbol{\theta}} \|\boldsymbol{\theta}\|_1, \quad \text{subject to:} \quad \mathbf{y} = \mathbf{\Phi}\mathbf{\Psi}\boldsymbol{\theta}, \tag{3}$$

From $\hat{\boldsymbol{\theta}}$, the reconstructed signal $\hat{\mathbf{x}}$ is obtained as follows:

$$\hat{\mathbf{x}} = \mathbf{\Psi} \cdot \hat{\boldsymbol{\theta}} \tag{4}$$

As demonstrated in [54], in the case of DBBD compression for ECG signals, the best choice for the dictionary matrix definition is the DCT matrix.

The solving of (3) is usually performed with the Orthogonal Matching Pursuit (OMP) algorithm, which exhibits a computational complexity $\mathcal{O}((N + M)S)$, where $S < N$ is the number of iterations. This step exhibits a high computational load that increases with N. Thus, the reconstruction step limits the use of CS in case of real-time systems or early warning implementations. For this reason, the idea underlying this paper is to detect anomalies on ECG signals directly in the compressed domain (i.e. by considering the vector $\mathbf{y}$ of compressed samples), removing the need of reconstruction.

3 Automatically Detecting Arrhythmia Conditions

In this section, we describe NEAPOLIS, an online detector of arrhythmia conditions based on the analysis of heartbeats signals that works both on uncompressed and compressed ECG signals. Figure 1 describes the workflow of NEAPOLIS.

First, NEAPOLIS receives as input a single lead digital ECG signal. A small portion of the signal is buffered until there are at least 11 R-peaks (*i.e.*, heartbeats). Follows a beat-to-beat segmentation and a 2-step median filter to get rid of baseline drifts. Next, the feature vector is generated and given to a machine learning model to perform the classification. As a result, NEAPOLIS provides a label for the most probable classification among N (Normal Sinus

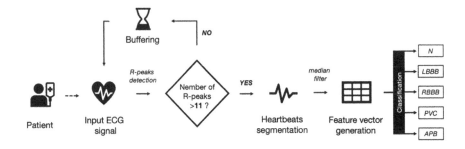

Fig. 1. The workflow of NEAPOLIS for online beat classification.

Rhythm), *RBBB* (Right Bundle Branch Block), *LBBB* (Left Bundle Branch Block), *PVC* (Premature Ventricular Contraction), and *APB* (Atrial Premature Beat). In the following sub-sections, we describe in detail each component of NEAPOLIS.

3.1 ECG Digital Processing

The digital signal processing embedded in NEAPOLIS is based on the one proposed by [52]. It can be conceptually divided in beat-to-beat segmentation and signal filtering. Both these procedures are triggered only when a long enough portion of a digital single lead ECG is buffered (*i.e.*, at least 11 R peaks). Once these two steps are completed, the features can be extracted from the obtained signal.

First, for the beat-to-beat segmentation, NEAPOLIS evaluates the position of the R peaks from all the buffered ECG segment using a QRS detector, such as the widely used algorithm proposed by [51]. As a result, the R peak positions in the buffered ECG are obtained, then the segmentation process can start. Evaluating a time window of 180 samples, centered on a R peak, all the the samples included in the window are selected. This leads to the definition of a single heartbeat signal, *i.e.*, a sample vector of length 180 centered on a R peak.

After, NEAPOLIS performs the baseline removal on the heartbeat signal. This means that two median filters are applied, where the first is a filter of 200 ms, applied on the raw signal, and the latter is a median filter of 600 ms applied on the signal resulting from the application of the first filter. At the end, a set of filtered heartbeat signals are obtained.

3.2 Heartbeat Features

Next subsections describe in detail the features extracted by NEAPOLIS.

After the previous steps, follows the feature extraction phase. In NEAPO-LIS we use a set of state-of-the-art features from the literature combined with morphological features. We select only the features that allow a real-time detection on the input signals, with the price of a limited buffered portion of the

ECG signal to be processed. Next, we describe in detail the feature used in NEAPOLIS.

- *Energy of Maximal Overlap Discrete Wavelet Transform.* The wavelet transform (WT) is a mathematical operator that can be used for the decomposition of time series signals into distinct subsignals. One of the two forms of WT is the DWT. The maximum overlap discrete wavelet transform (MODWT) is a modified DWT. In the MODWT, there is no process of subsampling, therefore leading to a higher level of information in the resulting wavelet and scaling coefficients, when compared to the DWT [22]. For our purposes, we evaluated the MODWT and then extracted the energy features according to the following steps: (i) selection of a mother wavelet function W and the decomposition level L; (ii) decomposition of the original heartbeat signals according to the specified W and L; and (iii) calculation of the energy of each coefficient in each node in the last level L. This procedure has also been partially considered in the feature extractor proposed by [41]. In our case, we used the *db2* Daubechies wavelet function and three levels of decomposition.
- *Autoregressive Model (AR).* As suggested in the method proposed by [70], we involved the calculation of the Autoregressive model (AR) coefficients of order 4. As outcomes, we evaluated the AR coefficients and the reflection coefficients, using the Yule-Walker estimator [21].
- *Multifractal Wavelet Leader.* The goal of multifractal analysis is to study signals that present a point-wise Holder regularity variable, *i.e.,* that may largely vary from point to point. When dealing with a signal, performing the multifractal analysis refers to the estimation of its spectrum of singularities. Therefore, the determination of the spectrum of singularities of a signal is important to analyze its singularities [40]. In case of a real-life signal, it cannot be numerically evaluated due to constraint like finite resolution and the sampling of signals [35]. To overtake this limitation, a multifractal formalism was introduced: the wavelet leaders [31]. In NEAPOLIS, we involved the multifractal wavelet leader estimates of the log-cumulants of the scaling exponents.
- *Fast Fourier Transform.* Our approach embeds the evaluation of the Fast Fourier Transform on the heartbeat signal. Indeed, FFT represents a method for extracting helpful information out of statistical features of ECG signal.
- *R-R interval descriptors.* These features have been selected from a larger set of R-R statistical descriptor proposed by Pandey et al. [52]. In detail, we selected only the features that can be computed with a limited buffering of the ECG signal. Thus, we excluded from our set o f features the *global-RR interval*, because it represented the average of all the pre-RR values present in the last 20 min. This would not allow NEAPOLIS to perform a real-time detection, even using ECG buffering. As a result, we select the following features:
  - *pre-RR interval*, that is the distance between the actual and previous heartbeat;
  - *post-RR interval*, that is the distance between the actual and next heartbeat;

- *local-RR interval*, that is the average of 10 previous pre-RR values.

Within this new study, we opted for removing the information related to the continuity of the R peaks. This choice was due to the considerations (i) that the R peaks are clinical features retrievable with a highly accurate QRS detector, which could impact on the low-complexity of the algorithm designed for this study and (ii) that the R peaks could not be always observed in a compressed domain.

- *Discrete Cosine Transform-based features.* Previous work showed that Discrete Cosine Transform (DCT) is the best choice for the reconstruction of the ECG signal from the compressed samples [54]. Therefore, we include features derived from the DCT when NEAPOLIS runs on compressed ECG signals. We used the same order we used for the FFT-based features.

3.3   Beat Classification

The last phase of NEAPOLIS is the beat classification. Once the previously described features are extracted, a normalization step and also data sampling (*i.e.*, SMOTE [8]) are applied. The first transforms the features in a predefined range of values, the latter helps to deal with unbalanced data.

Next, a machine learning model classifies the heartbeats as *N*, *RBBB*, *LBBB*, *PVC*, and *APB*. The only constraint that NEAPOLIS have for that phase is to use a supervised machine learning technique, thus different algorithms can be used. The best configuration of NEAPOLIS, as evaluated in the previous study, is represented by a machine learning pipeline composed of SMOTE sampling, min-max scaler and Random Forest algorithm.

4   The Study

In this section, a detailed description of the study is offered, concerning the study design, the context of the study and the final results.

4.1   Study Design

In this section we present the study designed to evaluate the applicability of our approach in the compressed domain. Specifically, when we first presented NEAPOLIS, we observed high classification performances in the classification of the heartbeat in N (Normal Sinus Rhythm), RBBB (Right Bundle Branch Block), LBBB (Left Bundle Branch Block), PVC (Premature Ventricular Contraction), and APB (Atrial Premature Beat). An important role were played by the features vector and therefore by the algorithms chosen to generate it.

In this work, the objective is to evaluate the applicability of such a set of features on a compressed version of the heartbeat signal, in order to assess the applicability of NEAPOLIS also in contexts of compressed data transmissions.

Thus, our new study is steered by the following research questions:

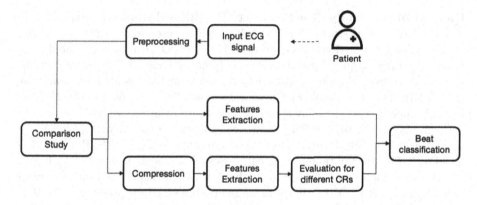

Fig. 2. The experimental workflow designed for this study.

RQ1: *What are the classification performances of* NEAPOLIS *when dealing with* **uncompressed** *ECG signals?*
RQ2: *What are the classification performances of* NEAPOLIS *when dealing with* **compressed** *ECG signals?*

With the first research question, we aim at evaluating the refined version of NEAPOLIS on the uncompressed signal with respect to the previous version of the approach [56].

With the second research question, we want to verify if NEAPOLIS—applied to compressed data—can reach a classification accuracy comparable to the versions of the approach that work on the uncompressed signal.

Experimental Workflow. The workflow of the experimented designed within this work is depicted in Fig. 2.

NEAPOLIS was designed to work in the time domain and the main processing steps were basically:

1. the buffering of an ECG single lead trace, according to a minimum amount evaluated on the number of R peaks;
2. the preprocessing aimed at segmenting the trace in heartbeats according to the R peaks and filtering the ECG from noise and artefacts;
3. the features extraction steps where the final features vector was generated to be used as input in the final classification stage.

The extension of NEAPOLIS is resulted in a comparison study between the classification performances of the model in the uncompressed and compressed domain. Therefore—in this study—the compression algorithm is applied right before the evaluation of the final features vector. In this way, it was possible to compare the usefulness of the different features both in the uncompressed than in the compressed domain.

Context of the Study. The Physionet MIT-BIH arrhythmia database [23,46] was involved in this study. It is a database widely used in the state of the art for the detection of arrhythmia conditions [46]. This DB contains 48 ambulatory ECG recordings, acquired 360 Hz sampling frequency and with 11-bit resolution. Cardiologists from Physionet worked to provide annotations for each heartbeat of this DB. The final number of hearbeats labeled are around 110,000 divided into 15 different categories. A standard procedure from the scientific literature [67] can be applied to this DB in order to: (i) remove record with paced beats and (ii) consider only 5 categories of beat annotations: N, LBBB, RBBB, APB and PVC. The distribution of such categories of hearbeats is depicted in Fig. 3.

The validation scheme involved in this work is the same used for the initial validation of NEAPOLIS. The scheme refers to a standard procedure [52] that needs an initial decomposition of the dataset into two sub datasets, namely *DS1* and *DS2*. According to the standard procedure, the first one is used as training set while the second as test set.

To guarantee the consistency of the experiment, we have repeated ×1000 the splitting process into *DS1* and *DS2*. This helped in avoiding any convenient split on a single run. The validation protocol was therefor applied ×1000 and the results were avareged accordingly.

Uncompressed Vs Compressed Domain. For uncompressed domain it is meant the original version of NEAPOLIS, where the features were evaluated directly on the uncompressed version of the heartbeat while for compressed domain it is meant the domain where the heartbeat is not considered in its entire length but in a compressed version. Indeed, we evaluated the applicability of the compression in NEAPOLIS for different compression ratios.

Specifically, the experiment was designed to compare the classification performances in the compressed domain for the compression ratios in the set 2, 4, 8, 16. This choice was due to:

- the length of the original heartbeat,
- the compression algorithm.

Indeed, the compression algorithm—chosen for this work—allowed to involve integer CRs, otherwise, the sensing matrix Φ cannot be defined (see (2)). For simplicity, in this work the *CRs* are chosen in forms of powers of 2 to experiment the maximum number of CRs, *i.e.,* four in this study. Thus, we opted for imposing an initial length of 176 (instead of 179) for each heartbeats. To do so, we performed a cutting of three samples at the extremities of the signal.

An example of a heartbeat signal represented in the uncompressed domain and in its four versions in the compressed domain is depicted in Fig. 4.

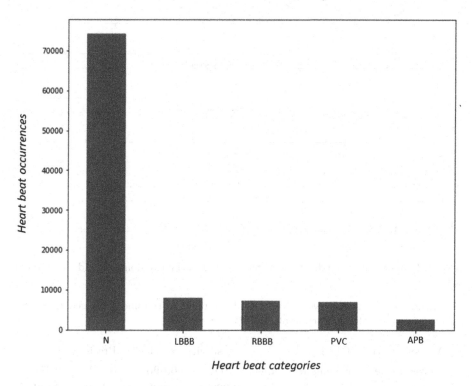

Fig. 3. Count of selected heartbeat types from the MIT-BIH arrhythmia database [46].

4.2 Study Results

This section reports the empirical evaluation we conducted to evaluate the classification performances of NEAPOLIS in the compressed domain.

The classification performances—obtained by NEAPOLIS applied to the uncompressed ECG signal and to the 4 versions of compressed ECG signal—have been compared by using the following class-level metrics:

- **Accuracy**, *i.e.*, the number of all the correctly classified instances divided by the total number of the instances. It is computed as $\frac{TP+TN}{TP+TN+FP+FN}$
- **Sensitivity**, *i.e.*, the number of positive instances the are correctly classified with respect to the sum between the number of correctly classified positive instances and wrongly classified ones as negative. It is computed as $\frac{TP}{TP+FN}$
- **Specificity**, *i.e.*, the number of negative instances that are correctly classified divided by the sum between the number of negative instances correctly classified and the wrongly classified positive instances, computed as $\frac{TN}{TN+FP}$
- **Precision**, *i.e.*, the number of positive instances that are correctly classified with respect to the total number of positive instances, computed as $\frac{TP}{TP+FP}$
- **F1**, *i.e.*, that represents the harmonic mean of precision and recall, computed as $\frac{2\times TP}{(2\times TP)+FN+FP}$

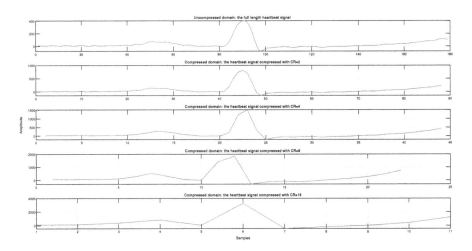

Fig. 4. Example of a heartbeat signal represented in the two domains and for different CRs.

Table 2. Comparison between NEAPOLIS applied to the uncompressed ECG and the previously published version of NEAPOLIS [56].

Version of NEAPOLIS	Sensitivity	Specificity	Precision	F1
Uncompressed - Previous version [56]	0,971	**0,995**	0,972	0,971
Uncompressed - This version	**0,989**	0,986	**0,989**	**0,989**

RQ1: NEAPOLIS for Uncompressed ECG Signals. To answer RQ1, we reported the global results — expressed in terms of the above classification metrics — in Table 2. This table compares the previously published version of NEAPOLIS with the refined version presented in this paper. Therefore, this table compares versions of the approach only in terms of application on uncompressed signal. From this results, it is possible to observe that the refined version of NEAPOLIS outperforms the previous version with respect to all the classification metric except for the specificity. These results demonstrate the advantage in refining the features vector to be used as input to the ML classification stage. Specifically, the new set of features—based on the evaluation of the cosine discrete transform—has revealed its impact on the classification performances of NEAPOLIS. The global accuracy achieved by this newly refined version of the NEAPOLIS is $0,989$.

RQ2: NEAPOLIS for Compressed ECG Signals. To answer RQ2, we reported the global results of NEAPOLIS in the compressed domain in Table 3. These achievements clearly highlight that the performances of NEAPOLIS on the uncompressed ECG signal are equals to the ones provided by NEAPOLIS when applied to the compressed signal.

Table 3. Comparison between NEAPOLIS applied to the uncompressed ECG and NEAPOLIS applied to the compressed ECG according to the specific CR.

Version of NEAPOLIS	Accuracy	Sensitivity	Specificity	Precision	F1
Uncompressed - This version	0,989	0,989	0,986	0,989	0,989
Compressed with CR = 2	0,992	0,992	0,987	0,992	0,992
Compressed with CR = 4	0,992	0,992	0,987	0,992	0,992
Compressed with CR = 8	0,992	0,992	0,989	0,992	0,992
Compressed with CR = 16	0,991	0,991	0,989	0,991	0,991

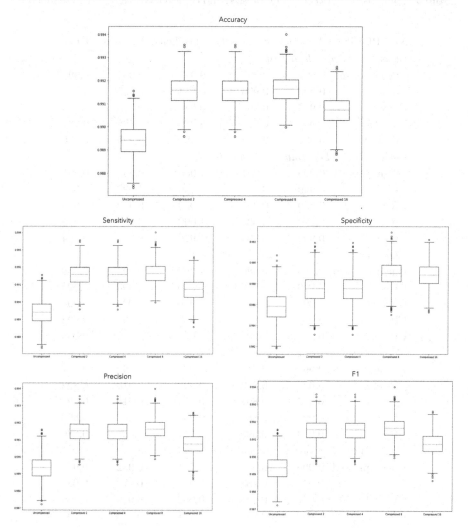

Fig. 5. The boxplots related to the global performances achieved by all the versions of NEAPOLIS.

Figure 5 contains the boxplots of the classification metrics for all the versions of NEAPOLIS, averaged among the 1,000 iterations.

To provide a complete overview of the results, Fig. 4 shows the classification performances detailed by class. These results are in line with the global ones, therefore — also in this case — it is possible to observe that NEAPOLIS shows comparable performances both in the uncompressed than in the compressed domain.

Table 4. Comparison between uncompressed and compressed NEAPOLIS detailed by class.

NEAPOLIS	Accuracy	Sensitivity	Specificity	Precision	F1
Class N - Normal heartbeat					
Uncompressed	0,991	0,995	0,981	0,994	0,994
CR = 2	0,993	0,996	0,984	0,995	0,995
CR = 4	0,993	0,996	0,984	0,995	0,995
CR = 8	0,993	0,995	0,986	0,995	0,995
CR = 16	0,992	0,994	0,986	0,995	0,995
Class LBBB - Left Bundle Branch Block					
Uncompressed	0,999	0,991	1,000	0,999	0,991
CR = 2	0,999	0,993	1,000	0,999	0,993
CR = 4	0,999	0,993	1,000	0,999	0,993
CR = 8	0,999	0,995	1,000	0,999	0,995
CR = 16	0,999	0,994	1,000	0,998	0,994
Class RBBB - Right Bundle Branch Block					
Uncompressed	0,998	0,986	0,999	0,992	0,989
CR = 2	0,999	0,993	1,000	0,995	0,994
CR = 4	0,999	0,993	1,000	0,995	0,994
CR = 8	0,999	0,991	1,000	0,996	0,994
CR = 16	0,999	0,991	1,000	0,995	0,993
Class APB - Atrial Premature Beat					
Uncompressed	0,993	0,845	0,997	0,892	0,867
CR = 2	0,995	0,868	0,998	0,918	0,892
CR = 4	0,995	0,868	0,998	0,918	0,892
CR = 8	0,995	0,883	0,997	0,902	0,893
CR = 16	0,994	0,890	0,997	0,883	0,886
Class PVC - Premature Vetricular Contraction					
Uncompressed	0,996	0,987	0,997	0,962	0,974
CR = 2	0,997	0,988	0,998	0,973	0,980
CR = 4	0,997	0,988	0,998	0,973	0,980
CR = 8	0,997	0,989	0,998	0,973	0,981
CR = 16	0,997	0,985	0,998	0,970	0,978

The only variations shown by all the results are mostly provided by the third decimal digit. This could mean that the difference is not significant and that the main result of this work is that NEAPOLIS shows the same potential for application in the uncompressed and compressed domain. However, this slight difference may be due to the filtering operation performed by the DBBD compression algorithm that reduces the effect of noise and distortion on the performed classification.

5   Conclusion and Future Work

In this paper we presented an extended version of NEAPOLIS, an approach originally designed to provide an accurate and real-time detection of arrhythmia conditions. Once satisfied these requirements, we focused on an extension of that work, with the aim at evaluating the potential of NEAPOLIS to be involved in contexts of compressed ECG.

To this aim, we slightly refined the set of features originally designed for NEAPOLIS and optimized it according to the chosen compression algorithm, *i.e.,* the one based on a Deterministic Binary Block Diagonal matrix as sensing matrix.

An extensive study was conducted to evaluate the potential of NEAPOLIS in the compressed domain; specifically, we evaluated the classification performances of our approach at varying of different Compression Ratios. The final results clearly showed that this new version of NEAPOLIS can work with highly compression ECG signal, by reaching a Compression Ratio of 16.

As future directions, we aim at performing a more extensive study focused on the impact of the features that compose the features vector of NEAPOLIS in relation to the different Compression Ratios. For example, if a specific feature loses its importance in relation of the compression ratio, it can be removed to lighten the classifier, too.

Furthermore, it could be necessary to conduct a comprehensive evaluation in the context of continuous machine learning, for example with a real-time monitoring IoMT system, to evaluate how the usage of a compressed ECG signal influence the prediction effectiveness and if it can be lead to the concept drift phenomenon.

Finally, we consider also the local prediction as a future line of work. Indeed, NEAPOLIS could be studied also in a local perspective, *i.e.,* with a refined training dataset in order to provide detections more accurate at patient level.

References

1. Amft, O.: How wearable computing is shaping digital health. IEEE Pervasive Comput. **17**(1), 92–98 (2018). https://doi.org/10.1109/MPRV.2018.011591067
2. Amir, M., Mappangara, I., Setiadji, R., Zam, S.M.: Characteristics and prevalence of premature ventricular complex: a telemedicine study. Cardiol. Res. **10**(5), 285 (2019)

3. Testing and reporting performance results of cardiac rhythm and ST segment measurement algorithms. Standard, Association for the Advancement of Medical Instrumentation, Arlington, VA (1998)

4. Atkins, J.M., Leshin, S.J., Blomqvist, G., Mullins, C.B.: Ventricular conduction blocks and sudden death in acute myocardial infarction: potential indications for pacing. N. Engl. J. Med. **288**(6), 281–284 (1973)

5. Baldasseroni, S., et al.: Left bundle-branch block is associated with increased 1-year sudden and total mortality rate in 5517 outpatients with congestive heart failure: a report from the Italian network on congestive heart failure. Am. Heart J. **143**(3), 398–405 (2002)

6. Balestrieri, E., et al.: Research challenges in measurement for Internet of Things systems. ACTA IMEKO **7**, 82–94 (2018). http://dx.doi.org/10.21014/acta_imeko.v7i4.675

7. Balestrieri, E., et al.: The architecture of an innovative smart T-shirt based on the internet of medical things paradigm. In: 2019 IEEE International Symposium on Medical Measurements and Applications (MeMeA), pp. 1–6. IEEE (2019)

8. Chawla, N.V., Bowyer, K.W., Hall, L.O., Kegelmeyer, W.P.: SMOTE: synthetic minority over-sampling technique. J. Artif. Intel. Res. **16**, 321–357 (2002)

9. Cheng, Y., Hu, Y., Hou, M., Pan, T., He, W., Ye, Y.: Atrial fibrillation detection directly from compressed ECG with the prior of measurement matrix. Information **11**(9) (2020). https://doi.org/10.3390/info11090436, https://www.mdpi.com/2078-2489/11/9/436

10. Clark, A.L., Goode, K., Cleland, J.G.: The prevalence and incidence of left bundle branch block in ambulant patients with chronic heart failure. Eur. J. Heart Fail. **10**(7), 696–702 (2008)

11. Col, J.J., Weinberg, S.L.: The incidence and mortality of intraventricular conduction defects in acute myocardial infarction. Am. J. Cardiol. **29**(3), 344–350 (1972)

12. Cosoli, G., Spinsante, S., Scalise, L.: Wearable devices and diagnostic apps: beyond the borders of traditional medicine, but what about their accuracy and reliability? IEEE Instrum. Meas. Mag. **24**(6), 89–94 (2021). https://doi.org/10.1109/MIM.2021.9513636

13. Curone, D., et al.: Smart garments for emergency operators: the ProeTEX project. IEEE Trans. Inf Technol. Biomed. **14**(3), 694–701 (2010)

14. De Vito, L., et al.: An undershirt for monitoring of multi-lead ECG and respiration wave signals. In: 2021 IEEE International Workshop on Metrology for Industry 4.0 & IoT (MetroInd4. 0&IoT), pp. 550–555. IEEE (2021)

15. Dias, D., Paulo Silva Cunha, J.: Wearable health devices-vital sign monitoring, systems and technologies. Sensors **18**(8), 2414 (2018). https://doi.org/10.3390/s18082414

16. Elhaj, F.A., Salim, N., Harris, A.R., Swee, T.T., Ahmed, T.: Arrhythmia recognition and classification using combined linear and nonlinear features of ECG signals. Comput. Methods Programs Biomed. **127**, 52–63 (2016)

17. Evans, A., Perez, I., Yu, G., Kalra, L.: Secondary stroke prevention in atrial fibrillation: lessons from clinical practice. Stroke **31**(9), 2106–2111 (2000)

18. Fahy, G.J., et al.: Natural history of isolated bundle branch block. Am. J. Cardiol. **77**(14), 1185–1190 (1996)

19. Figueroa-Triana, J.F., et al.: Acute myocardial infarction with right bundle branch block at presentation: prevalence and mortality. J. Electrocardiol. **66**, 38–42 (2021)

20. Franklin, R.G., Muthukumar, B.: Survey of heart disease prediction and identification using machine learning approaches. In: 2020 3rd International Conference on Intelligent Sustainable Systems (ICISS), pp. 553–557. IEEE (2020)

21. Friedlander, B., Porat, B.: The modified Yule-Walker method of ARMA spectral estimation. IEEE Trans. Aerosp. Electron. Syst. **2**, 158–173 (1984)
22. Ghaemi, A., Rezaie-Balf, M., Adamowski, J., Kisi, O., Quilty, J.: On the applicability of maximum overlap discrete wavelet transform integrated with mars and M5 model tree for monthly pan evaporation prediction. Agric. For. Meteorol. **278**, 107647 (2019)
23. Goldberger, A.L., et al.: Physiobank, physiotoolkit, and physionet: components of a new research resource for complex physiologic signals. Circulation **101**(23), e215–e220 (2000)
24. Haque, A., Ali, M.H., Kiber, M.A., Hasan, M.T., et al.: Detection of small variations of ECG features using wavelet. ARPN J. Eng. Appl. Sci. **4**(6), 27–30 (2009)
25. Hart, R.G.: Atrial fibrillation and stroke prevention. N. Engl. J. Med. **349**(11), 1015–1016 (2003)
26. Hart, R.G., et al.: Lessons from the stroke prevention in atrial fibrillation trials. Ann. Intern. Med. **138**(10), 831–838 (2003)
27. Huarng, K.H., Yu, T.H.K., fang Lee, C.: Adoption model of healthcare wearable devices. Technol. Forecast. Soc. Chang. **174**, 121286 (2022). https://doi.org/10.1016/j.techfore.2021.121286, https://www.sciencedirect.com/science/article/pii/S0040162521007204
28. Imanishi, R., Seto, S., Ichimaru, S., Nakashima, E., Yano, K., Akahoshi, M.: Prognostic significance of incident complete left bundle branch block observed over a 40-year period. Am. J. Cardiol. **98**(5), 644–648 (2006)
29. Ip, J.E., Lerman, B.B.: Idiopathic malignant premature ventricular contractions. Trends Cardiovasc. Med. **28**(4), 295–302 (2018)
30. Isin, A., Ozdalili, S.: Cardiac arrhythmia detection using deep learning. Procedia Comput. Sci. **120**, 268–275 (2017)
31. Jaffard, S., Lashermes, B., Abry, P.: Wavelet leaders in multifractal analysis. In: Qian, T., Vai, M.I., Xu, Y. (eds.) Wavelet Analysis and Applications. Applied and Numerical Harmonic Analysis. Birkhäuser Basel, pp. 201–246. Springer (2006). https://doi.org/10.1007/978-3-7643-7778-6_17
32. Julian, D.G., Valentine, P.A., Miller, G.G.: Disturbances of rate, rhythm and conduction in acute myocardial infarction: a prospective study of 100 consecutive unselected patients with the aid of electrocardiographic monitoring. Am. J. Med. **37**(6), 915–927 (1964)
33. Kleemann, T., et al.: Incidence and clinical impact of right bundle branch block in patients with acute myocardial infarction: ST elevation myocardial infarction versus non-ST elevation myocardial infarction. Am. Heart J. **156**(2), 256–261 (2008)
34. Kones, R., Phillips, J.: Bundle branch block in acute myocardial infarction. current concepts and indications. Acta Cardiol. **35**(6), 469–478 (1980)
35. Lashermes, B., Jaffard, S., Abry, P.: Wavelet leader based multifractal analysis. In: 2005 Proceedings (ICASSP'05). IEEE International Conference on Acoustics, Speech, and Signal Processing, vol. 4, pp. iv–161. IEEE (2005)
36. Laudato, G., et al.: ATTICUS: ambient-intelligent tele-monitoring and telemetry for incepting and catering over hUman sustainability. Front. Hum. Dyn. 3 (2021). https://doi.org/10.3389/fhumd.2021.614309, https://www.frontiersin.org/article/10.3389/fhumd.2021.614309
37. Laudato, G., et al.: Identification of R-peak occurrences in compressed ECG signals. In: 2020 IEEE International Symposium on Medical Measurements and Applications (MeMeA), pp. 1–6. IEEE (2020)
38. Laudato, G., Picariello, F., Scalabrino, S., Tudosa, I., De Vito, L., Oliveto, R.: Morphological classification of heartbeats in compressed ECG. SciTePress (2021)

39. Laudato, G., et al.: MIPHAS: military performances and health analysis system. In: 2020 13th International Conference on Health Informatics, HEALTHINF 2020- Part of 13th International Joint Conference on Biomedical Engineering Systems and Technologies, BIOSTEC, pp. 198–207. SciTePress (2020)

40. Leonarduzzi, R.F., Schlotthauer, G., Torres, M.E.: Wavelet leader based multifractal analysis of heart rate variability during myocardial ischaemia. In: 2010 Annual International Conference of the IEEE Engineering in Medicine and Biology, pp. 110–113. IEEE (2010)

41. Li, T., Zhou, M.: ECG classification using wavelet packet entropy and random forests. Entropy 18(8), 285 (2016)

42. Li, Z., Zhou, D., Wan, L., Li, J., Mou, W.: Heartbeat classification using deep residual convolutional neural network from 2-lead electrocardiogram. J. Electrocardiol. 58, 105–112 (2020)

43. Lin, C.Y., et al.: An observational study on the effect of premature ventricular complex burden on long-term outcome. Medicine 96(1), e5476 (2017)

44. Matias, I., Pombo, N., Garcia, N.M.: Towards a fully automated bracelet for health emergency solution. In: IoTBDS, pp. 307–314 (2018)

45. Melgarejo-Moreno, A., et al.: Incidence, clinical characteristics, and prognostic significance of right bundle-branch block in acute myocardial infarction: a study in the thrombolytic era. Circulation 96(4), 1139–1144 (1997)

46. Moody, G.B., Mark, R.G.: The impact of the MIT-BIH arrhythmia database. IEEE Eng. Med. Biol. Mag. 20(3), 45–50 (2001)

47. Mullins, C.B., Atkins, J.M.: Prognoses and management of venticular conduction blocks in acute myocardial infarction. Mod. Concepts Cardiovasc. Dis. 45(10), 129–133 (1976)

48. Newby, K.H., Pisano, E., Krucoff, M.W., Green, C., Natale, A.: Incidence and clinical relevance of the occurrence of bundle-branch block in patients treated with thrombolytic therapy. Circulation 94(10), 2424–2428 (1996)

49. Osowski, S., Hoai, L.T., Markiewicz, T.: Support vector machine-based expert system for reliable heartbeat recognition. IEEE Trans. Biomed. Eng. 51(4), 582–589 (2004)

50. Pal, A., Srivastva, R., Singh, Y.N.: CardioNET: An efficient ECG arrhythmia classification system using transfer learning. Big Data Res. 26, 100271 (2021)

51. Pan, J., Tompkins, W.J.: A real-time QRS detection algorithm. IEEE Trans. Biomed. Eng. 3, 230–236 (1985)

52. Pandey, S.K., Janghel, R.R.: Automatic arrhythmia recognition from electrocardiogram signals using different feature methods with long short-term memory network model. Sign. Image Video Process. 14(6), 1255–1263 (2020). https://doi.org/10.1007/s11760-020-01666-8

53. Picariello, F., Iadarola, G., Balestrieri, E., Tudosa, I., De Vito, L.: A novel compressive sampling method for ECG wearable measurement systems. Measurement 167, 108259 (2021). https://doi.org/10.1016/j.measurement.2020.108259, https://www.sciencedirect.com/science/article/pii/S0263224120307983

54. Ravelomanantsoa, A., Rabah, H., Rouane, A.: Compressed sensing: a simple deterministic measurement matrix and a fast recovery algorithm. IEEE Trans. Instrum. Meas. 64(12), 3405–3413 (2015). https://doi.org/10.1109/TIM.2015.2459471

55. Rizzon, P., Di Biase, M., Baissus, C.: Intraventricular conduction defects in acute myocardial infarction. Br. Heart J. 36(7), 660 (1974)

56. Rosa, G., Laudato, G., Colavita, A.R., Scalabrino, S., Oliveto, R.: Automatic real-time beat-to-beat detection of arrhythmia conditions. In: HEALTHINF, pp. 212–222 (2021)

57. Sahoo, S., Kanungo, B., Behera, S., Sabut, S.: Multiresolution wavelet transform based feature extraction and ECG classification to detect cardiac abnormalities. Measurement **108**, 55–66 (2017)
58. Scalise, L., Cosoli, G.: Wearables for health and fitness: measurement characteristics and accuracy. In: 2018 IEEE International Instrumentation and Measurement Technology Conference (I2MTC), pp. 1–6 (2018). https://doi.org/10.1109/I2MTC.2018.8409635
59. Shenkman, H.J., et al.: Congestive heart failure and QRS duration: establishing prognosis study. Chest **122**(2), 528–534 (2002)
60. Shindler, D.M., Kostis, J.B.: Electrocardiographic technology of cardiac arrhythmias. In: Sleep Disorders Medicine, pp. 182–187. Elsevier (2009)
61. Simpson, R.J., Jr., Cascio, W.E., Schreiner, P.J., Crow, R.S., Rautaharju, P.M., Heiss, G.: Prevalence of premature ventricular contractions in a population of African American and white men and women: the atherosclerosis risk in communities (ARIC) study. Am. Heart J. **143**(3), 535–540 (2002)
62. Surantha, N., Atmaja, P., David, Wicaksono, M.: A review of wearable internet-of-things device for healthcare. Procedia Comput. Sci. **179**, 936–943 (2021). https://doi.org/10.1016/j.procs.2021.01.083, https://www.sciencedirect.com/science/article/pii/S1877050921001149,. 5th International Conference on Computer Science and Computational Intelligence 2020
63. Villar, R., Beltrame, T., Hughson, R.L.: Validation of the hexoskin wearable vest during lying, sitting, standing, and walking activities. Appl. Physiol. Nutr. Metab. **40**(10), 1019–1024 (2015)
64. Wallmann, D., Tüller, D., Kucher, N., Fuhrer, J., Arnold, M., Delacretaz, E.: Frequent atrial premature contractions as a surrogate marker for paroxysmal atrial fibrillation in patients with acute ischaemic stroke. Heart **89**(10), 1247–1248 (2003)
65. Wallmann, D., et al.: Frequent atrial premature beats predict paroxysmal atrial fibrillation in stroke patients: an opportunity for a new diagnostic strategy. Stroke **38**(8), 2292–2294 (2007)
66. van Walraven, C., Hart, R.G., Singer, D.E., Koudstaal, P.J., Connolly, S.: Oral anticoagulants vs. aspirin for stroke prevention in patients with non-valvular atrial fibrillation: the verdict is in. Card. Electrophysiol. Rev. **7**(4), 374–378 (2003). https://doi.org/10.1023/B:CEPR.0000023143.98705.ee
67. Xu, S.S., Mak, M.W., Cheung, C.C.: Towards end-to-end ECG classification with raw signal extraction and deep neural networks. IEEE J. Biomed. Health Inform. **23**(4), 1574–1584 (2018)
68. Yildirim, Ö.: A novel wavelet sequence based on deep bidirectional LSTM network model for ECG signal classification. Comput. Biol. Med. **96**, 189–202 (2018)
69. Yildirim, O., Baloglu, U.B., Tan, R.S., Ciaccio, E.J., Acharya, U.R.: A new approach for arrhythmia classification using deep coded features and LSTM networks. Comput. Methods Programs Biomed. **176**, 121–133 (2019)
70. Zhao, Q., Zhang, L.: ECG feature extraction and classification using wavelet transform and support vector machines. In: 2005 International Conference on Neural Networks and Brain, vol. 2, pp. 1089–1092. IEEE (2005)
71. Zheng, Z., Chen, Z., Hu, F., Zhu, J., Tang, Q., Liang, Y.: An automatic diagnosis of arrhythmias using a combination of CNN and LSTM technology. Electronics **9**(1), 121 (2020)

DL-Assisted ROP Screening Technique

Vijay Kumar[1(✉)], Het Patel[2], Shorya Azad[3], Kolin Paul[1,2], Abhidnya Surve[3],
and Rohan Chawla[3]

[1] Khosla School of Information Technology, Indian Institute of Technology Delhi,
New Delhi, India
vijay.kumar@cse.iitd.ac.in
[2] Department of Computer Science and Engineering, Indian Institute of Technology Delhi,
New Delhi, India
[3] Dr. Rajendra Prasad Centre for Ophthalmic Sciences,
All India Institute of Medical Sciences Delhi, New Delhi, India

Abstract. Retinopathy of Prematurity (ROP) is the most common cause of visual impairment among premature babies throughout the world. The consequence of ROP impairment can be minimized by performing suitable screening and treatment. However, due to deficiency of health care resources, many of these premature infants remain unidentified after birth. As a result, ROP-induced visual impairment is much more prevalent in these babies. We propose a robust and intelligent approach based on deep artificial intelligence and computer vision to automatically recognise the optical disk (OD) and retinal blood vessels and categorise the severe severity (Zone-1) of ROP patients in this study. We report empirical evidence using premature infant retina images from a nearby hospital to evaluate and validate the proposed approach. The YOLO-V5 prediction model identifies the OD from premature infants retina images, according to our results. Furthermore, the preterm infants' fundus images were perfectly segmented by the computer vision-based system, which effectively separated the retinal vessels. Our system is able to obtain an accuracy of 82.5% in the Zone-1 occurrence of ROP.

Keywords: Fundus image · Retinopathy of Prematurity (ROP) · Computer Aided Diagnosis (CAD) · Image processing · Deep Learning (DL) · YOLO-v5

1 Introduction

Retinopathy of prematurity (ROP) is one of the most common causes of retinal disease in preterm newborns across the world [30]. This is caused by abnormal retinal vascular growth in preterm (born before 34 weeks of pregnancy) and light-weight (≤ 1750g) infants [5,45]. Worldwide, 53,000 infants out of 15 million preterm births require ROP treatment every year [37]. Out of this, more than 20,000 becomes permanently blind or severely visually impaired from ROP [24,30]. In India, 200,000 preterm babies out of 3.5 million are at high risk for developing ROP [17]. Furthermore, due to many difficulties, such as a lack of good health services and specialists, preterm deliveries in rural and remote areas of the country are high. In such situations, getting the proper diagnosis

C. Gehin et al. (Eds.): BIOSTEC 2021, CCIS 1710, pp. 236–258, 2022.
https://doi.org/10.1007/978-3-031-20664-1_13

and treatment for ROP-affected babies is extremely challenging. According to [4], in India, there are a large number of preterm babies. Therefore, it is not possible to get these infants under regular care and extensive screening for ocular conditions. Particularly in India, where more than 65% of the population lives in rural or small cities with inadequate medical services and coverage [3,43]. As a result, a high percentage of these premature infants remain undiagnosed after delivery. As a result, ROP-induced blindness is more prevalent in these newborns. Additionally, the neonatal care division and ophthalmologists have a finite amount of time to provide appropriate care and prognosis, making the problem even more difficult [43].

The human ocular system is highly sophisticated and complex, including the eye, optical nerves, and brain. The structure of the eye consists of two different sections. The first is the visible outer section, including the eyelid, pupils, cornea, iris, and lens. The second is the inner section of the eye, which comprises the retina, optical nerve head (ONH), blood vessels, and macular [3]. ROP is a condition that affects the retina, which is the inner portion of the eye. In this condition, retinal blood vessels develop abnormally on the baby's retina [24,37]. ROP was first seen by Terry as an infectious disturbance of the infant's eye in 1942 [15,37]. Since the development of ROP disease, physicians uses various pathological signs and retinal screening/diagnostic methods to investigate and detect the disease. Therefore, several devices and techniques for ROP screening have been developed over the past several decades that utilizes various clinical and pathological features of ROP and Plus disease. Plus disease means that the blood vessels themselves are twisted and enlarged [9].

The international classification of ROP (ICROP) classifies ROP based on anteroposterior location (area), severity (stage) and vascular characteristics (extent and presence or absence of disease) [7]. The extent of vascularization is one of these classification factors, and the disease is classified into three zones: Zone-1, Zone-2, and Zone-3, as illustrated in Fig. 1. The severity of the disease is classified into five stages, that is, from stage 1 to stage 5. Children with Zone 3 are sometimes affected by low ROP and often do not need treatment even when ROP develops [30]. However, it is essential to detect Zone 1 and 2 accurately. Specifically, Zone 1 is the high-severity state of ROP that causes the most ROP-induced blindness in children. Therefore, there is a need for an innovative solution to detect and classify Zone-1 ROPs accurately. Finding the Zone

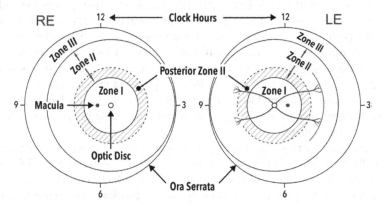

Fig. 1. ICROP based ROP disease classification into three Zones: Zone I, Zone II and Zone III [7].

requires identifying the optical disc (OD), macula, and blood vessels as the boundary of the blood vessels is used to diagnose and classify ROP [7]. The OD is the bright and elliptical region in the fundus image, whereas the macula is located in the center of retina, an area of high concentration of light sensitive cells.

Given its importance, the authors have recently developed many artificial intelligence (AI)-based ROP diagnosis and classification techniques. Image processing, computer vision, machine learning (ML), and deep learning (DL) are used to power these AI-powered CAD systems. At present, ML/DL-based approaches have significantly improved ROP diagnostic and classification applications' performance over time [13,48]. ROP can be successfully detected and classified with DL-based methods, but they do not provide a comprehensive and quantitative understanding of the disease. As a result, ophthalmologists are often unable to link the results of DL-based systems to clinical symptoms [5,39,40]. In this paper, we propose a solution taking this problem into account where, interpretation of results is considered a significant element in providing quality healthcare services in medical applications. In addition, DL-based systems are data-driven and require a large amount of labelled pathological data to train, test, and validate a model. In the case of ROP, obtaining a large number of fundus images is challenging, and the available datasets are not publicly available [36]. As a result, this limits the progress and use of DL-based techniques in medical applications.

In our previous study [25], we have proposed a DL-assisted system to detect and classify ROP disease. ROP classification is mainly based on the location and extent of vascularisation. It requires a retinal vessels map with the extent and location of the optical disk (OD). DL module YOLO-v5 is used for OD detection, while a computer vision-based technique is used for the segmentation of blood vessels. The ROP classification algorithm uses OD as a reference point to determine the degree and progression based on the extent of blood vessels. In addition, the ophthalmologist can utilise retinal features to determine the correlation between the ML/DL system results and pathological signs and symptoms.

This work is an extended version of the conference paper "Deep Learning Assisted Retinopathy of Prematurity Screening Technique" presented at the Proceedings of the 14th International Joint Conference on Biomedical Engineering Systems and Technologies-HEALTHINF. This version has new state-of-art content in related work in Sect. 2 and a more detailed view of the retinal data collection, processing and ROP screening algorithm used in Sect. 3. We need to point out that our previous work did not evaluate the performance of pre-processing and vessel segmentation techniques, which were directly estimated based on the subjective assessment only. However, in this version, we have evaluated their performance quantitatively. Furthermore, in this work, we have also considered the performance of ROP Zoning on a more comprehensive set of ROP image datasets compared to earlier ones. Besides, we also analysed the effect of the pre-processing step on the ROP image quality during the pre-processing stage to improve the image quality.

The remainder of paper is organized as follows. Sect. 2 presents the recent work related to ROP screening. Section 3 gives the design details of the proposed DL-assisted technique for ROP screening. Section 4 presents results, which comes at different stages of the proposed technique's pipeline. Finally, Sect. 5 concludes the papers and discuss some ways in which the work can be extended in future.

Table 1. Recent DL-based system for ROP diseases classification and grading.

Date/ Work	Network	Dataset size	Results
2020 [14]	ROPBaseCNN, ROPResCNN	959 images	Classification Se: 100, Sp: 96, Pr: 96, Ac: 98
2020 [8]	Hybrid (computer vision + CNN)	1199 images	Classification Pr: 62, Re: 62, F1: 62
2020 [31]	ResNet18 + Attention blocks	650 subjects (9794 images)	Classification Ac: 99.17% , Pr: 98.65%, Re: 98.31%, F1: 98.48% and AUC 99.84%.
2020 [19]	VGG-19	6710 images	Classification (Ac: 96%, Sen: 96.6%, Sp: 95.2%) and grading (Sen: 100% , Sp: 98.41%)
2020 [42]	ResNet and faster-RCNN	36,231 images	Classification Ac: 0.903, Identification Ac: 0.957
2020 [8]	Segmentation (Mask R-CNN + Resnet-101-FPN) and classifier (Inception v3)	2759 images	Classification Ac: 0.67 (Hybrid), 0.54 (classifier only), 0.47 (object segmentation)
2021 [44]	DeepSHAP (based on DeepLIFT and Shapley values)	52249 images	Classification F1: 0.718 to 0.981, Sen: 0.918 to 0.982, Sp: 0.949 to 0.992, and AUC: 0.983 to 0.998
2021 [1]	U-Net and Circle Hough Transform	1900 Retcam, 1100 Neo, 1000 OD and 250 BV images	Classification Ac: 98.0%
2021 [2]	Four CNNs modules: ResNet-50, Inception V3, Xception, and Inception-ResNet V2	8090 (cases)	Classification Ac: 93.2% and AUC: 0.98.
2021 [26]	ResNet50 and gradient-weighted class activation mapping class-discriminative localization technique	22,961 images	Classification with test set-1 (Sen: 94.84% Sp: 99.49 %) and test set-2 (Sen:98.03%, Sp: 94.55 %)
2021 [32]	Deep feature fuser (extractors are ResNet18, DenseNet121 and EfficientNetB2)	635 images	Grading Re: 0.9055, Pr: 0.9092, F1: 0.9043, Ac: 0.9827, and Kappa: 0.9786

(Sp: Specificity, Pr: Precision, Ac: Accuracy, Se: Selectivity, Sen: Sensitivity Re: Recall, F1: F1-score, CNN: Convoluted neural network), OD: Optical disc, VS: Blood vessels

2 Literature Review and Related Work

Ophthalmologists have adopted several ROP screening and diagnosis procedures over the decades. Manual screening is one of them. In this scenario, an ophthalmologist examines the symptoms of ROP disease in a retinal photograph. This is a biased and stressful approach. Since their decision is based on the color, texture, extent, and structure of the retinal vessels, it depends entirely on the ophthalmologist's skills and experience. As a result, the performances are highly individual-specific, leaving them vulnerable to inter-expert variability issues. Therefore, objective assessment is highly necessary with the Computer-Aided Diagnosis (CAD). Several methods have been developed to assist the clinician and ophthalmologist with CAD using different modalities for disease screening [10, 22]. For example, [28, 29] considered CAD to develop some traditional techniques to assist doctors in making objective decisions. The traditional techniques (based on image processing and computer vision) on the other hand, can only extract low-level features from fundus images which is insufficient to enhance the classification accuracy of normal and ROP images. As a result, fundus images are challenging to interpret, and lesion features are not prominent. The difference between the lesion and the normal area is comparatively insignificant when the illumination is uneven. Consequently, a method is needed to extract deep high-level information that allows automated ROP screening through machine learning, especially DL methods.

Deep Convolutional Neural Network (DCNN) (or DL) is well-known for the ability to analyze large image datasets [51]. Due to this feature of DL, the performance of computer vision applications has been improved significantly [20, 48]. The ability of DL to self-learn, along with their efficiency and accuracy, have drawn the interest of researchers. As a result, its applications in ophthalmology have been successful, especially for glaucoma, age-related macular degeneration(AMD), Diabetic Retinopathy(DR), Cataract and ROP, where retinal image features for these ailments are not identified [41]. These are data-driven methods in which the DL model is pre-trained using previous pathological datasets relating to the disease. ROP screening and diagnosis have also benefited from the development of many DL-based approaches. Table 1 lists some of the most recent DL-based ROP screening and diagnosis systems. To detect and categorise ROP and plus illnesses, it uses a unique form of the DCNN architecture. The performance of DL-based systems is better than that of traditional CAD applications. Furthermore, the DL-based screening technique eliminates the rule-based system's limitation of flexibility and adaptability.

DL-based systems require a large amount of data (labelled or unlabelled) for their training, testing, and validation [8,14,40,51]. Data collection (pathological, medication, and treatment history) and labelling are time-consuming processes for medical applications. In some contexts, the occurrence of a disease is limited, and its features are influenced by socioeconomic factors and regional boundaries, making it difficult to acquire high-quality critical information. The authors recently developed DCNN-based reinforcement pedagogical approaches for ROP in [40] that relieve the developer or researcher of the additional burden of labelling before training a DL model. The trained deep learning model's performance for a particular dataset is efficient and accurate, but its accuracy for any other dataset is uncertain. Furthermore, it is difficult for an expert to interpret and describe the link between the disease's clinical manifestations and the DL outcome [36].

Therefore, to address the issues mentioned earlier, we proposed a DL-assisted ROP screening technique that can be used in scenarios where large-scale historical datasets are unavailable and the interpretation of the DL-based system outcomes is highly relevant.

3   Methodology

Figure 2 depicts the proposed approach's detailed architecture. It consists of four functional units: fundus imaging (or retinal scanning), image preprocessing, feature extraction blocks, and ROP disease classification. The Fundus imaging unit is responsible for taking and managing retinal scan images, including videos for retinal disease detection and monitoring. Ophthalmologists commonly use the fundus camera to do retinal inspections. The fundus image is a colored picture taken with the fundus camera of the retinal surface of the eye. Irregular lighting, blurriness, and sudden and abrupt variations in the signal often lead to noise in scanned photos or videos. As a result, the image quality needs to be improved. A preprocessing unit is included in the system to deal with such kind of noise in the images or videos and improve the image quality. To limit the effects of noise, it employs a series of image reconstruction and enhancement methods, which are explained in the following sections.

The feature extraction unit extracts the preprocessed image's pathological characteristics associated with ROP. The feature extraction unit is comprised of two sub-units,

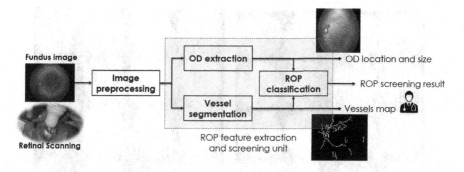

Fig. 2. DL assisted ROP feature extraction and disease screening system [25].

namely the OD extraction and the vessel extraction unit. The features associated with the ROP are extracted from a fundus image by both sub-units working simultaneously. Finally, the disease classification unit leverages these characteristics to identify ROP.

The proposed system in this study leverages the architecture and extent of retinal blood vessels to evaluate and classify ROP [9]. The classification unit then uses the extracted features to determine the severity of ROP disease. The feature set used for ROP is $\{OD, Vessel\}$. The classification unit follows ICROP guidelines (given in Fig. 1) [9]. The classification is done into three zones depending on the retinal vessel structure and its extent. As a result, the feature extraction unit is more crucial since the classification unit's performance is dependent on how well retinal features such as optical disk (OD), blood vessels ($Vessel$) are extracted from the fundus image [9]. The OD extraction unit employs a DL-based system, while the vessel extraction unit uses image processing and computer vision methods.

3.1 Neonatal Retinal Scanning

The ophthalmologist or clinician captured the premature babies' retinal images using the Retcam-3 fundus camera. The image of Retcam-3 has a resolution of 1600×1200 pixels.These images were taken from the posterior, nasal, superior, temporal, and inferior views (more than ten images) to scan an infant's eye entirely. Captured retinal images of premature infants are shown in Fig. 3b. It may be noted that the image quality is sometimes poor because of uneven illumination, motion blur, device miss-alignment, etc. Therefore, screening and monitoring pathological conditions related to neonatal retinal diseases using these images are difficult and require great effort. Neonatal ophthalmologists (experts) use these captured images for diagnosis and monitoring of progression of ROP and plus diseases.

3.2 Data Preparation

The proposed system will require a large number of pathological data points to train, test, and validate, especially for the DL-based module. As a result, depending on the availability of relevant data points (or images), we prepared a distinct set of fundus

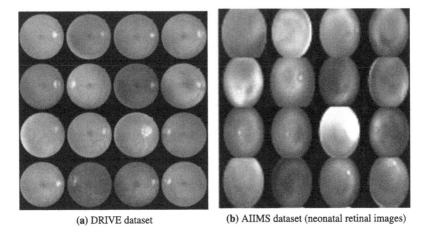

(a) DRIVE dataset   **(b)** AIIMS dataset (neonatal retinal images)

Fig. 3. Variation in quality of images in various data-sets [25].

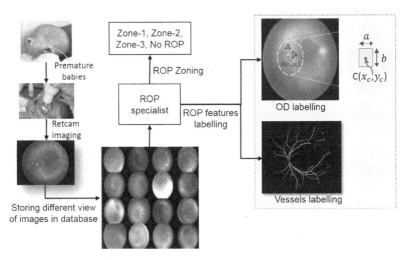

Fig. 4. Flow diagram for dataset preparation.

images for training, testing, and validation of various proposed system components. For the ROP disease, no fundus image datasets are available publicly. Therefore, we have collected a significant amount of premature infants fundus images datasets from the local hospital (AIIMS Delhi) for our study. Figure 4 explain the ROP data collection and labelling process used in this study. Premature infants' retinal images were captured by the ophthalmologist or clinician using the RetCam-3 fundus camera during their scheduled clinical examination of ROP progression. Table 2,summarized the AIIMS ROP dataset used in this study. Moreover, the size of ROP dataset is not sufficient for the DL-based application development alone. Therefore, we have also used publicly available fundus image datasets of elderly person related to DR, Glaucoma and AMD. Detail of all datasets are summarized in Table 3.

We have used datasets in two phases for the proposed system in this study. The first one was used for feature extraction during the first phase. We annotated a total of 1556 fundus photographs for this. As shown in Table 3, 990 labelled photos are taken for module training, 281 for testing, and 285 for validation. Image processing and computer vision-based methods are used in the vessel extraction module and it require no prior training. Premature newborns retinal images obtained by the ophthalmologist or clinician using the Retcam-3 fundus camera are used in this subsystem. These images are unprocessed and noisy, and vessel masks are not visible. On the other hand, assessment of its performance requires reference data or gold standards. Therefore, we manually annotated the blood vessels in a preterm baby retinal image to develop the vascular mask. The annotation activity is a time-consuming and intensive practice. As a result, only six blood vessels in each image have been labelled.

We used photos from the AIIMS dataset where the OD and blood vessels are visible in the image to validate our method in the final stage when we classify individual fundus images into the corresponding zones. A neonatal ophthalmologist collected and categorised these images into four groups: Zone-I, Zone-II, Zone-III, and normal, the ground truth.

3.3 Noise Reduction and Image Pre-processing

Various noises within the collected unprocessed image data, including blurriness, uneven lighting, and transient image signal disruptions, may lower the proposed system's performance accuracy. Hence, while using such data to detect and classify diseases, the quality of the image must be enhanced. Image pre-processing helps to alleviate the adverse effects of noise. We will discuss the image preprocessing approaches adopted by the proposed system to minimise the effect of noise in retinal scans (or images) in this section (Fig. 5).

The neonatal's fundus image is a pale yellowish color. There are three color channels in a color image or video frame: red (R), green (G), and blue (B). The R-channel is saturated, while the B-channel is underexposed. Therefore, detailed information from the R and B channels about vessels and OD is not visible. On the other hand, these features are visible and identifiable in the G-channel. Hence, we preferred the G-channel and used it in further image processing modules. We have also applied a median, average filter, and contrast-limited adaptive histogram equalization (CLAHE) to improve

Table 2. AIIMS ROP dataset [25].

ROP Zone	Total images	Total subject
Zone-I	105	6
Zone-II	217	16
Zone-III	41	5
Healthy	76	4
Total	439	31

Table 3. Fundus image datasets for OD detection [25].

Dataset	Total	Resolution	Training	Test	Validation
STARE	297	700×605	197	50	50
FIRE	224	2912×2912	144	40	40
DRIVE	40	565×584	30	5	5
HRF	45	3504×2336	25	10	10
IDRiD	511	4288×2848	361	75	75
AIIMS	439	1600×1200	233	101	105
Total	1556	–	990	281	285
%	–	–	63.62	18.06	18.32

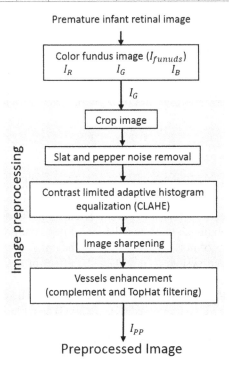

Fig. 5. Flow of image pre-processing.

the quality of the color photo and minimize the effect of illumination variations and blurriness [33]. However, the color image is used as an input in the DL system for feature extraction, disease identification, and classification. CLAHE is used to reduce the influence of uneven lighting on color image quality.

3.4 OD Detection

We used the standard approach specified by the ICROP [9] for ROP detection and classification. The reference circles (shown in Fig. 1) used in zoning are centred on the optical nerve in a retinal photograph, according to the ICROP classification of ROP.

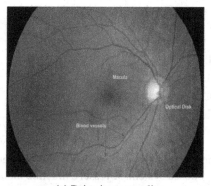

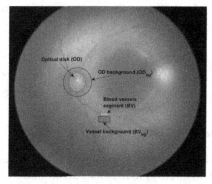

(a) Drive image quality   **(b)** Premature neonatal retinal image

Fig. 6. Retinal image quality comparison of elderly person and a neonatal retinal image and ROIs selection for image analysis.

The accuracy of an ROP classification is governed by how well the OD centre is recognized. Various researchers have proposed several simple non-data driven as well as data-driven techniques for this problem in the past [6,21,46,49], which leverage standard datasets like DRIVE [38] or STARE [18]. The fundamental problem with these methods is that they try to identify the optical disk in the fundus image using intensity variations, despite the fact that the optical disk is usually the brightest place in the image. The retinal camera RetCam is used to capture fundus images of premature infants in the AIIMS-ROP dataset. These pictures are not the same as those in the rest of the datasets. The difference between the grids may be shown in Fig. 3. It is also important to remember that these conventional datasets are significantly more uniform in quality, with low noise and high contrast. Hence, feature extraction can be performed using a non-data driven approach, but in ROP images acquired in a (standard) hospital setup, we have to deal with a wide range of image quality.

We utilize a DL module for ROP classification that can quickly and accurately perform OD detection. It also estimates the OD centre's location and size (bounding box length (a) and width (b)).

We developed an object detection module for the OD detection system based on the state-of-the-art DL-based object detection model YOLO-v5 [23], because this model provides better accuracy and prediction latency. To train these models, we have created one large dataset. We used a total of six datasets for this: five publicly available datasets and one from a local hospital. The details of all datasets are given in Table 3. Some fundus images do not have an OD in the newly created dataset. If OD is not present in an image, we need to ensure that we do not obtain a false-positive result (shown in Table 4). The YOLO predicts the object and provides information on its location and bounding box. As shown in Fig. 4, it identifies optical disk properties such as bounding box width (a), height (b), and center ($C(x_c, y_c)$) in the case of a fundus image.

Furthermore, the disease classification module and the expert directly use OD's attributes for disease monitoring and confirmation procedures. The detailed network architecture of the YOLO algorithm is described by Redd et al. in [34]. We labelled the compiled dataset as per the YOLO model's input and then trained the network with a 416×416 input pixel resolution.

Table 4. Training datasets for the OD detection (where, 0: without OD and 1: with OD) [25].

OD exist	0	1	% image with no OD
Train	115	875	11.62
Valid	10	275	3.51
Test	19	262	6.71

3.5 Vessels Extraction

The retinal blood vessel map is the second most significant retinal feature used by the ICROP-based ROP zoning algorithms in the proposed system. A vessel extraction module needs to provide accurate retinal vessel maps from retinal scans.

Many vessel extraction algorithms have been developed by different researchers over the last few years [12,20]. It performs well with the adult retinal image and generates accurate vasculature maps after segmentation. Preterm infants' retinal blood vessel systems do not fully mature, as shown in Fig. 6. Due to this, the blood vessels of the preterm infant retina are not distinguishable from the background. Therefore, conventional vessel segmentation methods, which perform well with publicly available retinal image datasets, do not work with an infant's retinal image.

Some researchers recently developed vessel segmentation techniques that can accurately segment the retinal vessel map of preterm infants [27,50]. The researchers used DL-based methods for vessel segmentation, which segmented the exact vessels map of the premature infants' retina images. The selection of the training dataset for the DL model is crucial because it influences the system's output. These DL systems use training data derived from specific demography affected by gender, race, age, and other factors. Therefore, these models are inconsistent with local datasets. However, the model

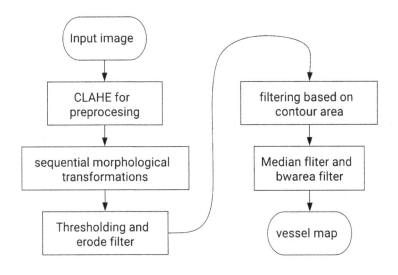

Fig. 7. Vessel extraction form retinal fundus images [25].

needs to be retrained before it can be used in specific demographics, which requires a lot of data. Notably, fundus image datasets for premature infants are not publicly available. On the other hand, retinal images of infants collected locally are insufficient, and their vessels are unlabelled. In the proposed system, we have used an algorithm from image processing and computer vision-based vessel segmentation that separates retinal vessels from fundus images. After that, we have used manually labelled vessels structure of neonatal images to validate the usefulness and correctness of vessel segmentation techniques used in the proposed system of ROP classification. Further, we have also verified the retinal vessels map obtained via the vessel segmentation approach with the neonatal ophthalmologist. The retinal vessels segmented by the vessel segmentation unit from the fundus image is sufficient for the ROP zoning application.

The vessel extraction algorithm pipeline is shown in Fig. 7. It consist of five stages viz; image preprocessing, sequential morphological operation, binarization, contour selection and filtering. The preprocessing stage performs essential processes to improve the retinal images' quality. We perform a series of morphological operations to strengthen and enhance the vessel map structure with respect to background. Further, the cluster thresholding generates barbarized structure of retinal vessels map. Finally, we have used various filtering techniques such as erode filter, filtering based on contour area and median filter to remove the shot noise and small vascular structures from the barbarized image to get an accurate vessels map.

3.6 ROP Classification

Using the modules as mentioned earlier, the proposed system provides an easy and efficient approach for zone classification. This study only considers a single fundus image for zone prediction. Therefore, we cannot cover the peripheral retinal regions needed

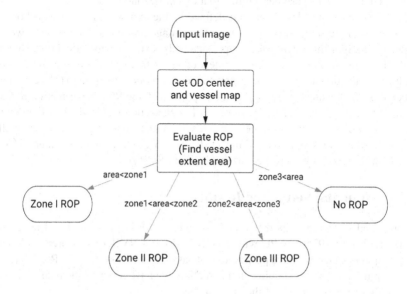

Fig. 8. Algorithm for ROP Zone classifier [25].

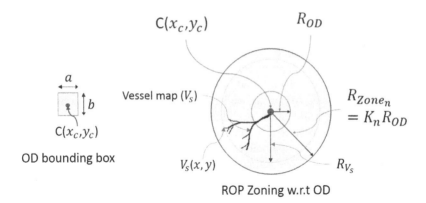

Fig. 9. ROP Zone radius calculation using OD information.

to detect Zone-2 or higher and classify an image as no-ROP. Because of the severity of Zone-1 ROP cases, our technique focuses on correctly identifying them. Figure 8 illustrates the flowchart for the proposed procedures. It classifies ROP into four different categories based on the extent of the blood vessels. During ROP classification, we used the ICROP rule to determine the extent of the blood vessel map. It uses the following equations to use the OD location ($C(x_c, y_c)$) and their sizes (a, b) as references for concentric rings for area/zone classification:

$$A_{Zone_n} = \pi \times (K_n \times d_{OD})^2 - A_{Zone_{n-1}}, \qquad (1)$$

where, $d_{OD} = max\{a, b\}$,, K_n is equal to the 5 and 7 for the corresponding Zone n equal to 1 and 2 respectively based on ROP classification proposed by the ICROP committee in March 2019 [7] and A_{Zone_0} is equal to zero. However, the A_{Zone_3} includes the residual crescent of peripheral retina that extent beyond the $Zone_2$.

The accuracy of the classification is defined by the two factors. The first is how well the vessels (V_s) are segmented from the retinal image and the second is, how well the OD detection algorithms detect the shape, size and location of an optical disk shown in Fig. 9. The radius of Zone-1 is approximately equal to the five times of the OD diameter. Finally, classification algorithm computes the retinal blood vessels map (V_s) extent with respect to the OD center ($C(x_c, y_c)$) and compares with the ROP Zone-n circumference of radius ($R_{Zone_n} = K_n R_{OD}$). Therefore, in Fig. 9, accuracy of ROP classifier depends on the how well the system computes the extent of vessels map (highlighted with yellow color) or farthest vessels point/end/tail ($V_s(x, y)$) in segmented vessel map (V_s) and compare their location with respect to the different ROP zones.

4 Experimental Setup and Results

The proposed system and its different DL modules are implemented and tested on a laptop with Intel i7-9750H CPU with 16 GB RAM and NVIDIA GeForce GTX 1660-Ti GPU. In this study, we have proposed a DL-assisted CAD system for ROP diagnosis and screening in premature babies. In this section, we have reported the results obtained in the study of various stages of the proposed system.

4.1 Evaluation Metrics

The qualitative and quantitative methodologies are used to detect the OD and analyse the effectiveness of vessel segmentation modules. Quantitative procedures express quality in terms of scores, with a higher score indicating higher quality and a lower score indicating lower quality. We use the evaluation metrics as accuracy, precision, recall and F1-score for the OD segmentation. It considers the true positive (TP), true negative (TN), false positive (FP), and false-negative (FN) classification conditions of each pixel in the segmented image with respect to the ground truth [52]. These metrics are calculated as:

$$Accuracy = \frac{(TP + TN)}{(TP + TN + FP + FN)} \tag{2}$$

$$Precision = \frac{TP}{TP + FP} \tag{3}$$

$$Recall = \frac{TP}{TP + FN} \tag{4}$$

$$F_1 = 2 \times \frac{precision \times recall}{precision + recall} \tag{5}$$

We use Intersection over Union (IoU) to evaluate the quality of the estimated OD boundary (bounding box), which is calculated as follows:

$$IoU = \frac{\text{number of common pixels between the target and prediction masks}}{\text{total number of pixels present across both masks}} \tag{6}$$

Further, to evaluate the quality of the segmented blood vascular map, we use the root mean square error (RMSE), peak signal to noise ratio (PSNR), and structural similarity index (SSIM) [16,35]. The RMSE measures the difference in predicted image pixels from the ground truth. PSNR, on the other hand, is used to evaluate the quality of reconstruction of a damaged blood vascular structure. We define RMSE and PSNR as follows:

$$RMSE = \sqrt{\frac{1}{N} \sum_{i=1}^{N} (y_i - \hat{y}_i)^2}, \tag{7}$$

$$PSNR = 20 log_{10}(MAX_I) - 10 log_{10}(MSE), \tag{8}$$

where, y_i = actual image pixel, $\hat{y}_i$ = predicted image pixel and N = total number of image pixels, MSE = mean square error = $(RMSE)^2$ and MAX_I = 255, as image pixel has max value of 255. The SSIM index is a perceptual metric used to measure the similarity between two images in terms of structure of segmented blood vessels . A detailed description of this metric can be found in [47].

Further, we also evaluate the absolute mean brightness error (AMBE), contrast (C) and contrast improvement index (CII) to analyze effect of image preprocessing on image quality [16]. AMBE is define as follows:

$$AMBE = mean(I_{original}) - mean(I_{enhance}), \tag{9}$$

where, $I_{original}$ and $I_{enhance}$ denotes the input (or original) and output (or enhanced) image. CII and C are evaluated [11, 16] as:

$$CII = \frac{C_{processed}}{C_{original}}, \tag{10}$$

$$C = \frac{m_f - m_b}{m_f + m_b}, \tag{11}$$

where, the terms $C_{processed}$ and $C_{original}$ are the contrast of the processed and original images, m_f and and m_b are the mean luminance values of foreground and the background.

In this work, we have utilized above all performance evaluation metrics to measure the quality of segmented OD, blood vessels map and ROP classification with respect to their corresponding ground truth.

4.2   Pre-processing of Fundus Image

We select the green channel (I_g) for analysis since it contains maximum contrast between blood vessels and background. Further, in preprocessing stage, we have to use a median filter to remove the effect of impulse noises. Impulse noise can be generated by sharp and sudden changes in image signal during acquisition. The averaging filter is used in the next stage, which reduces the effect of intensity variations across the neighbouring pixels. Further, sharping and CLAHE are used to enhance the image quality, as shown in the preprocessing results in Fig. 10. In the sharpening filter, we have used unsharp masking with the standard deviation of Gaussian low pass filter is 4 and strength of sharpening effect is 1.0. Contrast-limited Adaptive Histogram Equalization (CLAHE) is used to enhance the contrast of an image by transforming the values

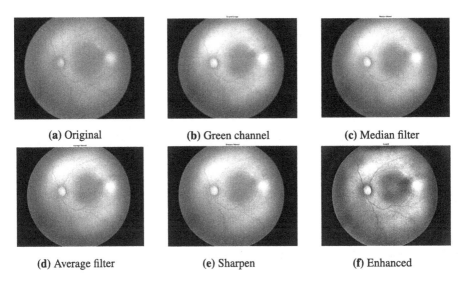

(a) Original   (b) Green channel   (c) Median filter

(d) Average filter   (e) Sharpen   (f) Enhanced

Fig. 10. Output images of different stages of preprocessing of original color (RGB) image.

Table 5. Effect of preprocessing on image quality.

Image processing	C_{vessel}	CII_{vessel}	C_{OD}	CII_{OD}	AMBE
Original Image (I_g)	0.0848	–	0.0697	–	–
Average	0.0847	0.9988	0.0696	0.9986	–0.15
Median	0.0851	1.0035	0.0697	1.0014	0.0253
Sharpen	0.0850	1.0024	0.0699	1.0029	0.012
Enhancement (or CLAHE)	0.1821	2.1474	0.1375	1.9727	14.97
Average + Median + sharpen + CLAHE	0.1990	2.3467	0.1394	2.0	24.5602

in the intensity image. Here, we have specified the number of tiles in a row, column and contrast enhance limit as 8×8 and 0.005 respectively and remaining all parameters such as the number of bins for histogram ($= 256$), output image intensity range ($= 0$ to 255), histogram distribution type ($= uniform$), and distribution parameters ($= 0.4$) are selected default value of MATLAB R2020b CLAHE[1] function.

We have chosen two regions of interest (ROIs) for the analysis of image preprocessing: the OD section and the blood vessel section, as shown in Fig. 6. It is challenging to isolate blood vessels, especially near the periphery of the fundus image. Therefore, to observe the effect of preprocessing, we selected the blood vessel structure region near the periphery of the image.Moreover, the spatial intensity level is unevenly distributed in an fundus images of premature neonatal. Therefore, in our evaluation of preprocessing of vessels/OD, we have selected background region adjacent to the ROIs to mitigate the effect of uneven illumination and intensity distribution. Table 5 summarizes the results of image preprocessing of neonatal fundus images. Image quality metrics, such as Image Contrast (C), Contrast Improvement Index (CII), and Absolute Mean Brightness Error (AMBE), showed advancement with image preprocessing. We have seen the effect of various filters in preprocessing on the original image (G channel). The CLAH filter significantly improves the image contrast of OD and vessels compared to all other filters. However, the result in the last row shows that the image quality metrics are at their maximum when using all the filter techniques one by one during the preprocessing of the neonatal retinal image. We have also tried multiple kernel sizes of the above filters for this study. The mean and median filters perform better with a kernel size of 3×3. For this, we have used Matlab 2020b inbuilt functions for image enhancement and sharpening with their default configuration.

4.3 OD Segmentation

We manually annotated the bounding box for OD in these images after collecting six different datasets (mentioned in Table 3) and then trained YOLO-v5 models. It took us about 10 h to train this model on our local machine with the earlier specifications and to predict OD from an image, and the result was always within 100 milliseconds. With train and validation datasets at different epochs, Fig. 13 depicts the performance measures of the generalised intersection over union ($GIoU$) loss, objective loss, and

---

[1] https://in.mathworks.com/help/images/ref/adapthisteq.html.

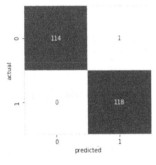

(a) AIIMS Train Dataset

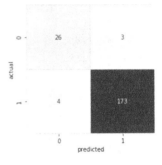

(b) AIIMS Test Dataset

Fig. 11. Confusion Matrix of OD detection (where, 0: without OD and 1: with OD) [25].

Table 6. Performance of YOLO-v5 on different datasets [25].

Dataset	Average IoU%		mAP@0.5 IoU		Accuracy@0.5		Accuracy@0.75	
	Train	Test	Train	Test	Train	Test	Train	Test
AIIMS	95.59	80.62	0.995	0.973	99.57	96.6	98.71	79.61
HRF	95.71	89.28	0.995	0.995	100	100	100	100
STARE	95.09	83.64	0.995	0.995	100	99	100	90
IDRiD	95.49	88.55	0.995	0.995	100	100	100	97.33
DRIVE	95.69	86.83	0.995	0.995	100	100	100	100
FIRE	89.93	86.31	0.995	0.995	100	100	100	98.75
Overall	**94.64**	**84.48**	**0.995**	**0.995**	**99.9**	**98.94**	**99.7**	**90.11**

* **IoU**: Intersection over union is the ratio of intersection of predicted bounding box and ground truth to the union of the both
* **mAP@0.5 IoU**: Mean Average precision at IoU threshold of 0.5
* **Accuracy@x**: Accuracy if we consider IoU>x as correct classification

confusion parameters (i.e., precision, recall, and mean average precision (mAP)) of the DL-module. The first two rows in that image show the $GIoU$ and objective function values that our model minimises for the training dataset in the first row and the validation dataset in the second row. Training loss lowers, and validation performance improves, indicating that the model has been successfully trained. We plotted several performance measures for the validation dataset in the last two columns as training progressed.

Table 6 summarizes the results obtained from the trained model. We have created this dataset to train YOLO models by merging multiple datasets. Hence, our model must perform well across all the datasets. We notice good accuracy figures for all of the datasets in this table. We can also see that it is easy for some standard datasets to get 100% accuracy,even for test datasets, and the consistency explains these results in images of the standard dataset.

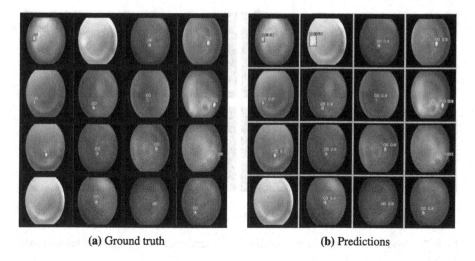

(a) Ground truth   **(b)** Predictions

Fig. 12. Results from YOLO-v5.

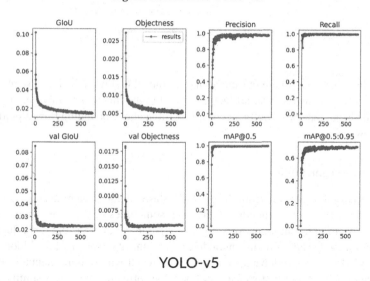

YOLO-v5

Fig. 13. Model training metrics plot with respect to the epoch number (where, GIoU: generalized intersection over union loss for training, Objectness: objective loss for training, Val GIoU: validation GIoU loss, Val Objectness: validation objective loss, and metrics are precision, recall, and mAP@x: mean average precision if we consider IoU > x as the correct classification) [25].

There were also some images in one dataset that did not have OD. So, if we consider the availability of OD to be a binary classification problem, we can generate the confusion matrix for this dataset using YOLO-v5, as shown in Fig. 11. This demonstrates that our model can also perform well in that task. Figure 12 has actual OD on one side and corresponding predictions on the other side to visualize the results. Here one can

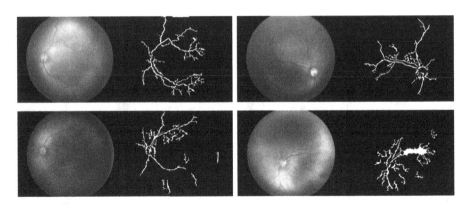

Fig. 14. Blood vessel extraction results [25].

Table 7. Blood vessels segmentation quality assessment result with premature babies fundus images.

Metrics	Accuracy	RMSE	PSNR	SSIM
Average value	94%	0.23	14.9	0.82

see that there is a case where our model has predicted OD whereas it is absent. This is because there is some OD like artifact generated in the image probably due to camera lens. And also in that case confidence value (written above bounding box of prediction) is very low.

4.4 Vessels Segmentation

The extracted blood vessels from the AIIMS dataset using our approach are shown in Fig. 14. These results show that this algorithm is sometimes susceptible to noise or over-exposure. We tried to fine-tune every algorithm parameter, but the dataset's fluctuation limits our method. Therefore, it cannot detect the thinner segments of the blood vessels accurately. Moreover, we have also compare our result with 6 more manually labelled ROP images dataset. For that we have got good performance metrics as summarized in Table 7. The results that we have got till now is acceptable for zone detection, which is the task in hand we need vessel extent for now.

4.5 ROP Zoning

The proposed solution is shown in Fig. 15; the blue circles indicate the boundaries of the zones centered on the optical disk in these images. In the earlier version of this work [25], only 12 images (from 5 distinct patients) were available for study, and the ground truth was labeled as zone 1 ROP. From that, the module correctly predicted results for ten images (83.33% accuracy image-wise) when using an image processing-based approach on these images for vessel detection. However, if the top-2 accuracy score is considered, it comes out at 100% patient wise as these two images belong to a patient with multiple images in the set. Another was correctly identified as Zone-1 ROP. In addition, if images of Zone-2 ROP are taken into account, the proposed method provides 72% accuracy.

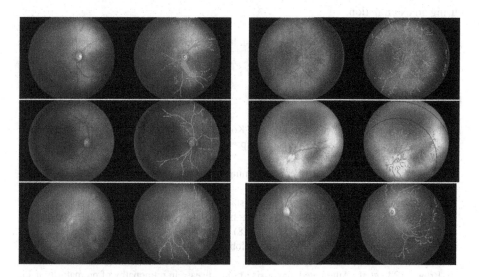

Fig. 15. ROP zoning results: blue line depict zone boundary (left side: original image, right side: ROP zoning based on vessels extent) [25]. (Color figure online)

In the next iteration of the dataset, larger dataset were obtained which had 52 Zone-1 images of 7 subject with good quality and OD visible. On this extended dataset when the same modules for the vessel extraction were used, the proposed approach gave the accuracy of **82.5%** which confirms that this method can generalize well on large datasets.

5   Conclusions

This paper presents proof of concept for the proposed DL-assisted retinal disease screening method. We investigated, designed, and implemented a new ROP screening and classifications system. We used image processing and computer vision-based technologies for Fundus image preprocessing and vessel segmentation while considering and testing YOLO-v5 DL-based algorithms to identify OD. It provides an integrated platform for working with both data-driven and rules-based systems simultaneously. As a result, even there are just not enough datasets, it can be done successfully. Also, in this approach, the doctors/clinicians may see the classification findings and visualization of detected OD and vascular systems, enabling them to understand and validate the system's choice.

We have also put our approach to the test by scanning the retinas of preterm infants at a local hospital. Our system's accuracy for the Zone-I ROP is around 82.5%. The retinal camera currently used for retina scanning has a narrow field of view (FOV). As a result, it will not acquire the retina's complete periphery in a single frame. However, a broader view of the retinal surface was essential for Zone-2 and Zone-3, which is not doable with the current arrangement. As a result, our system's accuracy in Zones 2 and 3 is poor, which we intend to increase significantly by using several photos or videos during an examination.

Acknowledgements. We acknowledge key insights received from Prof. P. K. Kalra in discussion that we have done related to this work.

References

1. Agrawal, R., Kulkarni, S., Walambe, R., Kotecha, K.: Assistive framework for automatic detection of all the zones in retinopathy of prematurity using deep learning. J. Digit. Imaging **34**(4), 932–947 (2021)
2. Attallah, O.: Diarop: automated deep learning-based diagnostic tool for retinopathy of prematurity. Diagnostics **11**(11), 2034 (2021)
3. Badarinath, D., et al.: Study of clinical staging and classification of retinal images for retinopathy of prematurity (ROP) screening. In: 2018 International Joint Conference on Neural Networks (IJCNN), pp. 1–6. IEEE (2018)
4. Blencowe, H., et al.: Born too soon: the global epidemiology of 15 million preterm births. Reprod. Health **10**(1), S2 (2013)
5. Brown, J.M., et al.: Automated diagnosis of plus disease in retinopathy of prematurity using deep convolutional neural networks. JAMA Ophthalmol. **136**(7), 803–810 (2018)
6. Budai, A., Bock, R., Maier, A., Hornegger, J., Michelson, G.: Robust vessel segmentation in fundus images. Int. J. Biomed. Imaging **2013**, 154860 (2013). https://doi.org/10.1155/2013/154860
7. Chiang, M.F., et al.: International classification of retinopathy of prematurity. Ophthalmology **128**(10), e51–e68 (2021)
8. Ding, A., Chen, Q., Cao, Y., Liu, B.: Retinopathy of prematurity stage diagnosis using object segmentation and convolutional neural networks. arXiv preprint arXiv:2004.01582 (2020)
9. Dogra, M.R., Katoch, D., Dogra, M.: An update on retinopathy of prematurity (ROP). Indian J. Pediatr. **84**(12), 930–936 (2017)
10. Doi, K.: Computer-aided diagnosis in medical imaging: historical review, current status and future potential. Comput. Med. Imaging Graph. **31**(4–5), 198–211 (2007)
11. Ema, T., Doi, K., Nishikawa, R.M., Jiang, Y., Papaioannou, J.: Image feature analysis and computer-aided diagnosis in mammography: reduction of false-positive clustered microcalcifications using local edge-gradient analysis. Med. Phys. **22**(2), 161–169 (1995)
12. Fraz, M.M., et al.: Blood vessel segmentation methodologies in retinal images-a survey. Comput. Methods Programs Biomed. **108**(1), 407–433 (2012)
13. Gensure, R.H., Chiang, M.F., Campbell, J.P.: Artificial intelligence for retinopathy of prematurity. Curr. Opin. Ophthalmol. **31**(5), 312 (2020)
14. Guo, X., Kikuchi, Y., Wang, G., Yi, J., Zou, Q., Zhou, R.: Early detection of retinopathy of prematurity (ROP) in retinal fundus images via convolutional neural networks. arXiv preprint arXiv:2006.06968 (2020)
15. Hellström, A., Smith, L.E., Dammann, O.: Retinopathy of prematurity. Lancet **382**(9902), 1445–1457 (2013)

16. Henry, A.G.P., Jude, A.: Convolutional neural-network-based classification of retinal images with different combinations of filtering techniques. Open Comput. Sci. **11**(1), 480–490 (2021)

17. Honavar, S.G.: Do we need India-specific retinopathy of prematurity screening guidelines? Indian J. Ophthalmol. **67**(6), 711 (2019)

18. Hoover, A.D., Kouznetsova, V., Goldbaum, M.: Locating blood vessels in retinal images by piecewise threshold probing of a matched filter response. IEEE Trans. Med. Imaging **19**(3), 203–210 (2000). https://doi.org/10.1109/42.845178

19. Huang, Y.P., et al.: Deep learning models for automated diagnosis of retinopathy of prematurity in preterm infants. Electronics **9**(9), 1444 (2020)

20. Islam, M., Poly, T.N., Walther, B.A., Yang, H.C., Li, Y.C.J., et al.: Artificial intelligence in ophthalmology: a meta-analysis of deep learning models for retinal vessels segmentation. J. Clin. Med. **9**(4), 1018 (2020)

21. Islam, M.M., Poly, T.N., Li, Y.C.J.: Retinal vessels detection using convolutional neural networks in fundus images. bioRxiv 737668 (2019)

22. Jefferies, A.L., Society, C.P., Fetus, Committee, N.: Retinopathy of prematurity: an update on screening and management. Paediatr. Health **21**(2), 101–104 (2016). https://doi.org/10.1093/pch/21.2.101

23. Jocher, G., et al.: ultralytics/yolov5: v5.0 - YOLOv5-P6 1280 models, AWS, Supervise.ly and YouTube integrations (2021). https://doi.org/10.5281/zenodo.4679653

24. Kim, S.J., Port, A.D., Swan, R., Campbell, J.P., Chan, R.P., Chiang, M.F.: Retinopathy of prematurity: a review of risk factors and their clinical significance. Surv. Ophthalmol. **63**(5), 618–637 (2018)

25. Kumar., V., Patel., H., Paul., K., Surve., A., Azad., S., Chawla., R.: Deep learning assisted retinopathy of prematurity screening technique. In: Proceedings of the 14th International Joint Conference on Biomedical Engineering Systems and Technologies - HEALTHINF, pp. 234–243. INSTICC, SciTePress (2021). https://doi.org/10.5220/0010322102340243

26. Lei, B., et al.: Automated detection of retinopathy of prematurity by deep attention network. Multimed. Tools Appl. **80**(30), 36341–36360 (2021)

27. Luo, Y., Chen, K., Mao, J., Shen, L., Sun, M.: A fusion deep convolutional neural network based on pathological features for diagnosing plus disease in retinopathy of prematurity. Invest. Ophthalmol. Visual Sci. **61**(7), 2017–2017 (2020)

28. Oloumi, F., Rangayyan, R.M., Ells, A.L.: Computer-aided diagnosis of retinopathy of prematurity via analysis of the vascular architecture in retinal fundus images of preterm infants. In: Doctoral Consortium on Computer Vision, Imaging and Computer Graphics Theory and Applications, vol. 2, pp. 58–66. SCITEPRESS (2014)

29. Oloumi, F., Rangayyan, R.M., Ells, A.L.: Computer-aided diagnosis of retinopathy in retinal fundus images of preterm infants via quantification of vascular tortuosity. J. Med. Imaging **3**(4), 044505 (2016)

30. Organization, W.H., et al.: World report on vision. Technical report, Geneva: World Health Organization (2019)

31. Peng, Y., Zhu, W., Chen, F., Xiang, D., Chen, X.: Automated retinopathy of prematurity screening using deep neural network with attention mechanism. In: Medical Imaging 2020: Image Processing, vol. 11313, p. 1131321. International Society for Optics and Photonics (2020)

32. Peng, Y., et al.: Automatic staging for retinopathy of prematurity with deep feature fusion and ordinal classification strategy. IEEE Trans. Med. Imaging (2021)

33. Ravichandran, C., Raja, J.B.: A fast enhancement/thresholding based blood vessel segmentation for retinal image using contrast limited adaptive histogram equalization. J. Med. Imaging Health Inf. **4**(4), 567–575 (2014)

34. Redd, T.K., et al.: Evaluation of a deep learning image assessment system for detecting severe retinopathy of prematurity. British J. Ophthalmol. **103**(5), 580–584 (2019)
35. Sara, U., Akter, M., Uddin, M.S.: Image quality assessment through FSIM, SSIM, MSE and PSNR-a comparative study. J. Comput. Commun. **7**(3), 8–18 (2019)
36. Scruggs, B.A., Chan, R.P., Kalpathy-Cramer, J., Chiang, M.F., Campbell, J.P.: Artificial intelligence in retinopathy of prematurity diagnosis. Trans. Vision Sci. Technol. **9**(2), 5–5 (2020)
37. Sen, P., Rao, C., Bansal, N.: Retinopathy of prematurity: an update. Sci. J. Med. Vis. Res. Foun. **33**(2), 93–6 (2015)
38. Staal, J., Abramoff, M., Niemeijer, M., Viergever, M., van Ginneken, B.: Ridge based vessel segmentation in color images of the retina. IEEE Trans. Med. Imaging **23**(4), 501–509 (2004)
39. Tan, Z., Simkin, S., Lai, C., Dai, S.: Deep learning algorithm for automated diagnosis of retinopathy of prematurity plus disease. Trans. Vis. Sci. Technol. **8**(6), 23–23 (2019)
40. Ting, D.S.W., et al.: Artificial intelligence and deep learning in ophthalmology. British J. Ophthalmol. **103**(2), 167–175 (2019)
41. Ting, D.S., et al.: Deep learning in ophthalmology: the technical and clinical considerations. Prog. Retinal Eye Res. (2019)
42. Tong, Y., Lu, W., Deng, Q.Q., Chen, C., Shen, Y.: Automated identification of retinopathy of prematurity by image-based deep learning. Eye Vis. **7**(1), 1–12 (2020)
43. Vinekar, A., Mangalesh, S., Jayadev, C., Gilbert, C., Dogra, M., Shetty, B.: Impact of expansion of telemedicine screening for retinopathy of prematurity in India. Indian J. Ophthalmol. **65**(5), 390 (2017)
44. Wang, J., et al.: Automated explainable multidimensional deep learning platform of retinal images for retinopathy of prematurity screening. JAMA Netw. Open **4**(5), e218758–e218758 (2021)
45. Wang, J., et al.: Automated retinopathy of prematurity screening using deep neural networks. EBioMedicine **35**, 361–368 (2018)
46. Wang, X., Jiang, X., Ren, J.: Blood vessel segmentation from fundus image by a cascade classification framework. Pattern Recogn. **88**, 331–341 (2019)
47. Wang, Z., Bovik, A.C., Sheikh, H.R., Simoncelli, E.P.: Image quality assessment: from error visibility to structural similarity. IEEE Trans. Image Process. **13**(4), 600–612 (2004). https://doi.org/10.1109/TIP.2003.819861
48. Wang, Z., Keane, P.A., Chiang, M., Cheung, C.Y., Wong, T.Y., Ting, D.S.W.: Artificial intelligence and deep learning in ophthalmology. Artif. Intell. Med. 1–34 (2020)
49. Yavuz, Z., Köse, C.: Blood vessel extraction in color retinal fundus images with enhancement filtering and unsupervised classification. J. Healthc. Eng. **2017**, 1–12 (2017). https://doi.org/10.1155/2017/4897258
50. Yildiz, V.M., et al.: Plus disease in retinopathy of prematurity: convolutional neural network performance using a combined neural network and feature extraction approach. Trans. Vis. Sci. Technol. **9**(2), 10–10 (2020)
51. Zhang, Y., et al.: Development of an automated screening system for retinopathy of prematurity using a deep neural network for wide-angle retinal images. IEEE Access **7**, 10232–10241 (2018)
52. Zhao, Z.Q., Zheng, P., Xu, S.t., Wu, X.: Object detection with deep learning: a review. IEEE Trans. Neural Netw. Learn. Syst. **30**(11), 3212–3232 (2019)

Author Index

Alves, Pedro 158
Azad, Shorya 236
Azzopardi, Joseph 18

Balbino, Marcelo 180
Baschirotto, Andrea 1
Böhlen, Conrad Fifelski-von 120
Bonfanti, Silvia 139
Brinkmann, Anna 120

Chawla, Rohan 236
Colavita, Angela Rita 213

De Matteis, Marcello 1
de Miranda, Débora 180

Ebejer, Jean Paul 18
Errachid, Abdelhamid 61

Folgado, Duarte 80
Franco, Rafael 158
Frickel, Jürgen 61
Fudickar, Sebastian 120
Fujão, Carlos 80

Gamboa, Hugo 80
Gargantini, Angelo 139
Gómez-Rodellar, Andrés 102
Gómez-Vilda, Pedro 102
Graça, Ricardo 158

Halima, Hamdi Ben 61
Hein, Andreas 120
Hellmers, Sandra 120
Heuberger, Albert 61
Hofmann, Christian 61

Jandre, Caroline 180

Kiwanuka, Achilles 202
Kumar, Vijay 236

Laudato, Gennaro 213

Moreira, Dinis 158

Nabukenya, Josephine 202
Nobre, Cristiane 180

Oliveto, Rocco 213

Palacios-Alonso, Daniel 102
Patel, Het 236
Paul, Kolin 236
Pfeiffer, Norman 61
Picariello, Francesco 213

Rodrigues, João 80
Rosa, Giovanni 213
Rosado, Luís 158
Russodivito, Marco 213

Santos, António 80
Santos, Sara 80
Scalabrino, Simone 213
Shibayama, Eri 45
Stevenazzi, Lorenzo 1
Surve, Abhidnya 236
Suzuki, Taira 45

Tsanas, Athanasios 102
Tudosa, Ioan 213

Vallicelli, Elia 1
Vasconcelos, Maria João M. 158
Vito, Luca De 213

Wachter, Toni 61

Zárate, Luis 180